MANAKA MADE SIMPLE

A Step-By-Step Guide to Dr Manaka's System of Japanese Acupuncture and Moxibustion

VOLUME 1

ORAN KIVITY, STEPHEN BIRCH,
MARIAN FIXLER, BRENDA LOEW,
PAUL MOVSESSIAN

Manaka Made Simple: A Step-by-Step Guide to Dr Manaka's System of Japanese Acupuncture and Moxibustion

Volume 1

Illustrations by Rebecca Wijesurya
Cover design and layout by 100Covers.com
Sayoshi Books, London, 2026

FREE CLINICAL QUICK-REFERENCE GUIDE

Thank you for purchasing Manaka Made Simple. Readers are welcome to download our free companion guide, **Manaka Made Simple: Abdominal Patterns at a Glance.**

This visual quick-reference presents the key diagrams for abdominal palpation from the main book, with all the visual information you need for pattern recognition in one place. The guide is designed for practical use in the clinic, to support you while palpating.

Download your free quick-reference guide.

Scan the QR code with your mobile camera to access the resource.

If you are unable to scan, simply visit the URL below.

https://sayoshibooks.orankivity.com/mms/

For Junko Ida

who has guided and inspired all of us

Everything should be made as simple as possible, but not simpler.

—attributed to Albert Einstein

WHAT'S POSSIBLE

We begin this book with a story that shows the power of Dr Yoshio Manaka's methods: a single treatment that transformed everything. Each of the co-authors has witnessed moments like this—quick, dramatic shifts in our patients when using Manaka System Acupuncture (MSA). Here, we share one such moment from the practice of Paul Movsessian.

> *The first time I used MSA was in 1989, treating a woman with a whiplash injury. For ten years, she had been unable to turn her head more than 10%. Nothing she had tried had worked, and she lived with constant pain, relying on painkillers.*
>
> *I applied Manaka's whiplash treatment, which involves needling the master and coupled points of the Yang Qiao Mai and the Yang Wei Mai bilaterally, and connecting them with ion-pumping cords.*
>
> *It was a winter evening in Upstate New York. I covered her with a blanket, dimmed the lights, and left her to rest. At the end of the treatment, when I removed the cords and needles, she sat up, turned her head without pain, and, crying with joy, thanked me.*
>
> —Paul Movsessian

After experiencing similar moments in our practices, none of the authors has ever looked back. Such experiences are life-changing. We hope that reading this book will be life-changing for you, too. The journey you are about to embark on may well become a defining moment in your practice. The rewards of MSA are profound, and its clinical efficacy so immediate that your patients will be forever grateful for your dedication and expertise.

Over the years, we have trained numerous students across the world, and they often tell us the same thing: Dr Manaka's work changed their understanding of acupuncture and gave them the confidence to build a successful practice.

—Oran Kivity, Stephen Birch, Marian Fixler, Brenda Loew, Paul Movsessian

CONTENTS

CHAPTER 6

CHAPTER 7

CHAPTER 8

CHAPTER 15

CHAPTER 16

CHAPTER 17

LIST OF TABLES

TABLE OF FIGURES

ACRONYMS AND ABBREVIATIONS

The following acronyms and abbreviations appear throughout this book. Here is a quick-reference list of the full terms.

Acronym	Full Name
ASIS	Anterior Superior Iliac Spine
CS	Cross Syndrome
EA	Electrostatic Adsorbers
EFT	Emotional Freedom Technique
EJOM	European Journal of Oriental Medicine
FIR	Far Infrared
IBD	Ion Beam Device
ID	Intradermal needle
IPC	Ion Pumping Cord
IUI	Intrauterine Insemination
IVF	In Vitro Fertilisation
JAAM	Japanese Acupuncture and Moxibustion
JCM	Journal of Chinese Medicine
KHT	Korean Hand Therapy
KMS	Kiiko Matsumoto Style
MSA	Manaka System Acupuncture
NAJOM	North American Journal of Oriental Medicine
PLF	Prone Leg Flexion (Sotai technique)
PPP	Pressure Pain Point
PSIS	Posterior Superior Iliac Spine
RA	Rheumatoid Arthritis
ROM	Range of Motion
RSI	Repetitive Strain Injury

Acronym	Full Name
SSP	Silver Spike Point (silver terminal)
TCM	Traditional Chinese Medicine
TEAM	Traditional East Asian Medicine
TRP	Transient Receptor Potential ion channel
YQD	Yang Qiao Du
YQR	Yin Qiao Ren
YWC	Yin Wei Chong
YWD	Yang Wei Dai

ON TREATING CHILDREN

This book describes treatment methods intended for adults only. The treatment of children with MSA is not covered in this book. This is a distinct subject, with its own specialised techniques, such as Shonishin in Japan.

If you want to use these methods with children, first master MSA with adults. Then take a paediatric acupuncture course, such as Shonishin, to understand the differences between treating adults and children.

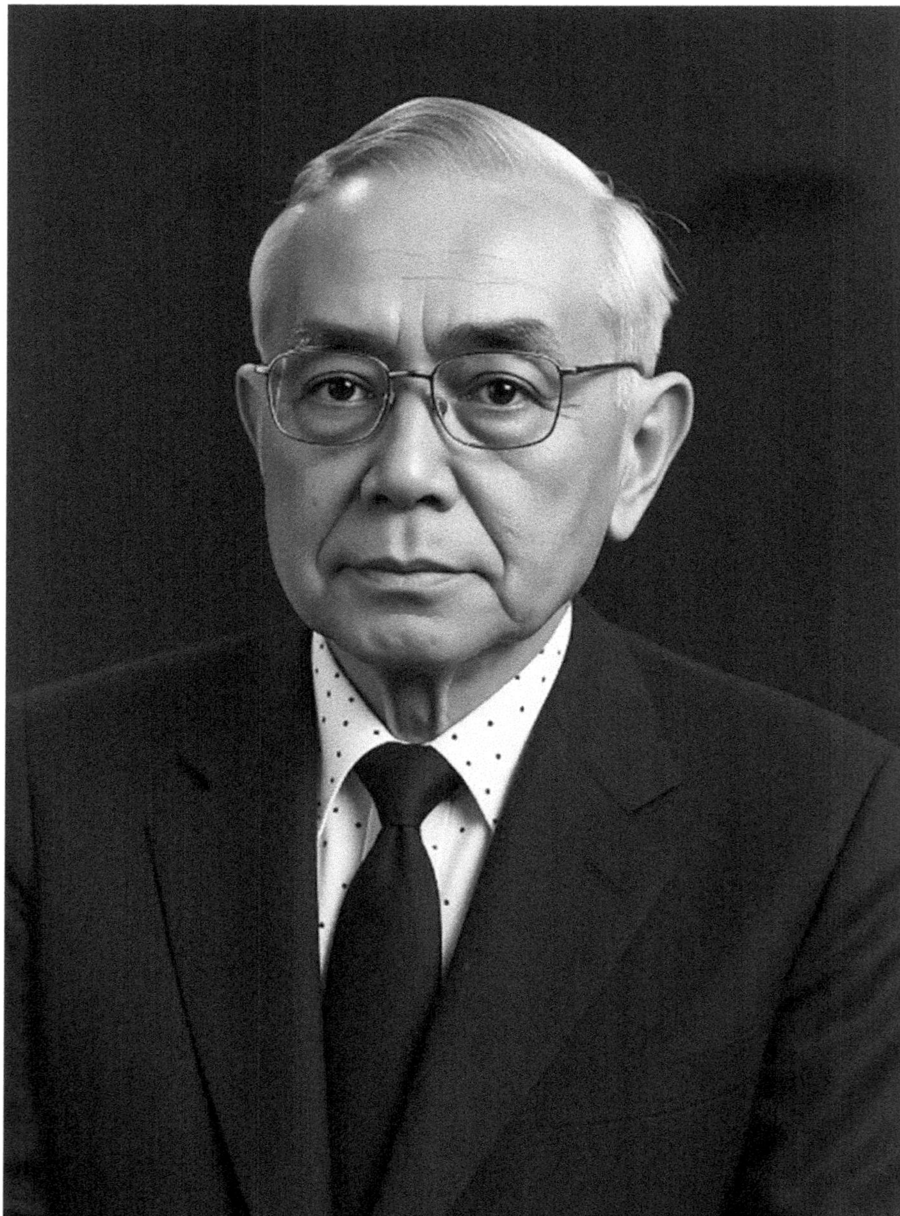

Dr Yoshio Manaka (1911–1989)

INTRODUCTION

When I begin to lecture an audience, regardless of who they are,
I often begin by saying, "Don't believe what I'm going to tell you."

—Yoshio Manaka

Dr Yoshio Manaka was a medical doctor who combined rigorous research with a fascination for traditional healing. Renowned in Japan, he achieved outstanding clinical results. He tested new ideas, kept what worked, and added his own innovations. One example was his use of Sotai bodywork: stretching a limb with one hand while applying direct moxibustion with the other—a unique application of moxibustion into physical therapy.

"Don't believe what I'm going to tell you" was more than a catchphrase. Dr Manaka wanted people to test his research and confirm it for themselves. He passed away in 1989, leaving behind a large body of books and papers on the meridian system, as well as a clear, effective system of acupuncture that Stephen Birch and Junko Ida introduced to the West.

Manaka was a true polymath: fluent in several languages, and a sculptor, poet, and painter. Birch once told me that Manaka was the only genius he had ever met. Studying with him was, in Birch's words, "mind-expanding" and like catching a "curiosity virus".

That infection led to the publication of *Chasing the Dragon's Tail*. However, when I came across the book in 1995, I put it back on the shelf, finding the graphs and mathematical formulae too dense and technical. It was only after studying with Birch that my mind opened up to Manaka's extraordinary thinking.

But Birch has continued to spread the so-called Manaka Meme, challenging students to look at acupuncture rationally and pragmatically, testing and adapting what works, and rejecting assumptions and dogma if they don't make sense. With a doctorate in acupuncture research and numerous books to his name, he has been a key link between Japan and the West, shaping how we study acupuncture.

Over the years, Birch has taught Manaka System Acupuncture (MSA) as a three-level course, each taught over three days. At my first Level 1 training, he promised: "By the end of this weekend, you will be able to practise this method." He was right—I started using MSA in clinic the following week and, like Paul Movsessian, never looked back.

Chasing the Dragon's Tail was published in 1995. It is full of reasoned theories and the evidence to back them up. Brilliant though it is, as a textbook to accompany the weekend trainings, it is unwieldy.

This book series is designed to fill that gap. Volume 1 covers Level 1, Volume 2 covers Level 2, and Volume 3 covers the final topics. By the end of this book, you will have everything you need to practise Level 1 MSA.

How to Use This Book

This book aims to present the material in *Chasing the Dragon's Tail* in a way that makes it not only more accessible and easier to digest but also more practical and comprehensible. MSA introduces a different perspective on the meridian system and, just like Traditional Chinese Medicine (TCM), requires its own terminology and language. Once you grasp the basic grammar, the system becomes far easier to understand. We've made it as simple as possible, but no simpler.

It's best to attend a course on MSA with one of the instructors—if you do, this book will save you from having to take too many notes. It has a dual structure:

1. Clinical aspects of MSA
2. Contextual essays on Japanese acupuncture and moxibustion

The clinical chapters follow the Four Steps protocol. The contextual chapters explore the distinctive features of Japanese acupuncture, palpation, and the theory of moxibustion. Easily identified by the word *Context* before the chapter title, they offer essential background for the clinical techniques covered in the book. If you're pressed for time or just want to get into the clinical aspects of MSA, these chapters can be skipped, though they are well worth revisiting.

Chasing the Dragon's Tail is more than thirty years old—a snapshot of how Manaka treated patients before he died in 1989. If he were alive today, he would almost certainly be treating differently. MSA has evolved since then: Stephen Birch and Brenda Loew have proposed new abdominal findings and treatment approaches; Indonesian and Brazilian practitioners have pioneered non-insertive methods using silver electrodes taped in place; and I have integrated Ontake Warm Bamboo moxa with Manaka's meridian frequencies. We have tried to make clear the distinction between the approaches from *Chasing the Dragon's Tail* and these contemporary adaptations.

The initial draft of this book was largely written by me, with a dedicated chapter from Stephen Birch and adapted lecture notes from Brenda Loew, Marian Fixler, and Paul Movsessian. This draft underwent extensive refinement, with each author adding new material, suggestions, and revisions. Occasionally, we've attributed contributions by quoting directly from the author to reflect our distinct styles, while other contributions have been left unattributed. As this book goes to print, it represents a shared consensus among us on how best to interpret Manaka's legacy and carry it forward. We all continue to learn and develop in our practice of Manaka System Acupuncture.

—Oran Kivity
Taiwan, 2025

PART ONE

MANAKA'S SYSTEM

CHAPTER 1

MANAKA'S OCTAHEDRAL MODEL

Let's start with a thought experiment. Have you ever blown up balloons for a birthday party? Imagine you're holding a single balloon in your hand. This balloon is a sphere, and (ignoring the nozzle where you blew in the air) it has neither up and down nor left and right. If you rub the balloon on your clothing, it builds up a static charge, and you can stick it to a flat surface. Let's imagine our balloons also stick together. Now take a second balloon, rub it, and attach it side by side to the first.

Immediately, we have a left balloon and a right balloon, separated by a longitudinal axis. Let's rub two more balloons and place them on top of the first pair. Now we have two storeys of balloons, with a horizontal axis separating the upper and lower levels. Let's repeat the entire process and attach four more balloons behind the first four. Now, there are eight balloons with a new vertical axis that separates the front four from the rear four. Our new structure has four quadrants at the front and four quadrants at the back. It's an octahedral shape.

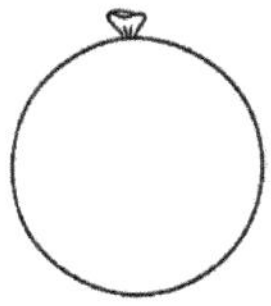

Figure 1-1: Single balloon with no axis.

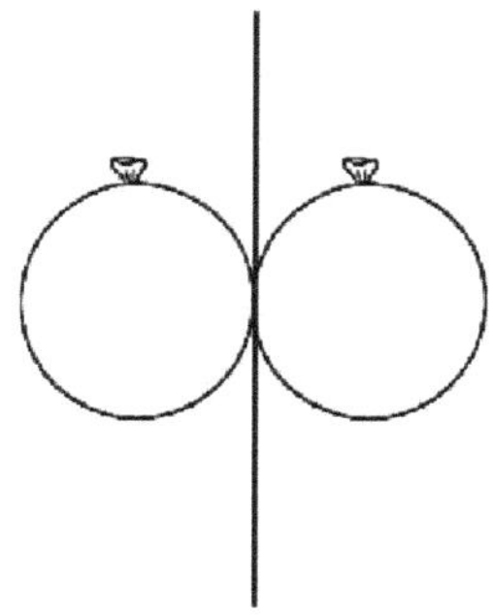

Figure 1-2: Vertical axis separates left from right.

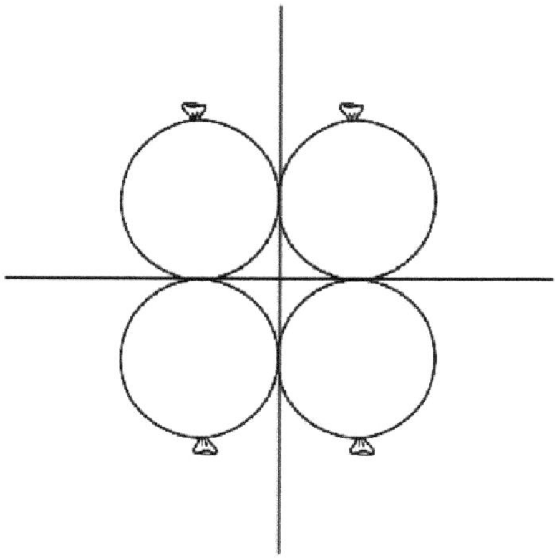

Figure 1-3: Horizontal axis separates top from bottom.

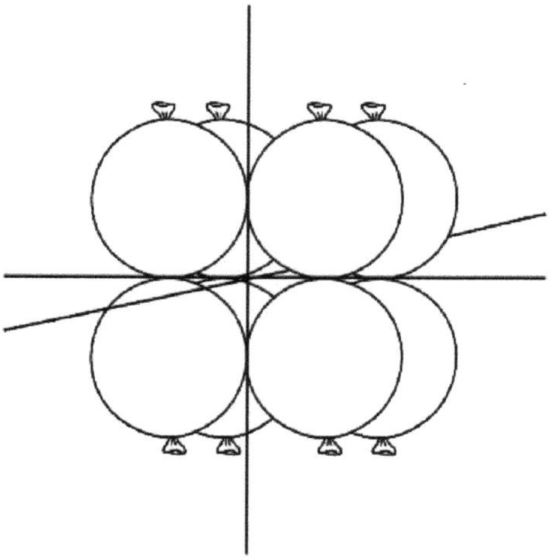

Figure 1-4: Third vertical axis separates front from back.

We've actually been incorporating concepts of yin and yang here. We've established the three axes of anatomy (left–right, superior–inferior, and anterior–posterior) and three anatomical planes (sagittal, transverse, and frontal). Dr Manaka observed that if you draw the axes and then connect the ends, they make a geometric shape: an octahedron.

Now let's run the same thought experiment again, this time considering biology and starting at conception. Let's imagine a zygote, which divides once, creating the first axis, separating left and right; again, creating a second horizontal axis, separating top from bottom; and again, creating the final third axis, separating front from back. Once again, we end up with eight cells, creating an octahedral structure.

Manaka was widely read in the sciences and was probably familiar with the work of the American engineer and architect Buckminster Fuller, renowned for his use of geodesic domes. Fuller studied and described the physical properties of geometric structures. He described the octahedron as one of the simplest and most stable structures in nature.

An octahedron is an eight-sided figure, but in classical acupuncture anatomy (i.e. the structure of the meridian system), the meridians are organised in sets of twelve. There are twelve collateral meridians (*luomai*), twelve sinew meridians (*jingjin*), twelve primary meridians (*jingmai*), and twelve divergent meridians (*jingbie*). In addition to these meridians, there is another system of eight vessels: the *qi jing ba mai* in Chinese, or *kikei hachi miyaku* in Japanese—the Eight Extraordinary Vessels. Over time, it was the Eight Extraordinary Vessels that drew Manaka's attention. Could the Eight Extras, in some way, relate to the octahedron enfolded within the body's three axes?

Manaka theorised that these early cell divisions could be the moments of creation for the Eight Extras. The first division creates Ren Mai and Du Mai, a vertical axis that separates left from right. Another division creates the Dai Mai, a horizontal axis separating superior from inferior, and the next division creates a line dividing anterior from posterior on the torso, which, for now, for simplicity's sake, we'll call the Yang Wei Mai. Manaka's thinking on this axis is more complicated, and we'll explore the Yin and Yang Qiao Mai and the Yin Wei and Chong Mai later.

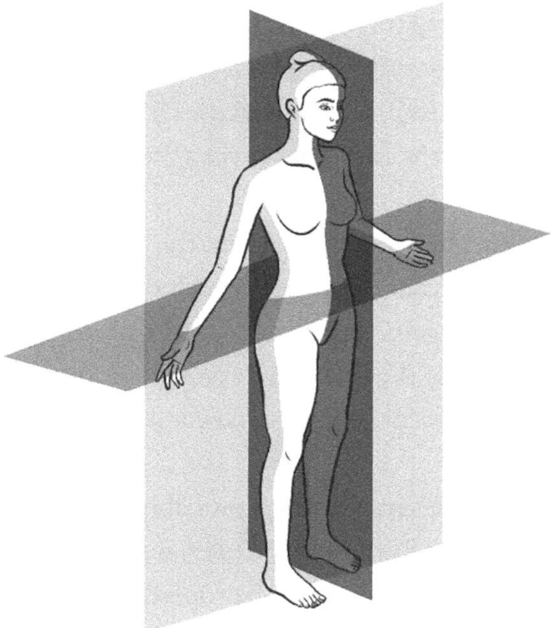

Figure 15: The three yin–yang axes generate the three anatomical planes: frontal, transverse, and sagittal, dividing the body into four anterior and four posterior quadrants.

What relevance does a pile of eight balloons with three axes have to a fully functional human body? After all, there are trillions of cells in the human body, and this process of cell division has yielded only eight.

Manaka considered this stage to be crucial, because it's at this very early point that the developing embryo can start to exploit properties associated with the three axes of left–right, upper–lower and anterior–posterior, each of which is traditionally defined as a yin–yang polarity.

He was also fascinated by topology, particularly in the context of evolution. As species evolve, there is a consistency of form.

> *Topology is the branch of mathematics dealing with three-dimensional geometric forms, both physical and imaginary. It deals with space—the topological space, the phase space—and the properties of solids. In particular, it is useful for describing those properties of solids which remain unchanged through a series of different deformations of an object. Some of these properties, such as connectedness, allow a description of how the whole*

system behaves. When an object is deformed by stretching, bending, etc., the old form and new form retain certain properties in common. The two forms are then homeomorphic to each other.[1]

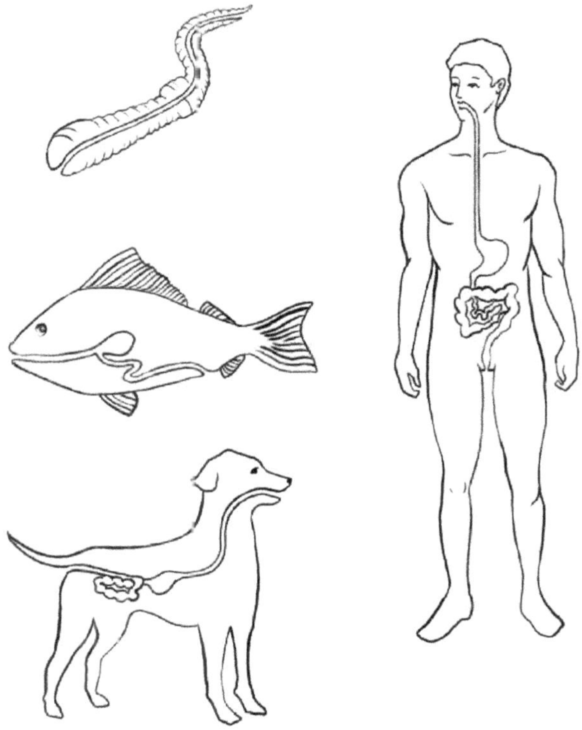

Figure 1-6: Topographical similarities in evolution.

A primitive life form, such as a worm, is essentially a long tube with a hole at each end. A fish is a long tube with a hole at each end, with the addition of fins on the sides. A quadruped, such as a dog, is a long tube with a hole at each end, but the fins have developed into four legs. Now we come to humans. A human is a long tube with a hole at each end, but two of those legs have developed into arms. In topographical terms, some of the properties of the more primitive structure persist. Bipedal humans are essentially more complex versions of their ancestors, retaining similar properties that can be described in the language of topography.

---

1 Manaka, Y., Itaya, K., & Birch, S. (1995). *Chasing the Dragon's Tail: The Theory and Practice of Acupuncture in the Work of Yoshio Manaka*. Brookline: Paradigm Publications. p. xxxvi.

Manaka believed the same topographical similarities play out in embryological development. In developmental terms, if the octahedron can be said to exist in the early stages of foetal development, then topographically it must still be there by the final stage and, therefore, in all stages of life, from birth and infancy into childhood and adulthood.

INHERITED FUNCTIONS

When there are only eight cells in the developing embryo, there is no nervous system and no endocrine system. How do these cells then coordinate their growth and development? Manaka theorised that the Eight Extras might provide a kind of communication network for the developing embryonic cells that helps guide later development. As the embryo develops, and other signalling mechanisms start to emerge through blood vessels and nerves, the role of the Eight Extras begins to be eclipsed by the more sophisticated and efficient mechanisms of the nervous and endocrine systems. Nevertheless, he proposed that the Eight Extras remain in place and active, slipping gradually into the background. They are enfolded within the body and lie *behind* the hormonal and neural regulation processes of the body. He hypothesised that although increasingly less active, they nevertheless exert a constant influence on the body, becoming more active as a therapy, such as acupuncture, is applied.

> *At the heart of his theoretical model lies the notion that the theories and rules of acupuncture—yin-yang, five phases, qi, meridians, acupoints, etc.—belong to a much broader, unobservable biological signal system that operates at very low levels of energy, and is very sensitive to 'tiny' stimulation.*[2]

In contemporary acupuncture, we refer to this original communication network as the Qi Paradigm or meridian network. However, as Manaka investigated it and tried to validate it, he began to refer to it as the X-signal system.

---

2 Birch, S. (2009). 'Dr Manaka Yoshio's Insights and Contributions to the Field of TEAM', *NAJOM* (Special Issue: In Memory of Dr Manaka Yoshio), 16(47). p. 19.

> *The older system now exists enfolded within the body, operating continuously at unobservable levels and clearly manifesting only with the correct stimulus energy input. This signal system works cooperatively with the other, less primitive systems and has the role of global regulation.*[3]

This X-signal system arose in the course of evolution and has been overshadowed by more efficient neurological, hormonal, and other signal systems. Nevertheless, it's still there, operating in the background.

Birch uses the analogy of memory to discuss this idea. When we are young, we have formative experiences that we later forget. These experiences still program us and influence the way we behave in adult life, even if we can't remember the original experiences.

> *At certain stages of evolutionary and/or embryological development, this information and its flow (meridians circuitry, qi movement, etc.) served specific biological functions. It exists in the body now, much like old childhood memories.*[4]

> *Both relate directly to the previous experiences but still exert influences now and in the future. They are mostly unobservable, but in specific circumstances, they can be recalled.*[5]

Much later, in adult life, this embryonic signalling system can still be accessed.

To use Bohm's terms, the information that is stored and not currently manifesting can be said to be 'hidden' or 'enfolded'.[6]

---

3 Ibid.

4 Ibid. p. 18.

5 Ibid.

6 Ibid. p. 20.

FROM THEORY TO APPLICATION

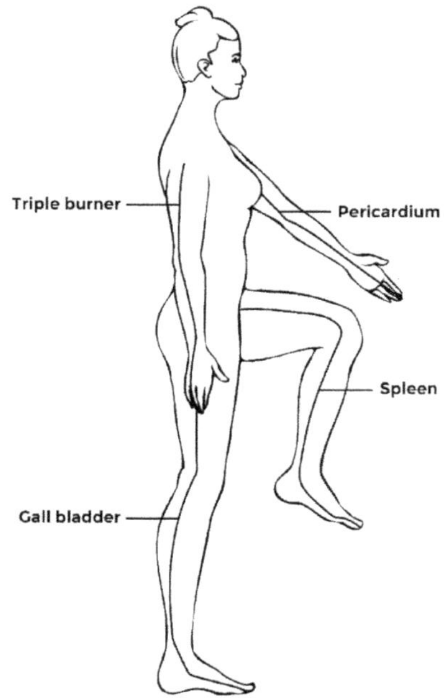

Figure 1-7: The shaoyang meridians divide the anterior and posterior aspects. The pericardium and spleen meridians separate anterior and posterior aspects of the limbs. On the trunk, GB 22, GB 26 and SP 21 are all on the mid-axillary line, separating the anterior and posterior halves of the body.

Let's go back to that anterior–posterior dividing line. We previously referred to it as the Yang Wei Mai. Still, it's good to remind ourselves that the Yang Wei Mai repeatedly intersects the trajectory of the foot *shaoyang* gall bladder meridian. When we look at that trajectory, we see that it roughly follows a line that separates anterior from posterior, both on the torso and on the yang lateral aspect of the leg. Similarly, when we look at the trajectory of its paired arm *shaoyang* triple burner meridian, when the arm is hanging naturally by the side of the body, it can be seen to follow a line that separates the anterior and posterior aspects of the arm on the yang lateral surface. Thus, the two meridians together separate the anterior and posterior aspects of the body.

Manaka also suggested that on the yin aspect of the leg, the leg *taiyin* spleen meridian separates anterior from posterior and, on the torso, ends on the sub-axillary line to separate anterior and posterior. When the arm is hanging naturally by the side of the body, however, it's the arm *jueyin* pericardium meridian that separates the anterior and posterior halves on the medial-facing yin aspect.

On the trunk, GB 22, GB 26 and SP 21 are all on the mid-axillary line, separating the anterior and posterior halves of the body.

Thus, some of the topological dividing lines of the octahedron fall on the gall bladder, triple burner, spleen, and pericardium meridians. Manaka postulated that this is why the master and coupled points of the Dai Mai, Yang Wei Mai, Chong Mai, and Yin Wei Mai fall on these meridians, namely GB 41, TB 5, SP 4, and P 6, respectively.

> *This nearly perfectly fits the pattern of four meridians dividing the front and back portions of the yin and yang aspects of the body. The exception is SP 4 on the spleen meridian, where the liver meridian would be more theoretically satisfying. In noting this variance, Manaka points out that the spleen meridian has a pathway very similar to the liver meridian on the inside of the legs. Even considering the theoretical variance, these four meridians do divide the front and back sides of the body and connect the upper and lower portions.*[7]

Finally, when looking at the meridian system, we see that the Ren Mai on the torso is closely flanked by the kidney meridian whereas, on the back, the Du Mai is closely flanked by the bladder meridian. We see this close relationship reflected in the master points of the Yin Qiao and Yang Qiao Mai, KID 6 and BL 62, which are also the coupled points of the Ren Mai and Du Mai.

Perhaps this sounds complicated? Indeed, Manaka's thoughts about the X-signal system and the octahedron drew on vast reams of scientific thinking and research. However, clinical applications of the octahedral model are far less complicated than the theory. Let's summarise the story so far and begin to flesh it out:

- Dr Manaka hypothesised that after the first three divisions of the zygote, the embryo has taken on specific properties associated with three dimensions, defined by the three axes.
- In anatomy, we refer to these as the sagittal, coronal, and transverse planes. The body is organised around these three planes throughout foetal development and after birth.

---

7 Matsumoto, K., & Birch, S. (1988). *Hara Diagnosis: Reflections on the Sea*. Brookline: Paradigm Publications. p. 363.

- The three axes of the body create an octahedral structure. Manaka correlated this structure to the Eight Extras. He saw them as an early information exchange and regulation system that is gradually overlaid by more complex and dynamic systems. They continue to function and regulate the body, operating behind other messenger systems, such as the nervous and endocrine systems.
- Manaka believed that in both evolutionary and foetal development, in topographical terms, life remains the same. This means that, just like our stack of balloons, the body can be divided into four anterior quadrants and four posterior quadrants. It's this mapping that's at the root of Manaka's method and allows his theory to flower into a coherent, pragmatic, and elegant clinical system.

Is there any evidence of all this in clinical practice? Are there, for example, diseases that manifest in quadrants or on one side of the midline? Or in the upper half or lower half of the body only? Yes. This evidence is presented in *Chasing the Dragon's Tail* and *Hara Diagnosis: Reflections on the Sea*. These include reports of experiments that observe sweating on one side of the body only, or in upper or lower quadrants, as well as harlequin syndrome, a neurological condition characterised by asymmetric sweating and flushing on only one side of the face, neck, and chest, often triggered by exercise or heat.

REGULATION

In *Restoring Order in Health and Chinese Medicine*, Birch and his co-authors document that the principal reason for the simultaneous development of metal tools for treatment and the construct of the *jingmai* was expressly for the purpose of regulating qi.[8, 9]

---

8 Birch, S., Cabrer, M., & Rodriguez, M. (2025). *Restoring Order in Health and Chinese Medicine: Studies of the Development and Use of Qi and the Channels*. 2nd ed. London: Sayoshi Books.

9 Unschuld, P. U., & Tessenow, H. (2011). *Huang Di Nei Jing Ling Shu: The Ancient Classic on Needle Therapy*. Berkeley: University of California Press.

The idea of regulating the flow of qi to cure disease is almost universal in Traditional East Asian Medicine (TEAM), including in meridian-based bodywork methods such as Shiatsu. For example, renowned Japanese Shiatsu practitioner Shizuto Masunaga (1925–1981) described a balloon model. When someone is ill, it's as if an inflated balloon (the energy system) develops a dent (*kyo*, or deficiency). This dent is mirrored by a corresponding bump elsewhere in the system (*jitsu*, or excess). The purpose of treatment is regulation: ironing out these dents and bumps.

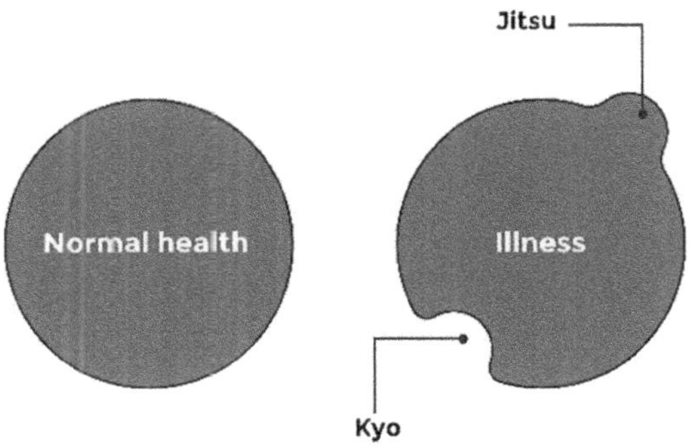

Figure 1-8: Dents and bumps.

One way to visualise this inner–outer relationship is to look at a commonplace DIY tool: a carpenter's contour gauge. Designed like a very dense comb but with movable pins, you can press it against an irregular surface such as a skirting board or the lintel of a door. The pressure depresses the pins at the points of contact on the inner-facing edge and pushes them out at the outer-facing edge, so they protrude symmetrically—a mechanical manifestation of yin and yang.

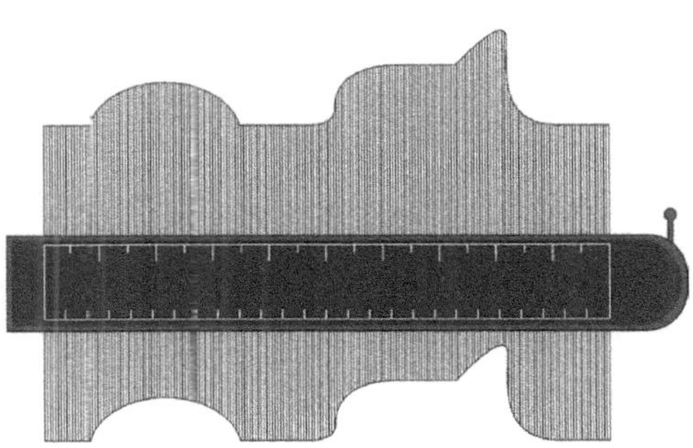

Figure 1-9: A carpenter's contour gauge shows in two dimensions how dents and bumps mirror each other.

We can observe the same compensatory process at work in the three-dimensional structure of the body, as seen, for example, in the lumbar curvature. If the lumbar curvature is too pronounced, as in anterior pelvic tilt, then the belly seems to protrude, even if the person is not overweight.

Since 2009, Birch has been developing a model of concentric circles—one that shows how the meridians, the organ/functional systems and the patient's vitality are interconnected.[10, 11, 12, 13]

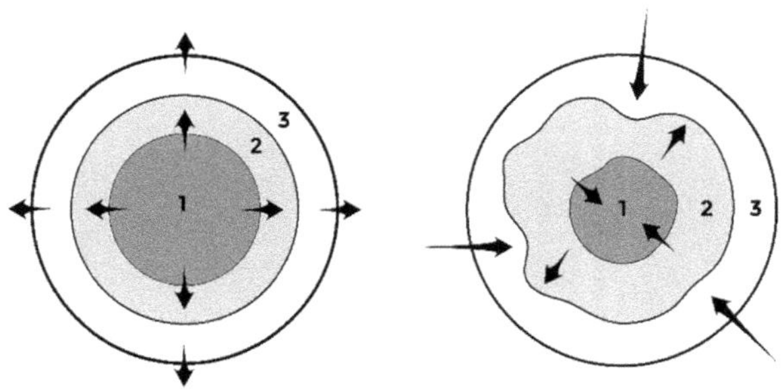

Figure 1-10: Birch model: 1) zangfu organs, 2) meridian systems, 3) overall vitality.

The inner circle (1) represents the *zangfu* organs, and the middle circle (2) represents the meridians on the exterior of the body. If you depress or distort the outer circle, like pressing on the contour gauge, corresponding protrusions may occur on the opposite side and the inner circle. These distortions affect the functioning of the inner circle. If you can correct the imbalances on the outside, you can improve the functioning of the organs on the inside. The outer circle (3) represents the overall vitality (in Chinese, e.g. *zhengqi*, *yuanqi*, *shengqi*). The more distorted the circles within it, the more weakened it can become. Treatment is aimed at balancing *kyo* and *jitsu* in the meridians so the functional systems can be repaired.

---

10 Birch, S. (2009). 'Filling the Whole in Acupuncture. Part 1: What Are We Doing in the Supplementation Needle Technique?' *European Journal of Oriental Medicine*, 6(2). pp. 25–35.

11 Birch, S. (2009). 'Filling the Whole in Acupuncture. Part 2: What Are We Doing in the Supplementation Needle Technique?' *European Journal of Oriental Medicine*, 6(3). pp. 18–27.

12 Birch, S. (2011). *Shonishin: Japanese Pediatric Acupuncture*. Stuttgart: Thieme Medical Publishers.

13 Birch, S., Cabrer, M., & Rodriguez, M. (2025). *Restoring Order in Health and Chinese Medicine: Studies of the Development and Use of Qi and the Channels*. 2nd ed. London: Sayoshi Books.

These models are excellent ways to represent the fundamental relationships between yin and yang, interior and exterior, and structure and function, and will inform our thinking about the purpose of applying acupuncture.

Manaka's octahedral model is no different. We can imagine an octahedron with similar dents and bumps that inhibit physiological function. By extrapolating that the body is composed of four anterior and four posterior quadrants, Manaka hypothesised a constantly interacting model, where the amount of qi flowing through each of the octants was regulated by the amount of qi flowing through the other seven. Illness and health depend on the circulation of energy through the eight octants.

Manaka's model has three practical principles:

1. The octahedron can be mapped out on the body.
2. Palpating the abdomen and associated points helps identify the appropriate treatment.
3. The Eight Extras can be used to regulate and adjust the octahedral structure.

Classical acupuncture had already produced mappings on the abdomen that reflected the condition of the five elements, the organs, and the meridians. Manaka further developed these classical *hara* palpation models, charting the influence of the Eight Extras on the abdomen. His model uses the Ren Mai and Du Mai to separate left and right; the Dai Mai, at the level of the umbilicus, to separate upper from lower; and the Yang Wei Mai to separate the anterior quadrants from the posterior ones.

If illness and health depend on the circulation of energy through the eight octants, then his treatment objective was to restore the overall balance within the meridian system between the inferior and superior, front and back, and left and right halves of the body. By regulating the meridian system on the outside of the body using the Eight Extras, he could regulate the functioning of the organs on the inside of the body.

> *Disorders manifesting symptoms on the posterior aspect of the body are often most effectively treated on the anterior aspect of the body, and vice versa. Lumbago back pain, for example, can be treated by stimulating*

> *the sensitive points of the thorax and abdomen.... In accordance with this 'principle of opposites', one should also treat complaints of the upper body by points on the lower body, and vice versa.*[14]

Manaka's system focuses on regulating the meridian system by applying all the principles of yin and yang, lower and upper, front and back, and left and right in his model to balance the octahedron, utilising various methods and modalities. He considered the flow of qi in the meridians in the eight octants of the body to be a key to rectifying the condition of the body and curing disease. What distinguishes it is the emphasis on the Eight Extras for doing so. In Manaka's model, we have to regulate the facets of the octahedron through the Eight Extras, the dividing lines or fulcra between yin and yang, either through their pathways or by the location of their master and coupled points.

Finally, and crucially, rather than using traditional methods for selecting the Eight Extras, such as differentiation of symptoms, Manaka devised a palpation-based diagnostic method, mapping out stiffness and pressure pain reactions on the abdomen and other related points. We'll be studying those mappings and points in detail soon. For now, what's important to understand is that this theory is intensely practical. **To diagnose the state of the octahedron, we must palpate the abdomen and meridians.**

ACUPUNCTURE DOESN'T 'CURE' ANYTHING

Patients often ask if there is an acupuncture point for a specific symptom. "Can you do a point for knee pain? Is there a point for headaches? Which point should I press for sleep?" In some ways, and at certain levels, the answer is yes, there are acupuncture points for specific symptoms. P 6 is used for nausea, LIV 3 is good for headaches, and Master Tung's DT.07 point is good for knee pain when bled.

14 Manaka, Y., & Urquhart, I. (1972). *The Layman's Guide to Acupuncture*. New York: Weatherhill. p. 121.

This was also true of the Eight Extras. Their original presentation was as a collection of symptoms. If a patient presented with one or more of these, the practitioner would choose that vessel. For example, for shortness of breath, they would needle the master and coupled points of the Ren Mai. We can refer to this approach as symptomatic acupuncture, and it has an important role in treatment.

Traditional acupuncture, however, is not just about needling the right point for a specific symptom. The regulatory models above suggest that by adjusting the body back to its optimum configuration, we improve its overall functioning. In other words, acupuncture doesn't 'cure' anything: instead, it signals the body to cure itself. We send a signal from the outside of the body to the inside, and this signal triggers mechanisms in the body that create shifts in body function and levels of pain.

We can use the analogy of going to visit a favourite relative. When you arrive at the front door, you ring the doorbell. Eventually, the door opens, and Grandma emerges to greet you. We can all agree that it was not the doorbell that opened the door: it merely sent a signal to the interior of the house, and that signal created movement within it.

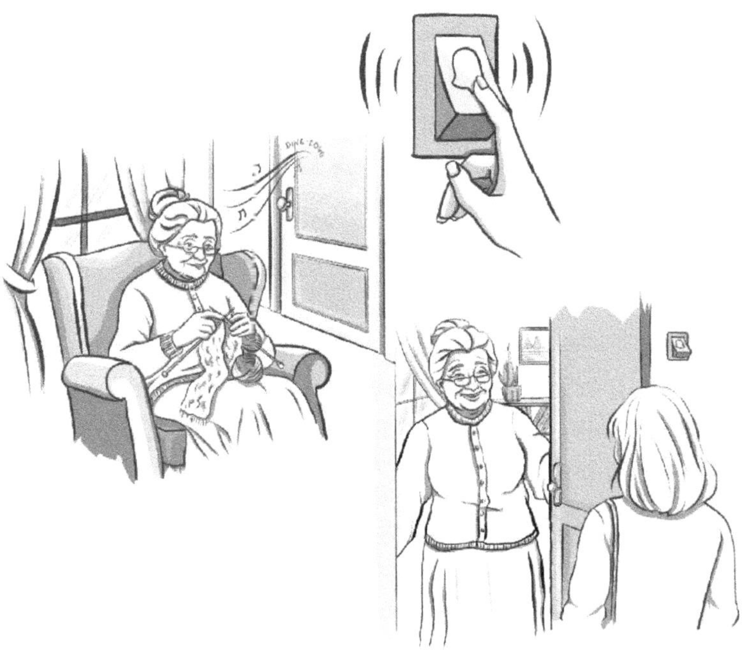

Figure 1-11: Acupuncture doesn't open the door; it merely sends a signal.

THE QI PARADIGM, OR THE X-SIGNAL SYSTEM

This signalling process is a core principle of traditional acupuncture, the so-called Qi Paradigm. The Qi Paradigm includes all traditional explanations for the mechanisms of acupuncture that refer to the Chinese concept of qi, often translated misleadingly or incompletely as 'energy'. As we have seen, Dr Manaka came up with an alternative name for this: the X-signal system. This term suggests meanings that are not present in the word *energy*. If we can think of qi as information and the meridian system as an information highway, conveying signals, then we may gain a clearer understanding:

> *There is a primitive signal (information) system in the body that has embryological roots, but is masked by the more advanced and complex control (regulation) systems. Thus, the original signal system is hard to find or see. This primitive system is able to detect and discriminate internal and external changes and plays a role in regulating the body by transmitting this information. This system serves as the modus operandi of acupuncture.*[15]

What's more, if we go back to the analogy of a doorbell, a doorbell typically uses minimal electrical current. While the results of ringing a doorbell may be dynamic, such as a teenager bounding noisily down the stairs to open the door, the doorbell remains a low-energy signalling system. Manaka had the same view of the meridian system. It first came into being after conception—it started as and remains a low-energy signalling system. Therefore, to access it, very low-energy stimulation is appropriate. This may seem obvious, but as much of modern acupuncture relies on high levels of stimulation, we should pause to explore this idea.

If you and one of the authors of this book were to go to a football match together (let's say it's Stephen Birch), when you want to communicate something to him, because of the noise the fans are making, you're going to have to put your mouth close to his ear and raise your voice. You might say, "I NEED TO GO TO THE TOILET. I'LL BE RIGHT BACK." For the situation and environment, this would be an appropriate level of signalling.

---

15 Manaka, Y., Itaya, K., & Birch, S. (1995). *Chasing the Dragon's Tail: The Theory and Practice of Acupuncture in the Work of Yoshio Manaka*. Brookline: Paradigm Publications. p. 18.

If, however, you were in a public library and you communicated the same message in the same manner, you would certainly get some disapproval, if not censure, from the people around you. The same rules apply to the X-signal system and the octahedral model. It doesn't like shouting—you have to whisper!

We can explain this in another, more mathematical way. If you take the numbers 2, 4, 8, 16, 32, and 64, what they all have in common is the smallest number, 2. If you now consider all the different kinds of acupuncture methods that exist—from the most subtle, such as contact needling or stroking with an *enshin* (a rounded rubbing tool described in the *Ling Shu*), to those that use the most stimulation, such as electroacupuncture or eliciting the strongest *deqi* sensations while entwining soft tissue fibres around the needle—what they all have in common is what happens with the most subtle. In other words, just as the nervous and endocrine systems overlay the subtle regulation of the embryological meridian system, strong stimulation acupuncture obscures the signals of the qi system, so that it's no longer possible to distinguish its effects from those of the nervous system.

> *It is important that we do not confuse the neurological and humoral effects of acupuncture, so thoroughly researched and described in needle analgesia and anesthesia research, with the signal system effects... While admittedly it is difficult to discriminate the clearer neurological and humoral effects of acupuncture from the subtler effects of the signal system, if we consciously try to use the signal system, we can produce remarkable results. This is because this system participates in the therapy regardless of whether we think about it or... If we can learn to control the signal system, which requires only the tiniest energy or signal input, we can produce dramatic effects throughout the information and energy systems.*[16]

Thus, our role is not to do something to the body to cure a symptom; our role is to signal, trigger, or induce changes in the body when it is imbalanced so it can find its own way to right itself. In traditional acupuncture, this process of signalling is called the 'regulation of qi and blood'.

---

16 Ibid. p. 35.

> *The goal of meridian-based* hari *therapy is the regulation of* ki *and* ketsu [qi and blood]. *Therefore, in this form of medicine, illness is seen as disturbances in the* ki *and* ketsu, *while health is recognised as their balance.*
>
> —Kodo Fukushima[17]

As Fukushima, the founding president of the Toyohari Association, stated, many practitioners in Japan would agree that this is all an acupuncturist does; in daily practice, our role is simply to regulate the flow of qi and blood. Manaka's goal was to regulate the flow of qi and blood in the octants—ringing the doorbell on the outside of the house to create movement within.

SUMMARY

- **Embryological origins:** The body's three axes (left–right, top–bottom, and front–back) form an octahedral structure that emerges early in embryonic development after the first three cell divisions.
- **The octahedral model:** Manaka theorised that this structure corresponds to the Extraordinary Vessels, which serve as a primitive signalling system predating nerves and hormones and continue to operate as a background regulatory mechanism throughout life.
- **A low-energy system:** As the system comes into existence in embryo, it's a low-energy system, so we need to stimulate it with low-energy mechanisms. It doesn't like shouting; it responds to whispers.
- **Topographical balancing:** Manaka's model is topological and regulatory: imbalances in one quadrant affect the others, like dents and bumps in a balloon. Treatment restores flow across the octahedron.
- **Root-level intervention:** Treatment of the Eight Extras addresses the root imbalance.
- **Diagnosis through palpation:** Clinical diagnosis relies on palpation, especially of the *hara*, to locate reactions and determine which Extraordinary Vessel requires treatment.

17 Fukushima, K. (1991). *Meridian Therapy*. Tokyo: Toyo Hari Medical Association. p. 37.

- **Signalling not curing:** The goal of treatment is regulation. Acupuncture doesn't 'cure' things; it signals the body to do the work, like ringing a doorbell and letting the system respond from within.

WHAT'S NEXT

Manaka's approach brings together root and branch treatments in a structured sequence. In the next chapter, we'll see how the Four Steps provide a clear framework for diagnosis, regulation, and symptom relief, while remaining flexible enough to adapt to each patient's needs.

CHAPTER 2

FOUR STEPS TO TREAT ROOT AND BRANCH

COMPARING ROOT AND BRANCH

Acupuncture treatment can be categorised into two primary modes of action: root treatment (*honchiho*) and branch treatment (*hyochiho*). Let's imagine a tall plant with a few wilting or brown leaves. We can use a pair of scissors to cut them off; this makes the plant look better, but it doesn't fix the problem.

If you take the opposite path—watering the roots and adding nutrients to heal the plant—it takes longer for the plant to grow new leaves, but it recovers fully. Treating the root means addressing the underlying causes of the disease, while treating the branch means addressing the symptoms. Fukushima described these two processes as fundamental healing and targeted healing.[18]

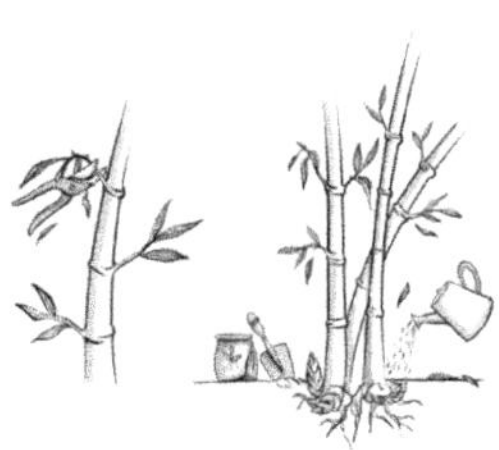

Figure 2-1: Branch treatment and root treatment—symptoms and cause.

---

[18] Ibid.

Some combination of root and branch treatment is necessary for effective outcomes. In acupuncture, there are purist schools that focus wholly on root treatment, and there are pragmatic approaches that focus wholly on branch treatment. Sadly, much current acupuncture research pays little attention to, or misunderstands, root and branch theory.[19] This research bias overlooks the importance of these two distinct approaches.

In most styles of acupuncture, assessing and correcting deficiency and excess are regarded as the most important tasks—and the most difficult. Treating the octahedron is similar, and the premise is the same. If we regulate qi in the octants, the body will regulate itself. As we will see below, Dr Manaka found that it was not necessary to focus on precise definitions of which meridians are deficient and which are excess—the octahedral model allows for a focus on qi regulation that simply exploits the natural balancing properties of yin–yang.

> *In the root treatment, a common pattern is discriminated with the aim of balancing the body as a whole and a common point selection strategy is used regardless of the complaint or disease. If the root treatment is fully successful, specific complaints or localised pain are resolved without symptomatic or local treatment (at least, that is the way it is supposed to work). Today, both aspects of treatment are considered necessary, like two wheels on an axle.*
>
> —Yoshio Manaka[20]

Manaka's parenthetical aside hints at a clinical reality: root treatment creates order, but it may not fully resolve stubborn symptoms or marked local pain. In these cases, branch treatment helps direct the body's newly regulated qi towards the areas that still need support. His axle analogy is useful here because it highlights the mutual importance of treating root and branch, although it does not specify the order in which to do so. Unless there is something very wrong with the vehicle, both wheels advance together simultaneously. In clinical practice, do you do root treatment before, after, or simultaneously with branch treatment? Manaka emphasised that his primary

---

19 *Japanese Acupuncture Today*. (2018). Episode 3: Hari-kyū Today [Video]. Available at: https://youtu.be/aoN3bwXmacY

20 Manaka, Y. (2009). 'The Concept of Meridians from a Systems Perspective', *NAJOM* (Special Issue: In Memory of Dr Manaka Yoshio), 16(47), p. 28.

focus was on root treatment, and he preferred to do it first, before branch treatment. This is because doing root treatment creates order when the system is in disarray. Once the system is more ordered, it is easier to do branch treatment.[21]

Additionally, from a practitioner's point of view, starting with root treatment and continuing to symptom relief creates a different kind of order—a helpful structure and routine for each session. This is like doing a *kata* in martial arts. Doing the same thing repeatedly leads to learning and mastery. Moreover, having a sequence and order is particularly useful with patients who have multiple symptoms clamouring for attention. In both Manaka System Acupuncture and Toyohari, a contemporary Japanese Meridian Therapy style, the root treatment quite often takes care of several symptoms, leaving only the most stubborn to be addressed by branch treatment. In rare cases in Toyohari, practitioners may begin with branch treatment when a patient arrives in such severe pain that they cannot lie down or settle sufficiently for root treatment.[22]

MANAKA'S ROOT TREATMENT

When we consider yin and yang in clinical terms, we look for relationships that are either harmonised or out of balance. We can imagine two children sitting on a seesaw. If the children are of equal weight, the seesaw is level. Put a heavier child on one seat and a lighter one on the other and you see an imbalance: the seat holding the lighter child goes up, and the seat holding the heavier child goes down. This is one way of representing the distribution between paired yin–yang halves in the body. Traditional Chinese Medicine (TCM) textbooks also represent these shifting balances with a series of column graphs. In all models, to treat a problem, we need to rectify an imbalance of yin and yang.

In Manaka's octahedral model, this simple yin–yang pairing expands into a larger system of eight facets that are in dynamic equilibrium. You can imagine this as four seesaws, all connected and moving in interlinked relationships, each child now representing one of the eight octants of the body. This is like having four seesaws, all connected and moving in interlinked relationships, each child representing one of the

21 Ibid.

22 Kivity, O. (ed.) (2007). 'Kikei Nuggets'. *Keiraku Chiryo—International* Toyohari News, 1(3). p. 39.

eight octants of the body. Upper balances lower, left balances right, front balances back, and vice versa. When teaching, Dr Manaka "often used a complex mobile to illustrate the multidimensionality of clinical reality".[23] Similarly, Stephen Birch has sometimes used a model octahedron made from coat-hanger wire or small magnets to illustrate the structural distortions that can occur throughout the model when pressure is applied to one of its eight facets. Treating just one of the seesaws affects all of them. Treating one octant affects all eight.

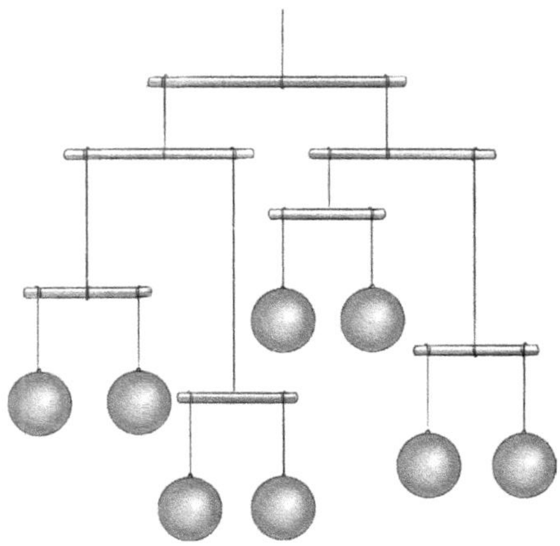

Figure 2-2: A hanging mobile can illustrate the multidimensionality of clinical reality.

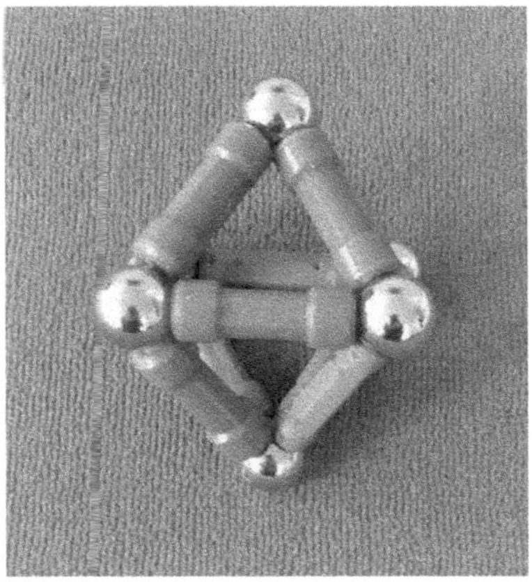

Figure 2-3: A magnetic octahedron.

---

23 Birch, S., & Felt, R. (1999). *Understanding Acupuncture.* Edinburgh: Churchill Livingstone. p. 139.

MAPPING OUT THE OCTAHEDRON

Let's map out Manaka's octahedron on the torso—it's a simple process. The Ren Mai and Du Mai run along the anterior and posterior midline, dividing the body into left and right halves. The Dai Mai (Belt Vessel) can be seen to run horizontally along the abdomen at the umbilicus, extending posteriorly to L2, giving us upper and lower halves. The anterior and posterior halves of the body on the trunk are defined by the Yang Wei Mai, sharing the trajectory of the gall bladder meridian along the median line of the lateral torso.

On the limbs, the dividing line between anterior and posterior is created by the triple burner paired with the gall bladder on the lateral aspects and the spleen paired with the pericardium on the medial aspects (see Figure 1-6 and Figure 2-4).

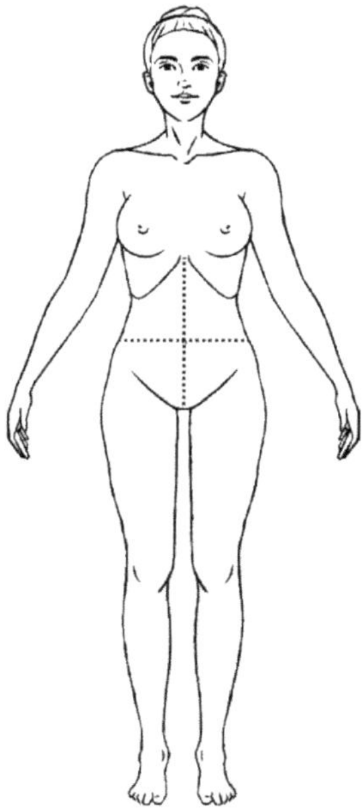

Figure 2-4: The four anterior quadrants on the torso.

It's worth emphasising the role of palpation here. We'll be returning to it often throughout the book since, in many Japanese therapies, the information gained through touch is considered paramount. Manaka systematically mapped out the abdomen, linking each of the anterior quadrants to the Eight Extras to develop a remarkably subtle diagnostic system. The reactive points on the abdomen provided clues for treatment, which aimed to clear those reactions.

These abdominal reactions are one of the delights of MSA, because not only do you, as the practitioner, feel them improving, but the patient also experiences the changes. And this process happens in seconds, not minutes.

> *Studying Dr Manaka's yin–yang balancing method brought acupuncture alive for me after ten years of TCM. It took me out of my head and into my hands, with dynamic changes occurring within a few seconds: tight, tender points on the abdomen relax; both patient and practitioner experience immediate feedback, also reflected in changes to symptoms.*
>
> —Marian Fixler

As you can see, Manaka's octahedral model of the body, like everything else in his work, is not an abstract theoretical concept but a clinical model with intensely practical applications. You can map it, touch it, and feel it changing under your fingers. Most importantly, your patients can feel these reactions as well, which helps them perceive and quantify their improvement.

THE FOUR STEPS

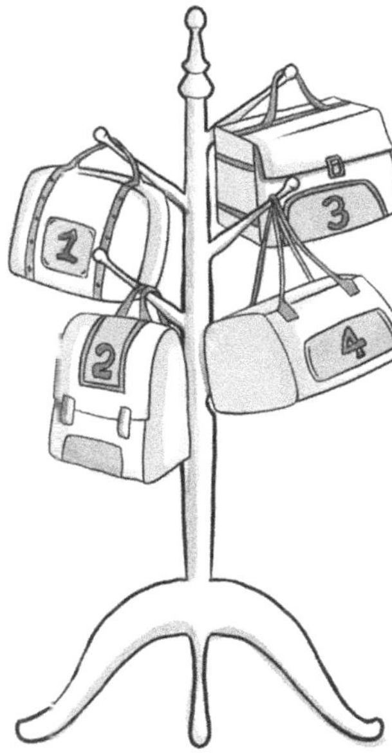

Figure 2-5: Dr Manaka's Four Step protocol provides us with four essential kitbags of options, each with a clear objective.

Dr Manaka's comprehensive and structured treatment approach applies the fundamental concepts of yin and yang to treatment. He created a Four Step protocol that works systematically to treat first the root, then the branch. He described this approach as "looking for the most significant paradox in the body".[24] The first two steps comprise the core root treatment. The third step addresses structural problems to support the root treatment, and the fourth step focuses on branch treatment (symptom relief). Some instructors list a further Step 5 which covers home therapy but, in this book, we focus on Manaka's core Four Step protocol; home treatment will be discussed in later volumes.

[24] Matsumoto, K., & Birch, S. (1988). *Hara Diagnosis: Reflections on the Sea*. Brookline: Paradigm Publications. pp. 349–375.

Table 2.1: Manaka's Four Steps.

	GOAL	**COMMONLY USED METHODS**
Step 1	Treat to reduce reactions on the yin anterior half of the body, focusing on the abdomen.	Usually applied with polarity agents such as ion-pumping cords, electrostatic adsorbers, or Manaka's ion-beam device placed on the master and coupled points of the Eight Extras. Other approaches to Step 1 will be explored in subsequent books.
Step 2	Treat to reduce reactions on the yang posterior half of the body, commonly associated with the abdominal findings.	Most commonly applied with *kyutoshin* (moxa on the needle) on the back-*shu* points related to the Step 1 treatment, though simple *chishin* (retained needle) and a heat lamp may be substituted.
Step 3	Adjust structural imbalances.	Neuromuscular re-education, with Sotai counter-resistance stretching movements. *Okyu* (small-cone moxibustion) can be applied simultaneously with the stretch.
Step 4	Control symptoms.	At this point, several options are available and can be applied, with moxibustion, additional retained needles, or intradermal needling. What is most important is to avoid overtreatment, tailoring these options to the specific needs and tolerances of the patient.

We can think of this Four Step protocol as a coat stand with four hooks. On each hook is a bag packed with a specific category of clothes: underwear in one, shirts and tops in another, and in the others, the things we wear on the lower half—skirts, shorts or long trousers. Every day, we rummage through each bag and take out one of each item, then we happily get dressed and go out. The order matters—we put on underwear before anything else—and the exact clothes we choose vary according to the circumstances, like the weather and the occasion. What's important is that each item fits its category and that the outfit works as a whole.

Manaka's Four Step protocol is similar. Our clinical kitbags contain a vast repertoire of techniques that may be used to treat our patients: ion pumping, needling, cupping, moxibustion, ear acupuncture, and bloodletting. Manaka organised his treatments into four basic categories with specific stated objectives. You can hang any method you want on these Four Steps, so long as it meets the objectives.

STEP 1: RELEASING THE YIN ASPECT OF THE BODY

The aim of Step 1 is to identify and release tightness and pressure pain findings on the abdomen, the anterior yin surface. Manaka's principal approach for this first step was his Eight Extras treatment. As we have seen in Chapter 1, the Eight Extras form an octahedral structure in the body. Treatment is designed to restore equilibrium between these sections or octants, thus creating balance in the overall meridian system. Manaka developed five basic patterns, which have been supplemented by patterns from instructors, such as Stephen Birch in Europe and Brenda Loew in the United States, resulting in eight to ten commonly used patterns. We'll examine these in more detail later.

Let's start by describing Step 1 in a few short lines:

- MSA identifies an affected Extraordinary Vessel pattern through abdominal palpation.
- Once the pattern is identified, the master and coupled points of that vessel are needled superficially without obtaining *deqi*. The needles are then connected using an ion-pumping cord (IPC), which is essentially a

polarity device that creates a microvoltage between the two points. This low-intensity stimulation is appropriate for treating the Eight Extras, which we have seen to be a low-intensity system.
- After application of the IPC, the tightness and pressure pain reactions in the abdomen should improve.

For example, if the midline of the abdomen feels tight and painful, relating to the Ren Mai, you will needle LU 7 and KID 6 bilaterally, then connect the points with an IPC. The abdominal reactions should improve rapidly, usually after roughly 30 seconds.

In addition to these basic patterns, several other patterns based on abdominal reactions can be applied. Manaka also used polar channel pairs (those meridians at opposite ends of the Chinese clock), treating the supplementing and draining points of both meridians with polarity agents. These are typically covered in the MSA Level 2 weekend trainings, and we will examine them in Vol. 2 of this book series.

Manaka had other rarely used fallback strategies for complex cases where nothing was working. These included whole-body moxibustion treatments. We'll look at these in Vol. 2. Essentially, anything goes, as long as it fulfils the goals of Step 1; namely, to release reactions on the abdomen.

AN ADDITIONAL GOAL FOR STEP 1

Step 1 is the patient's first contact with your treatment methods. They may often be a little stressed or anxious, perhaps because it is their first treatment or because they have been rushing to be on time for the appointment. Sitting in the waiting area, they may still feel connected to their work or family stresses through their mobile devices. They may be experiencing physical or emotional pain. Thus, Step 1 should be the time to bring them from this initial state of tension to a more relaxed and receptive state, allowing them to receive the information from the treatment.

When teaching, Stephen Birch has said he sometimes favours ion-pumping cords with needles over faster polarity devices such as electrostatic adsorbers—devices we'll describe and compare later. This is because the longer process required by needling 'pins down' the patient for ten minutes, and that stillness encourages them to relax. Thus, in addition to Manaka's goal for Step 1, we can add relax the body-mind as a secondary goal:

- Release the yin aspect of the body
- Relax the body-mind

STEP 2: RELEASING THE YANG ASPECT OF THE BODY

If the aim of Step 1 is to release the yin aspect of the body and relax the body-mind, the aim of Step 2 is to release the yang aspect of the body, principally the back. In historical MSA, Step 2 involves locating reactions at the back-*shu* points that relate to the pattern found in the abdominal diagnosis. For example, when treating the Yang Wei–Dai Mai pair with ion-pumping cords on the master and coupled points TB 5 and GB 41, the corresponding Step 2 treatment would be BL 19 and BL 22, the back-*shu* points of the gall bladder and triple burner. Usually, Manaka used *kyutoshin* (moxa on the needle; literally moxa placed on the needle handle) technique. If the patient is thin and unsuitable for the deeper needling required for *kyutoshin*, you can use *chishin* (shallow needling) and a heat lamp. The same approach applies when you cannot burn moxa because of clinic policies, smoke detectors, or inadequate ventilation.

STEP 3: TREATING STRUCTURAL IMBALANCES

Manaka described Step 3 as optional and did not routinely include it in the treatment flow for patients, reserving it only for cases where the patient showed clear structural imbalances. For example, when comparing the left and right sides, you might find scoliosis or differences in the level of the hip girdle, or the muscles on one side of the spine might be more swollen than those on the other.

SOTAI

Manaka studied, incorporated, and modified a series of neuromuscular re-education exercises known as Sotai. Sotai was first developed by the Japanese bodyworker and medical doctor Keizo Hashimoto (1897–1993) and involves using counter-resistance stretches to release restrictions of movement.[25] Manaka found ways to augment the therapy by incorporating the application of heat during the counter-resistance stretches. Sometimes he used fire needling, but usually small-cone moxibustion. He noted that the sudden pinch of heat from these tools greatly enhanced the effect of the exercises. This book will explore just one Sotai exercise, with more to come in later volumes.

It is worth mentioning that Sotai addresses the sinew meridians, and techniques from other disciplines of structural adjustment, such as osteopathy, chiropractic, Tuina, and Shiatsu, could also be added at this step.

STEP 4: SYMPTOM RELIEF

Step 4 is the final stage of Manaka's protocol. He used it to address the other wheel on the axle: to treat symptoms. Manaka had specific routines for symptom relief utilising combinations of local meridian points with hand acupuncture and ear acupuncture points. These combinations—what Dr Manaka called 'isophasal' treatments—are remarkably effective for treating symptoms and can also be taught in a simplified form for patients to use as home therapy. We recommend these techniques; however, for this step, any method that relieves the symptoms is permissible. For students of MSA coming from other styles, this is a big relief. You can still do what you do and what you know. These include needling symptomatic points, moxibustion, cupping, or bloodletting. However, we will see later that dosage is an essential component of treatment design. Other branch treatments can be considered, provided they don't exceed the patient's threshold for treatment. You don't want to overtreat your patient.

---

25 Hashimoto, K., & Kawakami, Y. (1983). *Sotai: Balance and Health Through Natural Movement*. Tokyo: Japan Publications Inc.

SUMMARY

- **Root and branch treatment:** MSA has two components: root treatment (addressing the octahedron) and branch treatment (addressing symptoms). Both are essential, like two wheels on an axle.
- **Structured clinical method:** The Four Step protocol is a structured approach that first treats the root imbalance (Steps 1 and 2), adjusts structural imbalances if necessary (Step 3), and treats symptoms (Step 4).
- **Step 1a. Diagnosing and treating the root:** The octahedral model provides the diagnostic focus of Step 1, with the abdominal pattern, diagnosed through palpation, determining treatment with the Eight Extras. The abdomen offers real-time feedback that both practitioner and patient can feel, often within seconds.
- **Step 1b. Yin polarity treatment:** Step 1 uses low-intensity stimulation with polarity devices such as ion-pumping cords to treat the anterior yin body and begins to restore the balance of the octahedron.
- **Step 2. Yang treatment via the back:** Step 2 addresses the yang posterior aspect through the back-*shu* points and techniques such as *kyutoshin*.
- **Step 3. Structural adjustment:** Step 3 uses Sotai, sometimes combined with moxa, to address structural issues.
- **Step 4. Symptom relief:** Step 4 focuses on symptom relief, using microsystems such as ear acupuncture. Other safe and appropriate techniques may be used, with the proviso that the patient isn't overtreated.
- **Flexibility of method:** The Four Steps are not tied to fixed techniques. Any method may be used if it achieves the objective of the step in which it is applied.

WHAT'S NEXT

In the first of our Context chapters, we'll explore the history of Japanese acupuncture and moxibustion. We'll look at its distinguishing features and its characteristic emphasis on palpation, minimal stimulation, and refinement. Unique though MSA is, it remains deeply rooted in its Japanese heritage.

CHAPTER 3

CONTEXT: JAPANESE ACUPUNCTURE AND MOXIBUSTION

You can skip this chapter if you want! Long ago, co-authors Marian Fixler and Oran Kivity completed a teacher training course with Eric Sotto, a trainer in education. Sotto maintained that most teachers like to start at what they consider the beginning of a topic. One of his most insightful pieces of advice was to start in the middle. Otherwise, by the time you've covered your topic's origins, history, and contemporary expressions, you've used up all your students' attention. When you get to the useful stuff, they're asking for a tea break. That's why the first two chapters of this book jump right into the gears and cogs of Manaka's system.

As we learn Manaka's Four Step protocol, we will occasionally step back from the clinical details to view the broader picture, exploring how his method fits within both Japanese Acupuncture and Moxibustion (JAAM) and Traditional East Asian Medicine (TEAM) as a whole. To this end, we include several chapters covering broader topics, which can be read at any time. These chapters are easily identified in the Table of Contents by the word *Context* before the chapter title.

Knowing that readers are rarely linear in the way they digest books, we can advise that if you're keen to get straight into the nuts and bolts of Manaka's system, you can skip the Context chapters for now. But if you want to practise MSA, you need to understand its place within the broader context of Japanese acupuncture history and culture, and you should definitely revisit these chapters. The focus of this one is on the unique, distinguishing characteristics of JAAM and how Manaka's system exemplifies them.[26]

HISTORY

Acupuncture first developed in China but, in 562 CE, knowledge of this and other technical subjects was introduced to Japan by a Buddhist monk named Chiso, who arrived bearing 164 books on acupuncture and herbal medicine—a truly immense cultural gift.[27] From written references to acupuncture in the *Ishitsu-ryo* (医疾令), which were ancient Japanese medical laws codified as early as 701 CE, it is clear that acupuncture immediately thrived in Japan, becoming an important pillar of public health care over the following 1,200 years.[28]

Initially, there were active exchanges of information between China and Japan; however, due to political factors, including wars and piracy, these exchanges were curtailed, ultimately coming to a complete halt in 1635. Japan then closed its borders to foreign influences for more than 200 years, until 1853.

One example of this is the very different relationship between herbal medicine theory and acupuncture theory in China and Japan. When the first training programmes were established in the Imperial Medical College, acupuncture and herbal medicine were regarded as distinctly different. Thus, from the outset, acupuncture and herbal medicine in Japan were always learned separately.

---

26 Much of the information in this chapter came from an online interview hosted by Oran Kivity with panellists Stephen Birch, Brenda Loew and Junji Mizutani. The interview later grew into an article for the *European Journal of Oriental Medicine*. Interview quotations have been lightly edited for clarity. See: Japanese Acupuncture Today (2018), Episode 3: 'Harikyu' [Video], available at https://youtu.be/aoN3bwXmacY and Kivity, O. (2018), 'Japanese Acupuncture: What's So Unique?', *European Journal of Oriental Medicine*, 9(2).

27 Fratkin, J. (1999). 'The Emergence of Japanese Style Acupuncture', *California Journal of Oriental Medicine (CJOM)*, 10(1), Winter.

28 Kobayashi, A., Uefuji, M., & Yasumo, W. (2008). 'History and Progress of Japanese Acupuncture', *Evidence-Based Complementary and Alternative Medicine*, 7(3), pp. 359–365. https://doi.org/10.1093/ecam/nem155

During the same period in China, acupuncture gained a reputation as a dangerous therapy and fell into disrepute. This allowed other therapies, such as moxibustion and herbal medicine, to become more popular. Then, in the early Song dynasty (960–1279), Emperor Renzong (Tiansheng), wondering if the harmful effects of acupuncture were due to poor point location, commissioned the Bronze Man text, which revitalised the study and practice of acupuncture in China. Shortly after this, renewed interest in classical theory led to major developments in herbal medicine, with four new schools emerging. Some of these schools described acupuncture and herbal medicine using the same theoretical frameworks and diagnostic approaches.

From this point onwards, acupuncture and herbal medicine in China often appeared in the same books using the same theoretical and diagnostic models—the modern expression of this trend is Traditional Chinese Medicine (TCM). In Japan, however, this was not the case. Herbal medicine theory and acupuncture theory remained separate. Thus, herbal theory had little or no influence on acupuncture in Japan. For example, few people in Japan today practise tongue diagnosis, as this arose from herbal medicine.

Japan ended its political isolation from the world after 200 years, in 1853. Interestingly, at about the same time, in another part of the world, the Galapagos Islands became famous for a different reason. This was the place where the British scientist Charles Darwin developed his theory of evolution. Observing the wildlife in this isolated archipelago, surrounded by ocean, led him to one of the central ideas of *On the Origin of Species*: when separated by natural barriers, such as mountains or oceans, species differentiate. The evolutionary biologist Richard Dawkins proposed the term *meme* to describe how ideas, behaviours, and cultural practices spread and evolve, analogous to genes in biological evolution. The same process of differentiation can occur in languages, religions, and technologies, and that is exactly what happened to acupuncture when it spread from China to Japan—it became isolated from its original source and underwent differentiation.[29]

In evolutionary terms, the physical isolation of the islands of Japan from China, compounded by its political isolation, allowed JAAM to develop in quite different directions from Chinese acupuncture. Moreover, discussing JAAM, it is important

29 Dawkins, R. (1976). *The Selfish Gene*. Oxford: Oxford University Press. p. 192.

to emphasise that it has had a thriving tradition for over 1,400 years, a longevity unparalleled by any medical tradition in the West and almost on a par with that of Chinese acupuncture itself.

WHAT IS JAAM?

> *When I say Japanese acupuncture, I'm using that as shorthand for a palpation-based, generally gentle, non-stimulatory or lightly stimulatory effect.*
>
> —Brenda Loew[30]

Acupuncture education in Japan differs from that in China, not least in that there is no unified national curriculum taught in universities and colleges nationwide. Instead, there is a huge diversity of styles, both old and new, including medical acupuncture and traditional acupuncture methods, as well as new or original styles, which are in constant competition and evolution. For example, it is estimated that "there are more than fifty Western medical subspecialities having physician-members who research and practise acupuncture and moxibustion. In addition, there are easily one hundred or more non-physician associations of acupuncture and moxibustion in Japan".[31]

> *In Japan, there's also a lot of other acupuncture that's done that's not based on traditional ideas; it's more based on anatomical thinking or other scientific models of the body, and I think that in China, you see less of this kind of diversity.*
>
> —Stephen Birch[32]

So, while one of the greatest cultural exports from China to the world is TCM, Japan has no single cultural equivalent. Instead, knowledge of different Japanese acupuncture styles is being transmitted to the West through a small group of Japanese emigrant

30 *Japanese Acupuncture Today.* (2018). Episode 3: Hari-kyū Today [Video]. Available at: https://youtu.be/aoN3bwXmacY

31 Birch, S., & Ida, J. (1998). *Japanese Acupuncture: A Clinical Guide.* Brookline: Paradigm Publications. p. 310.

32 *Japanese Acupuncture Today.* (2018). Episode 3: Hari-kyū Today [Video]. Available at: https://youtu.be/aoN3bwXmacY

teachers and other Western teachers who have trained in Japan or with emigrant teachers. We can see that MSA fits into this category through the educational work of Stephen Birch and Junko Ida.

The huge diversity of acupuncture styles in Japan, which includes medical acupuncture, electroacupuncture, and TCM acupuncture, could lead us to the position that there is no such thing as 'Japanese acupuncture' unless perhaps you are a Japanese national with a needle.[33]

We could make the same point about Japanese cuisine: there is so much diversity and adaptation in Japanese cooking styles that we can't really generalise about them; yet, clearly, there are internationally recognised dishes that are distinctly Japanese—sashimi looks and feels very different from British fish and chips. Thus, we can say that within the diversity of Japanese acupuncture styles, there are distinguishing features: for example, the historic invention and use of guide tubes that enabled the insertion of extremely fine filiform needles.

Although there are many styles of acupuncture within Japan, by JAAM we refer to those approaches that share certain distinguishing Japanese characteristics. It is these themes and commonalities that are the subject of this chapter.

Some of these themes were raised during a YouTube panel discussion with Stephen Birch, Brenda Loew, and Junji Mizutani, founder of the *North American Journal of Oriental Medicine*. Others are drawn from two papers published in 2017 by Benjamin Chant, Jeanne Madison, Paul Coop, and Gudrun Dieberg, who conducted four years of ethnographic fieldwork on the beliefs and attitudes of acupuncture practitioners in Japan.[34,35] As will become clear from the rest of the chapter, these themes overlap considerably.

---

33 Birch, S., & Ida, J. (1998). *Japanese Acupuncture: A Clinical Guide*. Brookline: Paradigm Publications. p. 21.

34 Chant, B., Madison, J., Coop, P., & Dieberg, G. (2017). 'Beliefs and Values in Japanese Acupuncture: An Ethnography of Japanese-Trained Acupuncture Practitioners in Japan', *Integrative Medicine Research*, 6(3). pp. 260–268. https://doi.org/10.1016/j.imr.2017.07.001

35 Chant, B., Madison, J., Coop, P., & Dieberg, G. (2017). 'Contact Tools in Japanese Acupuncture: An Ethnography of Acupuncture Practitioners in Japan', *Journal of Acupuncture and Meridian Studies*, 10(5). pp. 331–339. https://doi.org/10.1016/j.jams.2017.08.006

SHALLOW NEEDLING AND CONTACT TOOLS

One feature in particular distinguishes JAAM from other styles. Japanese acupuncture needles are much finer than those typically used in Chinese acupuncture. Moreover, even though the needles are much finer, insertion depths are much more shallow, often between 1–4 mm, as opposed to 1–2 *cun* in TCM.

Even more remarkably, in many styles (such as Meridian Therapy, Toyohari, and Shakuju), non-insertive needle techniques have been developed so that needles or blunt-tipped tools such as *teishin* are merely touched to or held lightly on the skin. No needle insertion takes place. These techniques are difficult to master and yet cause dynamic changes in the pulse and in the soft tissues that are being needled.

> *In China, I was taught to needle using mechanical techniques such as twirling, lifting, and thrusting, designed to create strong needle sensations, sometimes by entwining the tissues around the needle. When I told a teacher that there was a method in Japan called contact needling, he roared with laughter and told me not to be so gullible. Japanese touch needling is so different from Chinese needling that it is only recognisable as needling because a needle is being used.*
>
> —Oran Kivity[36]

In addition to non-insertive needling, the Japanese have also maintained and developed a range of other tools for treating the surface of the skin. These derive from the first three of the nine classical needles described in *Ling Shu*, Chapter 1.[37]

---

36 Kivity, O. (2018). 'Japanese Acupuncture: What's So Unique?' *European Journal of Oriental Medicine*, 9(2).

37 Birch, S., & Ida, J. (1998). *Japanese Acupuncture: A Clinical Guide*. Brookline: Paradigm Publications. pp. 39–40.

Table 3.1: Ancient needle types.

ENGLISH	CHINESE	JAPANESE	CONTEMPORARY APPLICATION
Sagittal (arrowhead) needle	*Chan zhen*	*Zanshin*	*Pressing, tapping*
Ovoid tip (roundhead) needle	*Yuan zhen*	*Enshin*	*Stroking, rubbing*
Blunt-tipped needle	*Shi zhen*	*Teishin*	*Touching, non-insertive point stimulation*

Benjamin Chant and his co-authors divide these contact tools into two categories: *teishin;* and friction tools, meaning tools that are used for stroking or pressing.[38] *Teishin* look like short knitting needles, usually with a tiny ball at one end and a blunt taper at the other. Rubbing and pressing tools, such as *enshin* and *zanshin,* can come in all sorts of shapes. *Enshin* look a little like a child's lollipop, but are made of various metals, including stainless steel, copper, and silver, and cost considerably more.

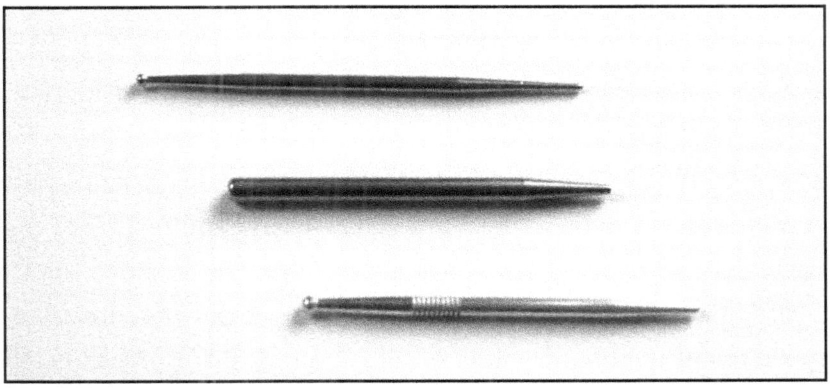

Figure 3-1: Teishin are blunt-tipped 'needles' that are used for non-insertive stimulation of acupuncture points.

[38] Chant, B., Madison, J., Coop, P., & Dieberg, G. (2017). 'Contact Tools in Japanese Acupuncture: An Ethnography of Acupuncture Practitioners in Japan', *Journal of Acupuncture and Meridian Studies*, 10(5). pp. 331–339. https://doi.org/10.1016/j.jams.2017.08.006

Of course, rubbing the skin is not unique to JAAM, as the Chinese also use *guasha* rubbing tools and blunt-tipped rollers; however, in JAAM, these tools are used in the same energetic way as for contact needling, to move qi in the meridians by applying a bare minimum of stimulation. In Toyohari, for example, if the skin turns red, the stimulation is considered to have been too much. This is the opposite of *guasha*, which prizes such reactions as evidence of effectiveness. Let's recall the mathematical analogy discussed in Chapter 1. If you take the numbers 2, 4, 8, 16, 32 and 64, what they all have in common is the smallest number, 2. JAAM, for the most part, focuses on the lightest of stimulation methods, which trigger effects common to all stimulation methods but can be overshadowed or rendered invisible by stronger stimulation.

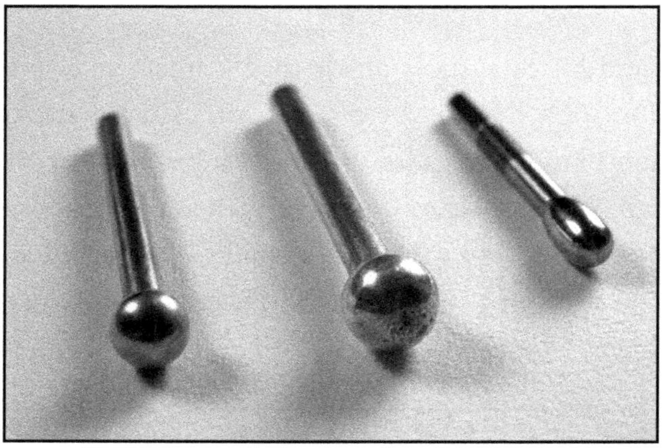

Figure 3-2: Enshin look like metallic lollipops and are used for very light rubbing of the meridians.

We have seen that Manaka considered the meridian system, his X-signal system, to be a low-energy system, which therefore required low-energy stimulation to engage with it. For that reason, when using his ion-pumping cords, he favoured shallow needle insertion, particularly in Step 1, with insertion depths of only 2–3 mm. We will look at polarity treatment methods in more detail later, but this approach is called 'plus-minus' needling—it uses polarities and extremely low voltages such as those created by different metals. This approach is common to many styles of JAAM. In Toyohari, for example, small pellets of copper and zinc are placed on the master and coupled points of the Eight Extras.

Moreover, Manaka developed skin contact tools called electrostatic adsorbers, another polarity device that bears a passing resemblance to *teishin* (see Figure 17-2). Other skin contact tools that he used were his ion-beam device and the *tenshin kyu*, a heated, spiked rolling device that he used to treat the Hirata Zones.[39]

ZEN BUDDHISM

As we can see from the present-day designs of the classical needle shapes, the Japanese have always been good at refining things and making them simple and elegant. This is in part due to the influence of Zen Buddhism, where simplicity and minimalism are highly regarded.

> *Zen concepts are so embedded in nonreligious beliefs and behaviours (including the practice of acupuncture) that they no longer retain religious meaning in these contexts.*[40]

Japanese history has been hugely influenced by concepts and beliefs in Zen Buddhism, so understanding this, first and foremost, is the key to understanding Japanese acupuncture. The truly Zen legend of Waichi Sugiyama (1610–1694), regarded as the 'Father of Japanese Acupuncture,' illustrates how these beliefs remain central to practice today. Sugiyama, a blind acupuncture student in the seventeenth century, was sacked dismissed first by one teacher and then a second, who, after years of trying to train him, despaired of him for being 'too dull' and 'without talent'. His needling was apparently clumsy and painful.[41] Eventually, after much struggle and meditation on the island of Enoshima, he tripped and fell, grasping a piece of bamboo in which lay

---

39 The Hirata Zones are a twelve-zone holographic mapping that repeat in different regions of the body. This mapping was developed by Kurakichi Hirata in the 1930s. See: Kivity, O. (2021). *Hirata Zone Therapy with the Ontake Method: Repurposing the Lost Art of Japanese Dermatome Moxibustion for Contemporary Practice*. London: Sayoshi Books.

40 Chant, B., Madison, J., Coop, P., & Dieberg, G. (2017). 'Beliefs and Values in Japanese Acupuncture: An Ethnography of Japanese-Trained Acupuncture Practitioners in Japan', *Integrative Medicine Research*, 6(3). pp. 260–268. https://doi.org/10.1016/j.imr.2017.07.001

41 Devitt, M. (2015). 'The Legend of Waichi Sugiyama, the Father of Japanese Acupuncture', *Meridians: The Journal of Acupuncture and Oriental Medicine*, 2(4). p. 26.

a pine needle.[42] From this, he was led, perhaps by divine inspiration or maybe by pure Zen pragmatism, to invent the *shinkan,* or guide tube. This simplest of inventions led to a transformation of Japanese acupuncture, enabling the insertion of even finer needles, including those made from soft metals like gold and silver. Sugiyama's guide tube, now in its plastic, disposable form, is still used worldwide today—and is probably sitting on your practice shelf.

He also became hugely influential in other ways, by setting up numerous schools for blind acupuncturists (*mojin-hari* 盲人鍼) and distilling the complexity of Chinese acupuncture into simpler, practical concepts that he could teach.[43] Part of this was because he was blind and had to have the classics read to him by a student, so he needed to disencumber himself from excessive theorising and make things simple. Still, this emphasis on practicality over theory is itself very Zen. This influence extends not only to the blind acupuncture communities, such as the Toyohari Association, but also serves as a general direction within Japanese acupuncture as a whole. Practical concerns overrule theoretical expectations.[44]

> *I asked* [Dr Manaka] *this question about this incredibly complicated, theoretical thing, something to do with the I Ching and all kinds of strange things I was interpreting, and he stood very politely, and he nodded, and he nodded, and when I'd finished, he turned to one of his assistants—he said "Toshi, lie down. Steve, show me your theory on Toshi!" and it was impossible!*
>
> —Stephen Birch[45]

Theory is often discarded for practical concerns. For example, according to *Nan Jing* theory, the tonification point of the spleen meridian should be SP 2; however, the Toyohari Association has discarded this point for SP 3, because SP 3 gets a better change on the pulse.

---

42 Some sources place the fall in Tokyo (then Edo), at the grounds of the shrine in Sumida-ku; most adhere to the Enoshima cave version. Both remain in circulation.

43 Yasui, H. (2010). 'History of Japanese Acupuncture and Moxibustion', *Journal of Kampo, Acupuncture and Integrative Medicine*, Special Edition. pp. 2–9.

44 Ibid.

45 *Japanese Acupuncture Today*. (2018). Episode 3: Hari-kyū Today [Video]. Available at: https://youtu.be/aoN3bwXmacY

Moreover, the emphasis placed on mindful practice and striving for mastery in Zen Buddhism is reflected in the teaching methods of Japanese acupuncture. In the Toyohari Association, for example, everyone in a group study session must practise basic needling techniques, even at the highest levels of the instructor corps, such as the president and vice president. Everyone has to practise the basics, time and again.

Again, Manaka exemplified this. He didn't create theories for their own sake. He was committed to creating theories that had practical, clinical value. His octahedral model is not an abstraction—it's a living model for clinical practice. Moreover, once he'd established his Four Steps, he could research and integrate many new methodologies for each step. We can see that his ever-expanding repertoire came partly from his understanding of ancient practice and partly from cultural adherence to this Zen idea of refinement.

> *Thus, ancient acupuncturists always observed the response to certain techniques or procedures and obtained feedback from the patient. Just as one modifies their technique in a chess game or fencing match, based on the reaction of the opponent, the ancients looked for ways to be flexible in changing their technique... He regrets that many practitioners limit themselves to only one system and neglect the many great systems developed by the Chinese throughout history... We should not forget them, because nothing is perfect, and thus we should always try to understand them all.*[46]

ROOT TREATMENT, OR WHOLE-BODY REGULATION

We've already seen that JAAM makes important distinctions between treating the root—regulating and harmonising the flow of qi throughout the body—and treating the branch—applying various techniques to address the presenting symptoms.

> *The root treatment is more general. I say it is a 'ground levelling'. If you have some rough ground, you have to make it flat. Then you will find some important part, some important point to dig to find something, so my idea is first just ground levelling, and then I find a good, good point to*

46 Ibid.

> *dig deeper and deeper and get some treasure from there. That's my idea of branch treatment. So, it varies. Two steps: the first step—just general treatment, then the second step, you focus on the most important point.*
>
> —Junji Mizutani[47]

> *When we're doing acupuncture, we're not keeping biological or chemical systems in mind, and we're not limited to symptom control; we're trying to regulate and harmonise the qi of the body.*
>
> —Brenda Loew[48]

> *Japanese traditional* [treatments] *are based on the regulation or harmonisation of qi. JAAM is essentially a wellness model versus the Western scientific model, which is a disease model—it's focusing on symptoms.*
>
> —Brenda Loew[49]

Root treatment, or whole-body regulation, is prioritised. It may be that, for effective root treatment, lighter techniques are more suitable.

> [Manaka] *suggested that the body has many different levels of regulatory systems involved, and there are certain kinds of regulatory systems that operate at very low energy levels in the body, sort of in the background... I think that maybe gentle needling techniques allow us to trigger this kind of regulatory effect in an easier way.*
>
> —Stephen Birch[50]

Manaka's octahedral model fits very comfortably into this idea of whole-body regulation. His core idea is to regulate the flow of qi and blood over the eight facets of the octahedron by treating the Eight Extras.

---

47 *Japanese Acupuncture Today*. (2018). Episode 3: Hari-kyū Today [Video]. Available at: https://youtu.be/aoN3bwXmacY

48 Ibid.

49 Ibid.

50 Ibid.

PALPATION

Palpation is part of the Four Examinations of Chinese medicine but has evolved very differently in China and Japan. Palpation in Japanese acupuncture can be seen, at least in part, as another legacy from Sugiyama, who made acupuncture a profession that blind people could enter. By necessity, blind acupuncturists (*mojin-hari* 盲人鍼) must rely on their other senses for diagnosis and have therefore elevated palpation to a fine art. For example, in the Toyohari Association, the blind practitioners talk about the lustre of the skin as something that can be palpated, rather than seen, often using the skin of the anterior forearm as an indicator of vitality. Reliance on palpatory findings for diagnosis and feedback, before and after treatment, is paramount.

Although *hara* diagnosis is mentioned in the *Nan Jing*, it plays no part in modern TCM diagnosis, where tongue diagnosis is prioritised. In Japanese acupuncture, palpation of the *hara* is much more important. Light stroking is used in some styles, such as Toyohari, and deeper palpation, looking for pressure pain reactions, is used in others, including MSA, Nagano, and Kiiko Matsumoto styles. Tongue diagnosis, by contrast, is considered part of herbal medicine, where it originated, and is therefore rarely used by acupuncturists in Japan.

It may also be true to say that Japanese practitioners have often looked back to the classics and tried to reproduce them closely, and that palpation is emphasised far more in the early classics than in many later Chinese texts. Cultural factors may also have played a part. In China, longstanding Confucian ideas about modesty made extensive hands-on examination less common, and the reform and standardisation of Chinese medicine during the Cultural Revolution shifted acupuncture towards a more conceptual, theory-driven diagnostic style.

By contrast, the clear separation of acupuncture and herbal medicine in Japan meant that practitioners were strongly influenced by their sister practice of massage, where palpation remains central. Combined with the more naturalistic attitudes associated with Daoist and Shinto traditions, this helped ensure that palpation retained a prominent place in Japanese acupuncture, while in China, as acupuncture became increasingly associated with herbal medicine, it gradually shifted from a palpatory approach to a more intellectual one.

Meridian palpation is also important. In China, this has been virtually ignored, with the exception of the late Wang Ju Yi.[51] Outside of TCM, other renowned Chinese practitioners such as Master Tung and Dr Tan certainly palpated the meridians. In Japanese acupuncture, meridian palpation is very common.

> *My treatment always starts from palpation. Why do I do that? I touch the skin right away. it's easy to feel energy: you can feel cold and heat or depression or induration, but through this information... you feel the energy very quickly. So once I've assessed the energy level of the patient, I decide how I can treat the patient... I don't think. like a diagnosis in my brain, my diagnosis is always from touch; I decide how to treat the patient, including qi or whatever. blood, everything comes from the touch.*
>
> —Junji Mizutani[52]

> *Junji said he immediately starts touching his patients—patients immediately relax—we're not robots, we're designed to respond to touch, and so that is an immediate part of the healing process as well.*
>
> —Brenda Loew[53]

INDURATION OR ABNORMAL TISSUE FINDINGS

Once palpation becomes the diagnostic focus, we should ask: What does it reveal? When palpating the belly or meridians, what are you looking for? What's normal? What's abnormal? Chant and his team identified a theme in JAAM that they called 'abnormal tissue findings'.[54]

---

51 Wang, J. Y., Robertson, J., & Van Buren, K. (2008). *Applied Channel Theory in Chinese Medicine: Wang Ju-Yi's Lectures on Channel Therapeutics.* Seattle: Eastland Press.

52 *Japanese Acupuncture Today.* (2018). Episode 3: Hari-kyū Today [Video]. Available at: https://youtu.be/aoN3bwXmacY

53 Ibid.

54 Chant, B., Madison, J., Coop, P., & Dieberg, G. (2017). 'Beliefs and Values in Japanese Acupuncture: An Ethnography of Japanese-Trained Acupuncture Practitioners in Japan', *Integrative Medicine Research,* 6(3). pp. 260–268. https://doi.org/10.1016/j.imr.2017.07.001

Our YouTube panel discussed these ideas, focusing on indurations and painful points, but the concept of abnormal tissue findings is much broader. In MSA, we focus on muscle tension, tightness, hardness, pressure pain, and jump reactions. In Toyohari, the palpation is much lighter, with an emphasis on excess and deficiency, such as hot and cold, swelling and puffiness.

What is critical to understand about JAAM is that whenever these findings are observed, treatment is given with the intention of changing them immediately. If the belly feels cool at the start of the session, it should feel warm by the end. If there are reactive points, they should become less reactive. If a muscle feels hard and swollen, it should relax.

In other words, an important part of the treatment in JAAM is not just about diagnosis at the level of *zangfu* or meridian differentiation, such as deciding to treat the liver organ or kidney meridian; it is also about identifying and rectifying abnormal findings on a tactile, palpatory level. These might be very specific findings—for example, that certain points on the belly feel painful or tight—or very general findings, such as the skin on the back feeling smoother or warmer. When applying moxibustion, the feeling of a point should change after the application of heat. For example, when treating Isaburo Fukaya's psychosomatic treatment points in the intervertebral spaces with small-cone moxibustion, the points should go from tender to less tender; otherwise, the treatment has not been successful (see Chapter 13).

What's more, these palpatory findings take precedence over theory. If theory indicates one thing, but there are no reactions at the points, then the diagnosis may be wrong.

> *So, I may have a very good diagnosis... and the diagnosis says, "Needle these points with these techniques." So I go to the point, and there's no reaction in the point! I can't find anything at the point! I don't doubt the theory—I think, "Oh, my diagnosis is probably wrong, I'd better go back and re-examine the patient." Maybe I've missed something or misjudged something, because the theory is that the palpable reaction at the point must be present—otherwise that point isn't relevant. And if I touch the same meridian and I still don't feel any reasonably good palpable reactions that indicate I need to tonify this meridian or drain this meridian, then I have*

to go back and say... "I must have missed something in the diagnosis." So, the palpable reactions in the patient actually play a very important part in bringing the theory to life.

—Stephen Birch[55]

Palpation is a crucial part of MSA, with a focus on the belly. In modern acupuncture, the twelve front-*mu* points of historical acupuncture have been ascribed a diagnostic function. Manaka developed his own so-called Manaka-*mu* points, different in location to the historical front-*mu* points but serving a similar purpose. He developed broad palpation categories to guide diagnosis and treatment: what he called primary reaction areas, primary reaction points, and secondary reactions.

FEEDBACK MECHANISMS AND RAPID CHANGE

In many traditions of acupuncture, there is an expectation of rapid change. For example, after inserting needles, many practitioners expect the pulse to change. Most Japanese acupuncture styles, relying as they do on palpation to such a high degree, make predictions about these rapid changes with each needle or point that is treated, and not just about the pulse, but about the tone of the soft tissues of the body, and changes in specific reaction points. For example, in MSA, if you needle KID 6 and LU 7 with ion-pumping cords, it should release tightness on the Ren Mai above the navel and pressure pain at KID 16. In Kiiko Matsumoto Style (KMS) acupuncture, if you find tenderness at left ST 25–27, you can release it by needling LIV 4 and LU 5.

Many of these reactions following needling occur on the abdomen, but others will be noted in reflex areas in other parts of the body. These reactions are predictable and repeatable; thus, many protocols in JAAM include reflex areas to check before and after treating specific points.

---

55 *Japanese Acupuncture Today*. (2018). Episode 3: Hari-kyū Today [Video]. Available at: https://youtu.be/aoN3bwXmacY

MINIMAL STIMULATION, DOSAGE, AND SENSITIVITY

We have already seen that JAAM is influenced by the Zen Buddhist concept of minimalism. The needles are finer, insertion depths are reduced, and non-insertive techniques have been developed. This concern with minimising stimulation is applied to all modalities, including cupping, moxibustion, and bloodletting. Cupping retention times are short, moxa cones are tiny, and moxa punk is manufactured to burn at lower temperatures. Bloodletting is researched so that the dosage (the number of drops squeezed out) matches the patient's strength.[56]

> *I use insertive needling, but my technique is getting lighter and lighter. When I was very young, there were no allergies, but today, there are many allergy patients. That means... people have become more sensitive so that we have to use lighter and lighter stimulation for sensitive people... Probably 100 years ago, 200 years ago, people were more tough, so we could use more stimulation, and then they changed. But today, even adults. have a light sensitivity, like a child, so I can use a child needle for adults now... In my thirty-five years of experience, my stimulation has become lighter and lighter.*
>
> —Junji Mizutani[57]

> *People's sensitivity, as I said, is changing, so that, you know, less heat works better now.* [In the past] *people burned the skin very severely; they made big scar tissue and keloid, but you don't need that today. If you use a tiny, tiny* shijohkyu[58] *(it's a string-type moxa), just one cone can change the condition very quickly, and with* chinetsukyu, *you don't burn the skin.*[59] *As soon as you feel the heat, then you take it off—then that works. So, moxibustion is changing... so is needling. Needles are becoming smaller and smaller,*

56 Birch, S., & Ida, J. (1998). *Japanese Acupuncture: A Clinical Guide*. Brookline: Paradigm Publications.

57 *Japanese Acupuncture Today*. (2018). Episode 3: Hari-kyū Today [Video]. Available at: https://youtu.be/aoN3bwXmacY

58 *Shijohkyu* (thread moxa): a moxa cone about the width of a piece of cotton thread placed vertically on the skin and burnt all the way down.

59 *Chinetsukyu* (cone moxa): sensing warmth moxibustion. A moxa cone is placed on the skin and allowed to burn until the patient feels the very first signs of warmth, then quickly removed, before the sensations feel hot. In Toyohari, the cone is removed when the pulse changes, often before the patient has felt any warmth at all.

> *smaller and very thin now, and then finally we don't have to insert the needle, we just touch the metal on the skin, or even if you don't touch, you just use quartz or whatever. And it still works. So, people's sensitivity is changing. Moxibustion heat sensitivity is changing.*
>
> —Junji Mizutani[60]

Dr Manaka, like many other JAAM practitioners, placed great importance on the issue of dosage, assessing the sensitivity of a patient, adapting treatment to their needs, and paying special attention to sensitive patients. We will explore these ideas in depth in Chapter 15.

SPECIALISATION

Specialisation in a single therapeutic approach is another historical feature of JAAM. For example, one of the most renowned practitioners of moxibustion, Isaburo Fukaya, was not licensed to perform acupuncture and treated with moxibustion alone.[61] Two other practitioners, Drs Kunimasa Kudo and Masao Murayama, practised for many years using *shiraku* (microbleeding) as their primary therapy.[62] Keizo Hashimoto, meanwhile, developed a unique bodywork system called Sotai. This trend in specialisation has allowed very sophisticated methodologies to develop in modalities such as cupping, microbleeding, and moxibustion, which in TCM training, particularly in the West, have been seen as more adjunctive or secondary.

Moxibustion is one area where this specialised knowledge has fed back into the acupuncture community and hugely elevated the role of moxibustion in clinical practice. It may also be true that moxibustion in Japan initially started and continued to be a 'people's medicine', something anyone can practise at home with their family,

---

60 *Japanese Acupuncture Today.* (2018). Episode 3: Hari-kyū Today [Video]. Available at: https://youtu.be/aoN3bwXmacY

61 Shudo, D. (1990). *Japanese Classical Acupuncture: Introduction to Meridian Therapy.* Seattle: Eastland Press. p. 201.

62 Birch, S., & Ida, J. (1998). *Japanese Acupuncture: A Clinical Guide.* Brookline: Paradigm Publications. p. 212.

whereas acupuncture first found its role with the wealthier classes.[63] Thus, in JAAM, moxibustion plays a crucial role, in parallel with needling, adding to the range and effectiveness of techniques available to the practitioner.

> *Moxibustion and acupuncture needle treatment are totally different kinds of stimulation. When we use a needle, the needle is metal, and we insert it into your skin, with the contact of the metal to your skin; but moxibustion is heat, and heat basically burns your skin, and it's a totally different stimulation. If you combine two different kinds of stimulation like that, if you have two different tools and if you connect two tools, two very good methods, you can make more efficiency. So, needle stimulation and moxa/heat stimulation don't conflict with each other; they help.*
>
> —Junji Mizutani[64]

> *When you burn moxa down to the skin and cause small tissue damage, it triggers these immunological changes, which happen on a larger scale and more diversely than you tend to see with simple needling alone, and if you understand how to use these... it gives you a very broad-ranging set of tools.*
>
> —Stephen Birch[65]

However, it is important to define here what we mean by moxibustion. If you search online for 'benefits of moxibustion', you will find all kinds of references to 'improving immunity and boosting white blood cell counts', but these references frequently confuse different kinds of moxibustion; for example, indirect moxa with a moxa stick, indirect moxa on the end of the needle, and Japanese small-cone moxibustion. These are three totally different therapies with very different effects. Moreover, even small-cone direct moxibustion in Japan is very different from direct moxibustion with small cones in China.

---

63 Young, M. (2023). *The Moon over Matsushima: Insights into Moxa and Mugwort.* 2nd ed. London: Sayoshi Books. p. 72.

64 *Japanese Acupuncture Today.* (2018). Episode 3: Hari-kyū Today [Video]. Available at: https://youtu.be/aoN3bwXmacY

65 Ibid.

This is kind of a speciality of moxibustion practice in Japan that you don't tend to see outside of Japan, except among other Japanese acupuncture practitioners... that the moxa is very different than the way it's done in China. I have seen a book. from modern China, describing the modern use of direct moxa, but they were making really large cones of moxa. and the burns that were produced were quite large. When we do Japanese-style okyu, as it's called, we don't create those kinds of burns; the burns we produce are very small.

—Stephen Birch[66]

My observations of small-cone moxibustion in China are that although the tip of the cone may be thread-like, the surface area of the base is relatively broad, and thus delivers much more heat than would be considered acceptable among practitioners in Japan. Moreover, the material used to make the cones is less refined and therefore burns hotter. Finally, my teachers in China used very tight rolling techniques that compressed the moxa, making it burn hotter.

—Oran Kivity[67]

The Japanese are very good at taking somebody's idea and kind of playing with it to make it better and more functional, so instead of making a round ball of moxa, you make your moxa shape like a grain of rice, so that the contact point on the skin is much smaller... and you don't roll it hard, you roll it softly, so it burns slowly, it's moulded softly to shape, so when it burns down—yes there's a pinch of heat but it's not the same kind of burning sensation or really, really hot sensations.

—Stephen Birch[68]

66 Ibid.

67 Kivity, O. (2018). 'Japanese Acupuncture: What's So Unique?' *European Journal of Oriental Medicine*, 9(2).

68 *Japanese Acupuncture Today*. (2018). Episode 3: Hari-kyū Today [Video]. Available at: https://youtu.be/aoN3bwXmacY

In conclusion, the underlying principles of Japanese *okyu* have developed to be quite different. The base is narrow, delivering less heat. The material is super-refined, also delivering less heat. Additionally, the traditional method of rolling cones emphasises leaving the moxa wool soft and uncompressed, resulting in even less heat. Thus, although *okyu* moxa treatment is considered stimulating, minimal stimulation is emphasised at all stages of the process, from manufacture to the favoured shape of the cone to the rolling technique, making it more suitable for contemporary patients while still achieving clinical results.

Dr Manaka treated many difficult conditions, but in his approach, he was a polymath and generalist. What he did was to take the work of specialists such as Fukaya, Hashimoto, Kudo, and Murayama, and slot their techniques into his Four Step protocol. We will see that Manaka was equally comfortable using large-cone moxa, small-cone moxa, moxa on the needle technique, bloodletting, and Sotai as alternative strategies at each stage, and this book will explore this extraordinarily versatile treatment system.

CONCLUSION

In summary, JAAM evolved very differently from acupuncture and moxibustion in China. We can use Darwin's idea of speciation as a way of explaining this. Japan was geographically and culturally isolated from China for more than 200 years. China was invaded by the Mongols, whereas Japan was not. China was overrun by Western colonial powers, whereas Japan was not. It was, however, profoundly influenced by Western colonialism, particularly in the scientisation of medicine.

Three major influences shaped JAAM's distinctive direction. First, Zen Buddhism encouraged both minimalism and theoretical simplicity. Second, practitioners in Japan continued to rely on palpation-based historical texts, a trend strengthened by the strong influence of blind acupuncturists, who became a significant segment of the acupuncture community. These factors combined to elevate the Japanese palpation-based approach to a fine art.

Palpation led to a greater emphasis being placed on abnormal tissue findings, such as indurations, and an expectation that these abnormalities could and should resolve quickly with treatment. JAAM makes very clear distinctions between whole-body regulation and the treatment of symptoms, as well as making allowances for different levels of sensitivity in patients. As a result, very light techniques were developed, including contact needling, stroking, and pressing with contact tools.

Other modalities, such as moxibustion, cupping, and bloodletting, due to a cultural trend towards specialisation, became increasingly significant not just as adjunctive therapies, but as primary therapies in their own right. These therapies, too, tended towards minimal levels of stimulation.

Putting all these factors together, this long and vibrant tradition of acupuncture in Japan has created not just one cultural export, like TCM, but many different styles of acupuncture and moxibustion. These different styles nevertheless share common themes of regulating the qi of the whole body with minimal intervention and a respect for the increased levels of sensitivity in contemporary urban patient groups. Innovative, brilliant, and unique as it is, Manaka's style is culturally very much within the mainstream of JAAM.

SUMMARY

- **Historical divergence from China**: Japanese acupuncture developed in isolation after 1635, leading to unique practices and theories distinct from those of China.
- **Separation from herbal theory**: Herbal and acupuncture traditions remained separate in Japan, unlike in China, where they became unified.
- **Palpation-based diagnosis**: Palpation, especially of the *hara* and meridians, is central to both diagnosis and feedback during treatment. Pragmatic applications take precedence over theory.
- **Immediate feedback**: Treatments aim to create tangible, real-time changes in tissue tone, temperature, or tenderness; if the point doesn't change, the treatment may not be appropriate or correct.
- **Root before branch**: The system prioritises whole-body qi regulation (root treatment) before addressing symptoms (branch treatment).
- **Zen Buddhist influence**: Simplicity, repetition, refinement, and practical mastery shape both treatment and teaching styles.

- **Specialisation and refinement**: Specialisation by experts in single modalities like moxa, bloodletting, or Sotai bodywork leads to refined stand-alone systems.
- **Moxibustion refinement**: Japanese moxibustion uses ultra-refined wool, rolled softly into rice-grain-sized cones that burn slowly and relatively gently—distinct from Chinese methods.
- **Minimal stimulation**: JAAM emphasises shallow or non-insertive needling, soft moxa, and cupping or bloodletting tailored to patient sensitivity.
- **Contact tools**: Tools like *teishin* and *enshin*, derived from the classical nine needles, are used non-insertively to move qi with minimal stimulation.
- **Manaka's alignment with JAAM**: Although innovative, Manaka's system reflects core JAAM principles: light touch, feedback-driven adjustments, whole-body regulation, and minimal dosage.

WHAT'S NEXT

The next chapter takes us from theory into palpation. Touch underpins diagnosis and point location, guides treatment, and provides the feedback we need at every step.

CHAPTER 4

CONTEXT: PALPATION

WHY PALPATION MATTERS

We've seen that palpation is a key feature of JAAM. In this chapter, we'll explore the basics of differing palpation methods, comparing them and their uses in relation to treatment, using examples from Keiraku Chiryo (Meridian Therapy) and MSA.[69] Once again, this is a Concept chapter, so you can skip ahead if you're in a hurry to get to the practicalities of MSA, but there's significant and foundational material here. Do come back to it when you are ready to deepen your knowledge of MSA palpation within the broader context of JAAM.

CLASSICAL ROOTS AND JAPANESE OFFSHOOTS

The preliminary descriptions of palpation, especially of the pulses, were given in the *Huang Di Nei Jing*, and then pulse and abdominal palpation were systematically described in the *Nan Jing*.[70] These texts, especially the *Nan Jing*, remain the

---

69 The bulk of this chapter comes from a Manaka course handout by Stephen Birch. See: Birch, S. (1997). *An Introduction to the Use of Palpation Methods in the Practice of Acupuncture and Moxibustion in Japan, with a Focus on Hara Diagnosis/Abdominal Palpation*. Course handout. Anglo-Dutch Institute for Oriental Medicine.

70 Unschuld, P. U. (1986). *Medicine in China: Nan Ching, the Classic of Difficult Issues*. Berkeley: University of California Press.

cornerstones for the practice of tradition-based acupuncture and the historical origins of the theory of systematic correspondence, which laid the foundations for traditional medical practices in China and many systems of acupuncture.[71]

It is also important to reinforce that acupuncture in Japan was and continues to be strongly influenced by the traditions of massage therapy and by the work of blind practitioners (mojin-hari, 盲人鍼), both of which have helped place a strong emphasis on the role of palpation and touching diagnosis. In China, the more intellectually-based systems of herbal therapeutics were a strong influence on acupuncture, but in Japan, the influence of herbal medicine was not brought to bear on acupuncture to the same degree. In fact, the two therapies were licensed and practised separately. What developed instead was a much stronger emphasis on hands-on approaches.

KEY FUNCTIONS OF PALPATION IN JAAM

PALPATION FOR FEEDBACK

As we saw in the last chapter, feedback mechanisms are a key feature of JAAM. In Meridian Therapy, the pulse is checked after each stage of treatment. If certain predicted changes do not occur, the practitioner receives rapid feedback about the effectiveness of the treatment just applied. The nature of the pulse change or a lack of change can reveal issues with the needling technique, whether qi was obtained and moved, or whether the point location was accurate. In other words, palpation can provide immediate and direct feedback about the patient's overall condition and the effectiveness of the treatment procedure applied.

Manaka developed his own sophisticated feedback system using abdominal and acupoint palpation. This provides immediate or near-immediate information about the effectiveness of the treatment. In MSA, once the ion-pumping cords (IPC) are applied, we expect to see a clear improvement in the abdominal findings. If that improvement is observed, it suggests the step was well executed. If not, it offers immediate feedback about issues with point location or treatment selection.

---

71 Ibid.

Manaka designed this method not only as a clinical tool but also as part of a more systematic, investigative approach to understanding the qi and meridian systems. In *Chasing the Dragon's Tail*, he describes how palpation and feedback were used as study tools for exploring the nature of acupoints, meridians, Extraordinary Vessels, and more. His genius did not stop there. It was through this palpation approach that, for example, he determined which acupoints are *reliable* indicators of the condition of each meridian. Applying a small stimulus to the associated meridian, such as needling in one direction, could increase pressure pain at the reflex point, while applying the opposite stimulus, reversing the direction of the needle, could reduce the reactivity.

PALPATION TO DETERMINE THE PATTERN

In MSA, palpation of reflex areas and points on the abdomen is used to determine the primary treatment pattern and point selection. Once a candidate pattern is found, additional reflex points on the torso, limbs, or neck can confirm the choice. This method, developed by Manaka and his colleague Kazuko Itaya, simplifies diagnosis by offering immediate tactile confirmation, making it suitable even for those without advanced pulse skills. Other Japanese systems also rely on abdominal palpation to guide treatment decisions.

Reflex point palpation elsewhere on the body, such as the limbs or neck, can further support or confirm the chosen pattern. For example, Meisho Honda and Kenji Miyawaki used palpation to identify the principal meridians to treat, while Koichi Ito applied it to determine the appropriate Extraordinary Vessels.[72, 73] In MSA, this broader palpation approach can confirm the main Extraordinary Vessel combination or guide the selection of meridian-based treatments.

---

72 Miyawaki, K. (1990). 'Abdominal Diagnosis of the Extraordinary Vessels', *Keiraku Shinryo*, 242(3–4). pp. 7–20.

73 Matsumoto, K., & Birch, S. (1986). *Extraordinary Vessels*. Brookline: Paradigm Publications. pp. 157–164.

ASSESSING THE PATIENT'S ENERGY

Palpation of the abdominal muscles also provides immediate insight into the overall status of the patient's qi. This is based in part on the *Nan Jing* and is described in detail in *Hara Diagnosis*.[74, 75, 76] If the muscles feel springy and relatively soft, this is a positive sign. Tension is less favourable, while hard, tight areas suggest deeper imbalances. The least favourable finding is a complete lack of muscle tone, when the abdomen feels soft with no springiness at all.

This kind of palpation offers a direct, non-intellectual assessment of the qi. Other styles of acupuncture often rely on more intellectual and analytical methods, interpreting signs and symptoms to determine the patient's qi condition.

DIFFERENT STYLES, DIFFERENT METHODS

Acupuncture is what we can call a 'naked-sense observation-based method of practice'—in other words, we don't use any tools or mechanical aids to diagnose. Thus, a variety of palpation methods has evolved.[77] Palpation in Japan is much more than simply pressing to see if it hurts—palpation typically covers a broader range of approaches, from using a light touch (assessing at the skin level) to using deeper pressure (assessing at the muscle level).[78] We also differentiate between what we feel as practitioners when palpating and what the patient feels.

Different systems of practice utilise different methods of palpation. Within specific systems of practice, palpation will also change depending upon the goal of treatment. In Meridian Therapy, when correcting problems of deficiency of qi, a light touch can

---

74 Ibid. pp. 130, 219–221, 499–501.

75 Matsumoto, K., & Birch, S. (1988). *Hara Diagnosis: Reflections on the Sea*. Brookline: Paradigm Publications.

76 Birch, S. (1997). 'Forming a Prognosis—Perspectives from the Works of Japanese Acupuncturists: A Preliminary Compilation of Ideas', *NAJOM*, 4(10). pp. 4–8.

77 Birch, S., & Felt, R. (1999). *Understanding Acupuncture*. Edinburgh: Churchill Livingstone.

78 *Ido-no-Nippon* (1986). 500th Special Issue, 45(4

be used to help decide the diagnosis, and even lighter for treatment point location.[79] However, in MSA and other meridian-based therapies, when palpating a point to relieve a specific symptom, pressure is often applied to find tight points (sometimes referred to as indurations) and elicit distinct feelings of pressure pain.[80,81] This approach is essential in *okyu*, the application of small-cone moxibustion.

A practitioner who uses thicker, deeply inserted needles with electrical stimulation—targeting sore spots on spasming muscles that align with motor or trigger points—typically applies strong pressure to locate the treatment point. In contrast, a blind acupuncturist practising *Keiraku Chiryo* (Meridian Therapy) with super-fine needles that barely penetrate the skin may diagnose and locate points using only the lightest touch. While the methods of palpation vary between and within systems, what does not vary is the underlying basis of these methods: they are all empirically rather than theoretically based. Each system uses what skilled practitioners have found useful and passed on to students or colleagues. Differences between approaches typically reflect personal preferences and the constraints of specific practice systems, with practitioners often aiming to replicate their teachers' methods rather than follow any overarching theoretical framework.

STROKING LIGHTLY: ASSESSING THE SURFACE OF THE SKIN

In Meridian Therapy, meridians are believed to circulate on or just beneath the surface of the skin. Accordingly, light touch is preferred to assess the condition of qi circulation. This approach evolved from the direct observation that simple touch provided sufficient diagnostic information and that surface needling methods were effective. The belief about the meridians' depth appears to have emerged from these clinical observations, rather than preceding them.

---

79 Fukushima, K. (1991). *Meridian Therapy*. Tokyo: Toyo Hari Medical Association.

80 Shudo, D. (1990). *Japanese Classical Acupuncture: Introduction to Meridian Therapy*. Seattle: Eastland Press.

81 *Ido-no-Nippon (1986). 500th Special Issue, 45(4).*

The Toyohari system is a style of Meridian Therapy. It was developed by the Toyohari Association, which was originally founded as an organisation for blind practitioners. The founders began by using inserted needles, as described in Kodo Fukushima's book.[82] Over time, however, they evolved techniques, known as contact needling, where more powerful and precise treatment effects could be produced without needle insertion.[83] This was not a theoretically driven change, but a direct observation based on study and clinical experience.

PRESSING DEEPER: ASSESSING THE MUSCULATURE

This approach is important for both point location and diagnostic assessment of reflex points or areas. Most schools of acupuncture and moxibustion in Japan employ palpation methods that seek pressure pain points (PPP). It is relatively easy to find pressure pain on palpation, and the feedback from the patient can be helpful as confirmation.

> *As an observer of many experienced practitioners in Japan—and through my own clinical experience—I've found that the more experienced the practitioner, the lighter their palpation when eliciting reactions. For me, this developed over time. When I began, I used strong pressure to avoid missing pressure pain points. But gradually, I started noticing other reactions—changes in texture, tone, and tension in the skin and muscles. These observations allowed me to find the same points with less pressure, relying on subtle tactile feedback rather than the patient's exclamation of discomfort. This isn't to say that using pressure pain is unsophisticated; only that it isn't always necessary.*
>
> —Stephen Birch

82 Fukushima K. (1991). *Meridian Therapy*. Tokyo: Toyo Hari Medical Association.

83 Birch, S. (2013). 'Traditional Needling Techniques as Practical Constructions from Reading Historical Descriptions', *European Journal of Oriental Medicine*, 7(3). pp. 26–33.

PULSE PALPATION

Pulse palpation is used to assess the status of the primary twelve meridians and the overall status of the qi and blood. This is derived from *Ling Shu*, Chapter 10, which instructs us to palpate the pulses to understand deficiency and excess of the twelve meridians.[84] The *Nan Jing* then develops radial pulse palpation as the focus for this, a focus that is a key feature for more traditional forms of acupuncture in Japan such as Meridian Therapy.[85, 86]

Dr Manaka did, of course, take the pulse, but interestingly, he considered pulse palpation too difficult to teach, and MSA is designed to function without it. **Accordingly, this book does not address pulse diagnosis.** That said, many practitioners, including the authors, still take the pulse during MSA treatment, as it aligns with their previous training. However, for those new to MSA, pulse palpation is not required for effective practice, which makes the system significantly easier to learn.

PALPATION FOR DIAGNOSIS

In MSA, palpation starts broadly on reflex areas to identify the treatment pattern, then narrows to identify reactive treatment points. It requires a combination of light and deep palpation techniques, applied primarily to the abdominal wall, as well as to select areas such as the torso, neck, and shoulders.

Palpation typically begins with light pressure on the abdomen, followed by deeper pressure. What are we looking for? Light pressure is used to assess the texture and tone of the abdominal muscles. Specifically, we investigate:

- Is there tension?
- Are there tight, hard areas?
- Are there regions that feel unusually soft or hypotonic?

---

84 Unschuld, P. U. (1986). *Medicine in China: Nan Ching, the Classic of Difficult Issues*. Berkeley: University of California Press.

85 Ibid.

86 Shudo, D. (1990). *Japanese Classical Acupuncture: Introduction to Meridian Therapy*. Seattle: Eastland Press.

- Does light pressure already provoke pressure pain?
- Are there jump reactions in certain regions?

With deeper pressure, the degree of tension, hardness, and tightness becomes more apparent. To evaluate the relevance of these findings, we pay close attention to:

- Pressure pain reactions
- Jump reactions

These responses are less commonly triggered with light pressure, so if they appear at that stage, they likely indicate more significant findings. When several tight or hard areas are found with deeper pressure, those that elicit pain or jump reactions are usually the most clinically relevant. In general, the stronger the reaction, the more significant the finding.

PALPATION FOR FINDING POINTS

The initial focus of palpation is on broad areas rather than discrete points. These general regions help establish evidence for the diagnostic pattern to be identified. Specific acupoints are then palpated as part of the diagnostic process for selecting a treatment pattern.

At this point, acupoint palpation transitions into a different function: it serves to locate the specific treatment points, with the technique focused on the reactive location. In MSA, as in many Japanese acupuncture traditions, acupoints are not viewed as fixed anatomical structures. This contrasts with modern interpretations influenced by anatomical science in recent centuries. Instead, we follow the spirit of the earliest descriptions, such as those found in *Ling Shu*, Chapter 1, which define points not by anatomy, but by the movement of qi.[87]

---

[87] Birch, S., Cabrer, M., & Rodriguez, M. (2025). *Restoring Order in Health and Chinese Medicine: Studies of the Development and Use of Qi and the Channels*. 2nd ed. London: Sayoshi Books.

In this view, acupoints are dynamic and movable. The standard anatomical location simply serves as the starting point for palpation, from which we search for the actual point. These reactive sites, referred to since at least the early twentieth century as 'live' points, are places where clear reactions due to internal changes are present, and when treatment is applied there, they directly influence those imbalances.[88]

In MSA Steps 1 and 2, treatment points are selected according to the diagnostic pattern found on the abdomen. The most reactive locations at those points are then used for treatment. In MSA Step 4, points are selected to target symptoms. These points are first palpated to assess reactivity, and the most reactive are then chosen for treatment. For example, in skin conditions such as eczema, we palpate and compare LI 4, LI 10, LI 11, and LI 15 on both arms, selecting the most reactive pair from the four pairs for treatment with *okyu*.[89] This principle is important in the practice of moxibustion, *hinaishin* (intradermal needles), and *empishin* (press tack needles). The type of reactivity in this context differs slightly from diagnostic palpation, as the reactions are more localised and often quite subtle.

We palpate the point using a larger portion of the thumb or finger pad. Once we identify an area of hardness, we refine our search using a smaller surface, such as the tip of the finger or thumb, to pinpoint the most reactive spot. Treatment points typically present as areas of hardness, often concentrated like a small knot. They are usually painful on palpation and may elicit a jump reaction.

CATEGORIES OF ABNORMAL TISSUE FINDINGS

The abnormal tissue findings described below are not things we should try to grasp intellectually. These are kinaesthetic concepts we understand through doing. Just as a dancer repeats movements until they become fluid and the instructions feel natural, or a piano student practises until the fingers know where to go, landing in the right places and sequences at the right time, palpation is an art that develops through repetition.

---

88 Ibid.

89 Birch, S. (2011). *Shonishin: Japanese Pediatric Acupuncture*. Stuttgart: Thieme Medical Publishers.

Reading the information in this chapter is one kind of learning—and an important one. But like dance, the best environment for this material is a practical setting, working with fellow students. It's best to practise as much as possible first, ideally with feedback and confirmation from an experienced practitioner.

MUSCULAR TENSION (TIGHTNESS)

The term muscular *tension* refers to a slight hypertonicity of the muscle, like tight shoulders. Even when the person is relaxed, the muscle remains subtly contracted. This is usually a mild finding and often less clinically relevant, meaning it is less useful for deciding the treatment. Some relatively healthy individuals may present with a well-toned abdominal wall and lack the more pronounced signs of muscular *hardness* (see below). In such cases where there is no obvious hardness, areas of increased muscular tension may take on greater clinical relevance.

MUSCULAR HARDNESS

Muscular *hardness* occurs when the abnormal tension in a muscle, described above, becomes severe and/or chronic. Thus, muscular hardness is seen as a progression from muscular tension.

This has two implications. First, when comparing two points for treatment, we usually select the one that shows more hardness. If two points or areas feel equally hard, we differentiate by checking for additional reactions, such as pressure pain or jumpiness.

Second, a high degree of hardness in a reflex area can act as a prognostic indicator, suggesting the condition may be more difficult to treat. In such cases, we look for further prognostic signs to support our judgment.

In Japan, *kori* is the lay term for this type of muscular hardness. *Kata kori* refers to the stiff, sore shoulders commonly seen there. While *kori* is beginning to appear in acupuncture usage, it should not be confused with the broader range of muscle-related palpable findings described above.

Manaka discussed the relationship between pressure pain and muscle tone in *Chasing the Dragon's Tail*. For example, he described a progression when palpating the right subcostal region. A little tension without pressure pain is less severe than a combination of tension and pressure pain. The presence of hardness alongside these findings indicates a further progression towards a more advanced or chronic condition.

HYPOTONIC MUSCLES

The progression of hardness described above can eventually result in its opposite: a reduction in muscle tonus, sometimes to the point of flaccidity—*hypotonia*. When palpating, if the muscle feels lax and the fingers sink in with little or no resistance, it suggests a more advanced condition, typically one of deficiency. In MSA, this finding in specific regions of the abdomen may be sufficient to determine the treatment pattern (see below).

PRESSURE PAIN

As we saw at the start of this section, palpation is used for diagnosis and for point location. *Pressure pain* is a useful finding in both processes, as there is a clear response from the patient, which helps to reduce the subjectivity of your palpation.

Many points or areas become reactive as a reflection of bodily changes associated with imbalances in the meridians. Thus, pressure pain responses in these reflex areas or points will aid diagnosis. In MSA, the finding of pressure pain in a number of related areas and acupuncture points is sufficient to determine where and how to apply the IPC at Step 1.

Treatment points also show pressure pain reactions. This is common in the selection of points for moxibustion, intradermal needles, press tack needles, *chishin*-retained needle techniques, and IPC needling. When applying *okyu* (direct small-cone moxibustion), the primary treatment points are usually those that show the most pressure pain (see Induration below).

It is important to distinguish between pressure pain that is felt when we press lightly and when we press forcefully. It is also important not to press too hard, as with enough pressure, it is possible to make even the most stoic patient feel pain. Moreover, pressing hard can act as a form of treatment in itself, or obliterate clues that a lighter touch will reveal. Here are two helpful palpation strategies that can elicit clearer reactions.

INDURATION (FIBROUS, PAINFUL KNOTS)

Induration refers to a hard, fibrous point that is typically very painful under pressure. The renowned Japanese practitioner Denmei Shudo described this reaction clearly, and it is often considered when selecting points for symptom relief.[90] Indurations are also a typical feature of reactive points for *okyu* (direct moxibustion). The influential Japanese practitioner Isaburo Fukaya even stated that a point is not suitable for direct moxibustion unless both induration and pressure pain are present.[91]

TWO USEFUL TECHNIQUES

1. CROSS-FIBRE PALPATION

Once we've located a tight area through general palpation, we can assess its level of reactivity by palpating *across* the muscle fibres with the fingertips while maintaining steady pressure. This technique helps to highlight the hard knot within the muscle and often makes the pressure pain more noticeable. The patient's response is often involuntary, with a clear *jump reaction* (see below).

---

90 Shudo, D. (1990). *Japanese Classical Acupuncture: Introduction to Meridian Therapy*. Seattle: Eastland Press.

91 Caudet, F. (2023). *Isaburo Fukaya: The Master of Japanese Moxibustion*. Tarragona: Okyayasan Books.

2. CIRCULAR PALPATION

When we find a hard area at an acupoint—such as a knot—and want to identify the most reactive spot for treatment, we can zone in by using circular palpation around and over the knot. By applying steady pressure while moving in small circles, we can often highlight the exact point that is most reactive, frequently eliciting pressure pain or a jump response.

READING PATIENT REACTIONS

Patients may indicate pressure pain through verbal responses or sounds. However, patients have widely varying pain thresholds influenced by factors such as personality, type of work, and life experience. Some patients may even exhibit a kind of hyposensitivity and feel no pressure pain, not vocalising at all. This lack of feedback can be misleading for beginners, as it's natural to feel more confident when a patient verbally confirms your assessment. We can address this lack of vocal response by observing other bodily reactions, as discussed below.

Jump reactions refer to involuntary body movements during palpation, often as a protective response. This is common in clinic and can be a helpful clue when the patient does not vocalise. Taking the anterior superior iliac spine (ASIS) as an example, we may find that both sides are equally hard. The patient is silent as we palpate, and we need to distinguish whether one side is more reactive than the other. Suppose we use cross-fibre palpation with equal force over each ASIS, and there is a jump response on one side, but not the other. In that case, the side with the additional jump response is the stronger reaction, and this information informs the diagnostic decision.

However, some people do not show even a jump response. For example, a large male patient in his mid-fifties who has spent a hard life as a farmer may not be expressive at all. Our palpation elicits neither vocalisation nor clear bodily reactions. In such cases, it is important to expand our visual field to take in the whole person, allowing us to observe more subtle responses, such as raised eyebrows, flexing toes, or a slight grimace.

Finally, some patients show no vocal or bodily responses at all. This form of hyposensitivity can result from medication. Manaka observed that drugs such as antidepressants, antihypertensives, and analgesics can blunt sensitivity. He also suggested that this kind of muted response may reflect a more advanced state of illness and can serve as a prognostic indicator.

In such cases, we may feel hardness, tightness, or knots, but receive no confirmation from the patient. We must then rely more on our own judgment, assessing which areas are most reactive based on qualities such as greater hardness or more pronounced knots.

Making diagnostic decisions or selecting treatment points in these situations can be more difficult. However, a key sign of improvement is the return of normal sensitivity. If, after a month of treatment, a previously unresponsive patient begins to react to palpation, they may believe their condition has worsened. We need to explain clearly and confidently that this renewed sensitivity is actually a positive sign—the body's ability to respond is being restored.

STRENGTHS OF PALPATION

PATTERN SELECTION

In MSA, effective root treatment can be determined through abdominal palpation alone, without needing to rely on the other aspects of the Four Examinations. In other words, we can decide the primary treatment pattern, treatment points, and methods simply from palpating the belly.

COMBINING WITH OTHER DIAGNOSTIC METHODS

Palpation findings can be integrated with other diagnostic information gathered through the Four Examinations. Sometimes these correlations are clear and decisive; at other times they may seem less obvious or contradictory. In these cases, the palpatory findings are weighed within the broader clinical picture. When abdominal palpation is difficult, due to pregnancy, strong abdominal musculature, or patient immobility, Manaka suggested alternative ways to select treatment patterns that relied less on palpation.

BETTER POINT LOCATION

Palpation allows for more precise point location. Point locations can vary slightly from patient to patient, and even day to day. Simply relying on anatomical locations is not precise enough for the more delicate needling techniques typically employed in Japanese acupuncture. Palpation enables fine-tuning and helps identify the live point.

IMMEDIATE FEEDBACK

Palpation provides fast, real-time feedback on the patient's condition and the effectiveness of the treatment procedure just applied.

LIMITATIONS OF PALPATION

SUBJECTIVITY

Palpation relies on subjective input from both the patient and the practitioner. Of course, this introduces the possibility of error. It's important to balance these findings with more objective data where possible. In the Toyohari system, the Kozato method provides a consensus-building approach to improve inter-rater agreement and increase diagnostic reliability. In MSA trainings, a similar teaching approach is used that builds consensus during practice sessions.[92]

Despite the limited number of scientific studies exploring palpatory decision-making, existing research has shown that palpatory findings can be consistent and reliable, particularly when practitioners undergo repeated training.

[92] Developed by Katsuyuki Kozato, this is a structured group-practice approach for refining needling technique, point location, and diagnostic skills. Practitioners work in small groups, diagnosing and treating together, giving real-time feedback as one person performs an action and another monitors the pulse, allowing immediate adjustment. This systematic, hands-on method accelerates skill development and helps practitioners fine-tune their approach.

IMPROVING RELIABILITY WITH PRACTICE

Subjectivity and diagnostic variability among individuals can be addressed through proven strategies that develop skills, reliability, and confidence. These include:

- Repetitive practice and structured feedback (e.g. the Kozato method, and the modified form used in MSA trainings)
- Manaka's experimental protocols for clarifying ambiguous reactions, many of which will be explored in this book
- Group practice sessions where all participants palpate the same areas, followed by open discussion. Over time, this approach builds skill, consensus, and confidence.

Earlier, we likened this to learning to play the piano or dance: the more we practise under the watchful eyes of others—in a supportive, non-judgmental environment—the more we can develop our palpatory sensitivity.

CONCLUSION

Hands-on practitioners in any tradition develop specialised knowledge and refined techniques. In JAAM, palpation has generated a rich body of clinically useful methods and observations. In Japanese systems such as MSA and Meridian Therapy, these techniques are central to the practice.[93]

In MSA, patterns identified through abdominal palpation form the basis of treatment. We palpate to decide the pattern. We palpate to find the treatment points. When the polarity agents are in place, we palpate again to see how the reactions have changed.

In Meridian Therapy, palpation plays a key confirmatory role. But even outside these systems, palpation offers a powerful way to augment acupuncture and moxibustion practice. The ability to quickly and accurately assess a patient's overall condition through touch is an invaluable clinical skill.[94]

---

93 Birch, S. (1997). 'Forming a Prognosis—Perspectives from the Works of Japanese Acupuncturists: A Preliminary Compilation of Ideas', *NAJOM*, 4(10). pp. 4–8.

94 Ibid.

SUMMARY

- **Palpation is central to JAAM:** It is used to assess the state of the *hara*, meridians, and pulse, and to confirm treatment effects in real time.
- **It has deep historical roots:** Mentioned in classical texts like the *Nan Jing*, it has evolved through hands-on traditions in Japan, especially among blind practitioners.
- **MSA uses palpation to both diagnose and treat:** The palpation sequence starts with a broad assessment of abdominal reflex areas to identify the pattern and narrows focus to reactive treatment points.
- **Light and deep pressure are both used**:
    - Light touch assesses muscle tone, texture, and surface sensitivity.
    - Deeper pressure reveals pressure pain, jump reactions, and muscular hardness.
- **Tissue findings guide diagnosis and treatment. These include:**
    - Muscular tension (mild tightness)
    - Muscular hardness (chronic or severe tightness)
    - Hypotonicity (soft or flaccid muscle tone)
    - Pressure pain
    - Jump reactions
    - Induration (fibrous, reactive knots)
- **Reactions vary by patient:** Some individuals provide clear verbal or physical feedback, while others may be muted due to personality, medication, or chronicity. Even subtle signs such as eyebrow flicks or toe twitches can offer diagnostic clues.
- **Palpation confirms treatment success:** A change in abdominal findings after IPC suggests the step was correctly applied. If not, point location or selection may need adjusting.
- **Different systems use different palpation styles:** Toyohari used a feather-light touch, whereas MSA used stronger pressure to locate points. The techniques may vary, but all are grounded in clinical observation, not theory.
- **Palpation isn't foolproof, as it's partly subjective:** Inter-rater training, structured feedback, and repeated practice improve reliability and confidence.
- **Like any physical skill, palpation must be practised:** Palpation sensitivity is learned through hands-on practice, not just by reading, and ideally under supervision from an experienced teacher.

WHAT'S NEXT

Next, we move to the *hara*, the main focus of MSA diagnosis. We'll explore Manaka's abdominal map and the five basic patterns it reveals, along with his categories of primary reflex areas and points for making a diagnosis and the secondary reactions that help refine it.

CHAPTER 5

STEP 1 PATTERNS: DIFFERENTIATION

THE *HARA*: PALPATING THE ABDOMEN

> *What is important is the need for, and utilization of, a creative and consistent research methodology and methods of assessing the effects of treatment. We can take nothing at face value because, without clinical tests and confirmation, we have no real idea of what these simplifications mean.*
>
> —Dr Yoshio Manaka[95]

We have seen that abdominal palpation started in the *Nan Jing* (circa 100 AD) and that it plays an important role in the practice of JAAM. In *Hara Diagnosis*, Kiiko Matsumoto and Stephen Birch, following the *Nan Jing*, speculated that there is a core centre to the qi systems in the body located in the lower abdomen.[96] This centre was called the "moving qi between the kidneys" and was described both as a dynamic centre and as "fundamental to the five yin and six yang organs, the root of the twelve meridians, the gate of breathing. It is the source of the triple burner".[97] This idea of a

---

95 Manaka, Y., Itaya, K., & Birch, S. (1995). *Chasing the Dragon's Tail: The Theory and Practice of Acupuncture in the Work of Yoshio Manaka*. Brookline: Paradigm Publications. p. 12.

96 Unschuld, P. U. (1986). *Medicine in China: Nan Ching, the Classic of Difficult Issues*. Berkeley: University of California Press. p. 130.

97 Matsumoto, K. & Birch, S. (1988). Hara Diagnosis: Reflections on the Sea. Brookline, MA: Paradigm Publications, Chapters 5–6.

core centre in the lower abdomen may provide the theoretical basis for palpating there to understand the primary disruptions in the qi systems of the patient (these concepts are discussed at length in *Hara Diagnosis*).[98] Certainly, this idea helps us understand how palpation of the *hara* can give specific prognostic information about the overall condition of the patient. It has also led to the development of systematic methods for assessing specific problems in the patient.

Chapters 16 and 56 of the *Nan Jing* outlined a basic method of abdominal palpation in relation to the Five Phases and their meridians and *zang* organs.[99] This method has become central in the use of abdominal palpation in Japanese Meridian Therapy. It has also encouraged the development of numerous other abdominal palpation mappings. Dr Manaka's Extraordinary Vessels mapping on the abdominal region is but one of these, but we will see that in his own inimitable way, as mentioned above, he took the historical category of front-*mu* points and developed it further.

THE FIVE-PHASE REFLEX AREA

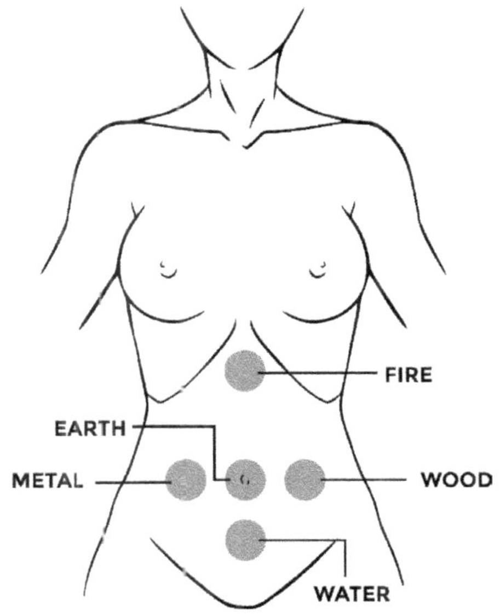

Figure 5-1: The earth element is at the centre, with the other four grouped around it.

---

98 Ibid.

99 Unschuld, P. U. (1986). *Medicine in China: Nan Ching, the Classic of Difficult Issues*. Berkeley: University of California Press. pp. 219–221; pp. 499–509.

The *Nan Jing* describes how each of the Five Phases and their corresponding meridians and organs are reflected in a pattern around the navel. The water/kidney area was below the navel, the earth/spleen area around the navel, the fire/heart area below the sternum, the wood/liver area to the left of the navel and the metal/lung area to the right. In modern practice, this map has been elaborated in various ways, depending in part on the methods of palpation.[100, 101, 102]

While useful for Meridian Therapy diagnosis, this mapping is not used or considered relevant in MSA.

MANAKA'S MAPPINGS

Each of the Eight Extraordinary Vessels is 'opened' by a master and coupled point, of which there are eight. This means that one pair of points corresponds with two of the Eight Extras. For example, LU 7 and KID 6 relate to both Ren Mai and Yin Qiao Mai. For this reason, Manaka referred to them as pairs; in this case, the Yin Qiao–Ren Mai pair. These can be abbreviated as shown in Table 5.1.

---

100 Shudo, D. (1990). *Japanese Classical Acupuncture: Introduction to Meridian Therapy*. Seattle: Eastland Press.

101 Matsumoto, K., & Birch, S. (1988). *Hara Diagnosis: Reflections on the Sea*. Brookline: Paradigm Publications.

102 Fukushima, K. (1991). *Meridian Therapy*. Tokyo: Toyo Hari Medical Association.

Table 5.1: Eight Extras pairing abbreviations.

EIGHT EXTRAORDINARY VESSELS	PAIRING NAME	ABBREVIATION
Yin Qiao Mai Ren Mai	Yin Qiao–Ren Mai pair	YQR
Yang Qiao Mai Du Mai	Yang Qiao–Du Mai pair	YQD
Yin Wei Mai Chong Mai	Yin Wei–Chong Mai pair	YWC
Yang Wei Mai Dai Mai	Yang Wei–Dai Mai pair	YWD

Manaka's octahedron is mapped out on the abdomen with dividing lines that run along vertical and horizontal axes. These axes intersect at the navel, around GB 26, and on the spine. As the navel is an intersection point of these axes, it allows for the examination of reaction patterns either along the primary axes or in the upper and lower quadrants of the abdomen defined by these axes. Manaka's diagnostic areas correlate to pairs of the Extraordinary Vessels. Reactions found along the vertical axis indicate the YQR (Yin Qiao–Ren Mai) pattern; reactions along the horizontal axis indicate the YWD (Yang Wei–Dai Mai) pattern; reactions in the subcostal regions (upper right quadrant and upper left quadrant) indicate the YWC (Yin Wei–Chong Mai) pattern; reactions at the anterior superior iliac spines indicate either the YWD (Yang Wei–Dai Mai) or YQD (Yang Qiao–Du Mai) pattern.

Manaka referred to these diagnostic areas as primary reflex areas. These reflex areas correspond to an eight extra vessel pair and show reduced reactions when the relevant pair of points is treated.

MANAKA AND THE *MU* POINTS

In addition to these primary reflex areas, Manaka also researched what he called primary reflex points, bilateral points that reliably indicate the status of the twelve meridians. These points are often referred to as the Manaka-*mu* points.

In classical acupuncture, the front-*mu* ('alarm') points are a group of twelve points, all distributed on the chest or abdomen. The points have been considered to reflect the condition of the related organ or meridian.

Peter Deadman describes the term *mu* as meaning "to gather or collect, and the front-*mu* points are where the qi of the *zangfu* gathers and concentrates on the anterior surface of the body".[103]

Another common way of thinking about the *mu* points was articulated by Kodo Fukushima: "Yang diseases travel through the yin region", so these points "manifest signs such as stiffness and bumps during yang illnesses".[104] The stiffness and bumps cause pain on palpation, and this pressure pain is used diagnostically.

Although the clinical uses of front-*mu* points include treating their related organs directly or treating local problems on the anterior, Manaka was more interested in how they could be used diagnostically. Historically, many have suggested that when there is a problem with a meridian, the related front-*mu* point can show a reaction on palpation. When the meridian is correctly treated, the reaction should reduce or disappear. Manaka tested this assumption systematically and found it *not* to hold true consistently.

Moreover, the twelve classical front-*mu* points are all located on the chest and abdomen, close to their related organs. LU 1, LIV 14, and GB 24 are the front-*mu* points for the lungs, liver, and gall bladder meridians, respectively, but the other nine front-*mu* points are not on their related meridian. Interestingly, the front-*mu* points for the pericardium, heart, stomach, triple burner, small intestine and bladder are all on the midline, at REN 17, REN 14, REN 12, REN 5, and REN 4, and REN 3, respectively.

---

103 Deadman, P., Al-Khafaji, M., & Baker, K. (1998). *A Manual of Acupuncture*. East Sussex: Journal of Chinese Medicine Publications. p. 44.

104 Fukushima, K. (1991). *Meridian Therapy*. Tokyo: Toyo Hari Medical Association. p. 173.

As Manaka's octahedral model is very concerned with, among other things, assessing left and right balances, he felt that these classical midline points were unable to give him the information he needed. We can easily detect differences between LU 1 on the right and left that reflect the condition of the right and left lung meridians. However, if we palpate REN 12, the front-*mu* point of the stomach, which is on the midline, we have no way to differentiate the condition of the left and right stomach meridians. As he developed his octahedral model and treatment system, Manaka subjected the classical *mu* points to a set of empirical tests.

> *What is important is the need for, and utilisation of, a creative and consistent research methodology and methods of assessing the effects of treatment. We can take nothing at face value because, without clinical tests and confirmation, we have no real idea of what these simplifications mean.*[105]

He researched and identified other reactive points on the torso that are located bilaterally. Placing magnets to the *yuan*-source points on the left and right meridians, he observed which torso points became more reactive or less reactive when north or south poles were applied. If one polarity made the test point more reactive and the other polarity made it less reactive, it demonstrated a relationship between the test point and the status of the corresponding meridian.

He also used simple meridian-stretching techniques: if stretching a meridian made tenderness disappear from one location and reappear at a candidate point, this confirmed a functional relationship. Finally, he needled the *yuan*-source point of the meridian and checked whether tenderness at the abdominal reflex point diminished or vanished. Through these procedures, performed with patients in a relaxed, supine posture, he found that various non-classical abdominal points behaved more reliably and more consistently than the traditional *mu* points.[106]

---

105 Manaka, Y., Itaya, K., & Birch, S. (1995). *Chasing the Dragon's Tail: The Theory and Practice of Acupuncture in the Work of Yoshio Manaka*. Brookline: Paradigm Publications. p. 12.

106 Manaka, Y., Itaya, K., & Birch, S. (1995). *Chasing the Dragon's Tail: The Theory and Practice of Acupuncture in the Work of Yoshio Manaka*. Brookline: Paradigm Publications. pp. 74–75.

In the example of REN 12 above, he explored a horizontal line lateral to it, connecting both ST 21 points, and this expanded line became his preferred diagnostic area. In the case of LU 1, he expanded the diagnostic area to include LU 2. This empirical thinking was applied to all twelve meridians and is the origin of the Manaka-*mu* points, a set of twelve diagnostic points with several key properties essential to Manaka's research and clinical work, including:

1. When there are problems in the related meridian, the Manaka-*mu* points feel tight or painful on palpation.
2. When the meridian is treated, this tightness or pain changes swiftly.
3. The Manaka-*mu* points are not on the midline, so each pair can be used to differentiate left and right meridian flow.

Table 5.2: Traditional and Manaka-*mu* points.

MERIDIAN	TRADITIONAL FRONT-*MU* POINT	MANAKA-*MU* POINT
Lung	LU 1	LU 1 to LU 2
Large Intestine	ST 25	ST 27 (can be slightly more lateral)
Stomach	REN 12	ST 21, including from left to right over REN 12
Spleen	LIV 13	Mid-axillary line from SP 21 to GB 26 (especially the points SP 21 and GB 26)
Heart	REN 14	KID 23 + sides of REN 14
Small Intestine	REN 4	ST 26 (can be slightly more medial)
Bladder	REN 3	KID 11
Kidney	GB 25	KID 16
Pericardium	REN 17	P 1 + REN 17[107]
Triple Burner	REN 5	ST 25 (can be slightly more lateral)
Gall Bladder	GB 24	ASIS (sometimes GB 24 can be used as well)
Liver	LIV 14	Subcostal region from LIV 13 to ST 19

Thus, when palpating, Manaka would first examine the abdomen for the primary reaction areas, using the vertical and horizontal lines that define the anterior quadrants. If a primary area showed a reaction, he would then confirm it by palpating the corresponding primary reflex points.

For example, if the primary area for the YQR pattern was reactive (see Figures 5.2 and 5.3), since the master and coupled points for this pattern are LU 7 and KID 6, he would palpate the lung and kidney reflex points (LU 1 to LU 2, KID 16).

107 Since P 1 lies slightly lateral and superior to the nipple, it is not feasible for many female patients to be palpated there, especially by male practitioners; thus, on female patients, only REN 17 is appropriate.

Likewise, if the primary areas for the YQD pattern were reactive, since the master and coupled points are SI 3 and BL 62, he would palpate the small intestine and bladder reflex points (ST 26, KID 11).

THE SECONDARY REACTIONS

Palpating for the primary reflex areas is the first stage of palpation, and palpating for the primary reflex points is the second. Manaka had a third differentiating palpatory sequence, usually deployed when the findings from the first two stages led to two or more candidate patterns of diagnosis with reactions at both the primary areas *and* primary points. This sequence consists of palpating a group of related points or areas, some on the abdomen, others on the chest, upper back, neck, arms, and legs. These are called secondary reactions.

These secondary reactions are used as tiebreakers—to differentiate two or more patterns that show reactions at their primary reflex areas and points. We select the pattern that has secondary reactions or the most prevalent reactions. However, in many patients, the primary areas and points are enough to make a clear diagnosis.

Discussing these secondary reactions in detail at this stage will over-complicate the picture, so we'll come back to them when we've fully covered the primary reflex areas and the primary reflex points. What's most important for now is learning the terminology of these three palpatory classifications:

- Primary reflex areas
- Primary reflex points
- Secondary reactions

THE BASIC FIVE PATTERNS

We're finally getting to the nuts and bolts of MSA: finding the primary reflex areas and the primary reflex points of the Eight Extras on the abdomen. And we will also encounter the first contemporary departures from historical MSA theory. Manaka developed five basic abdominal patterns, but we will also learn three contemporary iterations. Let's map out the reaction areas and then look at how we could go about palpating them and what we might find. Note that the primary reflex areas lie either along one of the dividing lines of the octahedron (e.g. Ren Mai, Dai Mai) or within abdominal quadrants defined by the anterior sections of the octahedron: along the subcostal margin, anterior to the anterior superior iliac spine (ASIS), and to the left or right of the navel in the lower quadrants along the stomach meridians.

HISTORICAL MANAKA: THE ORIGINAL FIVE PATTERNS

The diagrams below show the primary areas and primary points for Manaka's original five patterns. A pattern is diagnosed when there is a clear reaction in both the primary area and its corresponding primary points—whether those reactions appear unilaterally, bilaterally, or contralaterally.

YQR

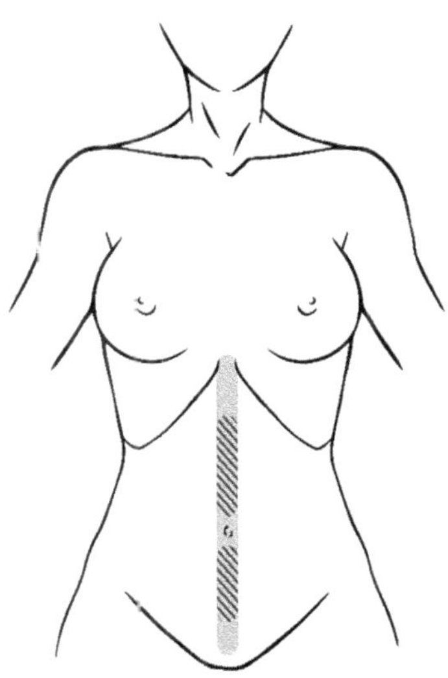

Figure 5-2: YQR primary area.

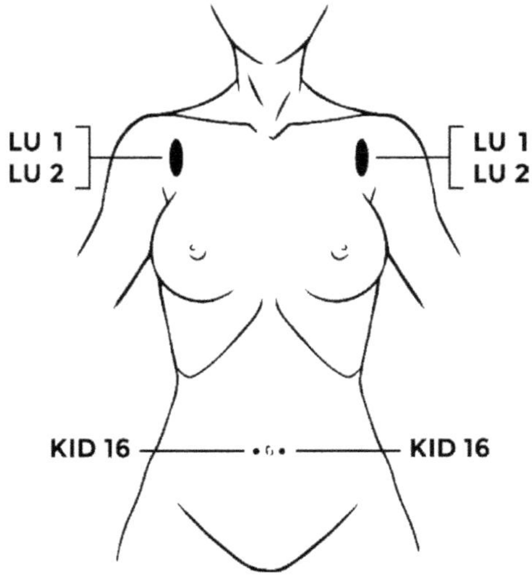

Figure 5-3: YQR primary points.

Going back to the balloon analogy of Chapter 1 to understand the octahedral model, the vertical line separating left and right in the embryo remains in the human body on the abdomen as a pivotal dividing line for autoregulation of the left and right halves—the Ren Mai. Look for reactions along the midline.

PRIMARY REFLEX AREA

- Midline

PRIMARY REFLEX POINTS

- LU 1–LU 2 area, KID 16

Reactions can show anywhere along the midline but are most common from REN 14 down to REN 4. The area above the navel often feels stiff or painful, while the region below the navel may feel soft or lacking in tone. The upper reactions usually centre around REN 10–REN 12, whereas the lower reactions tend to appear between REN 4 and REN 6.

Sometimes the whole abdomen is soft and weak, for example in postpartum women or the elderly. This global loss of tone can serve as a shortcut for diagnosing YQR. Tenderness or reactivity below the navel during menstruation is quite normal. However, if the same finding appears outside the menstrual period, it becomes a priority sign for YQR or a related pattern (see Chapter 14).

YWC

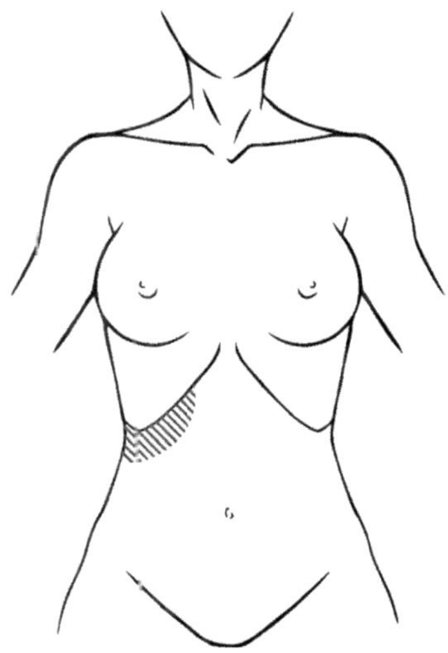

Figure 5-4: YWC primary area.

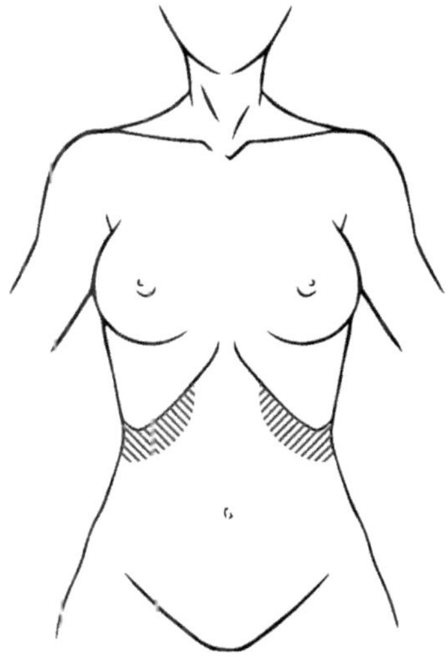

Figure 5-5: YWC primary area (more progressed).

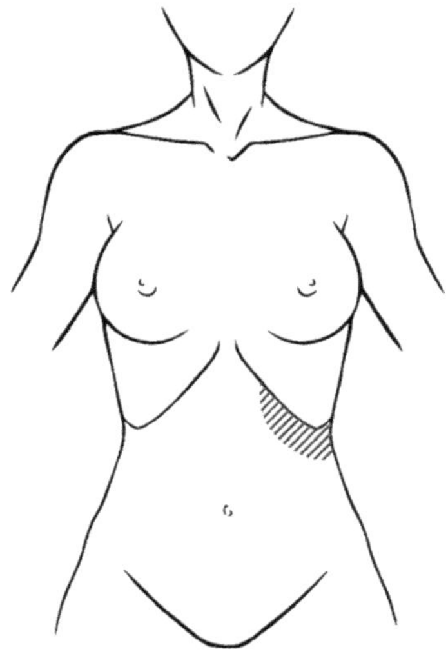

Figure 5-6: YWC primary area (most progressed).

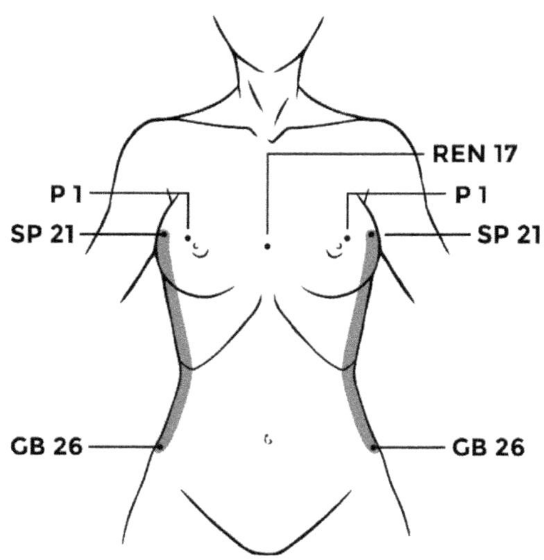

Figure 5-7: YWC primary points.

Why does the subcostal area relate to the YWC? In Japan, LIV 14 is located in the subcostal region, directly below the nipple. LIV 14 is also on the pathway of the Yin Wei Mai, and the liver is associated with the Chong Mai. LIV 14 and the subcostal regions are in the upper right and upper left quadrants and thus became a natural area for investigation.

PRIMARY REFLEX AREA

- Subcostal area, either on the right, bilaterally, or less commonly, only on the left. This shows a progression in severity: bilateral reactions can be a bit more stubborn to change and a reaction only on the left is considered potentially more serious.

In addition, Stephen Birch adds:

> *In the 1980s, when we were writing about MSA, we took 'subcostal' to mean the whole subcostal margin. When I helped write Manaka's book, I maintained that same definition, as long as it included LIV 14. However, in clinical practice over the years, I have come to define this reaction area more precisely: it extends laterally from ST 19 to LIV 13 on both sides, but not medially to ST 19.*
>
> *When there is a clear reaction only in the medial subcostal region, on the kidney meridian, it usually indicates Ren Mai involvement. If there are substernal reactions, and the main subcostal reaction is medial to ST 19 and lies on the kidney meridian, and the lateral subcostal area feels healthy, this presentation will often respond better to a YQR treatment.*[108]

PRIMARY REFLEX POINTS

- REN 17, P 1, the mid-axillary line between SP 21 and GB 26 (especially the points SP 21 and GB 26)

Look for a single reactive point along the mid-axillary line; don't expect the entire line to be tender.

P 1 is easy to palpate on men. With female patients it may be awkward, especially for male practitioners, so approach with sensitivity and use REN 17 if more appropriate.

---

[108] Kivity, O. (2023). Notes from authors' meeting.

YWD

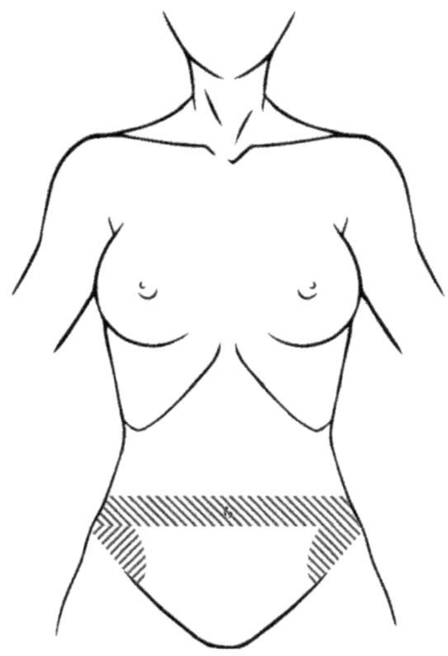

Figure 5-8: YWD primary area.

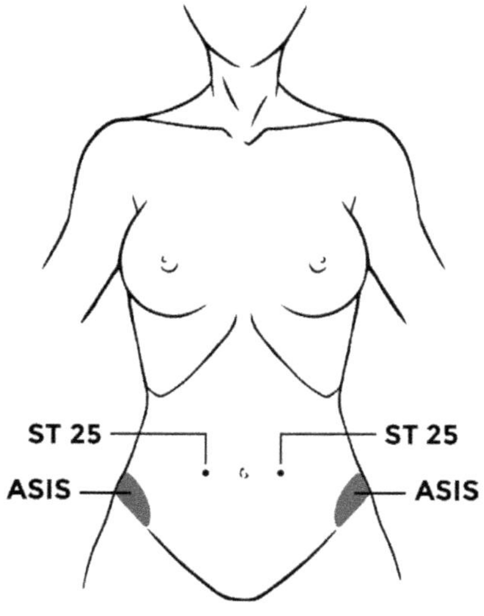

Figure 5-9: YWD primary points.

Once again returning to our balloon analogy, the horizontal line separating superior from inferior is still a pivotal line in the human body and on the abdomen, helping in the autoregulation of areas above and below it—this is the Dai Mai. Look for reactions along this horizontal line and also at the anterior superior iliac spine (ASIS). Dr Manaka, citing historical texts, interpreted the ASIS as GB 29 but as this differs from most descriptions of GB 29, we refer to this gall bladder primary reflex point only as the ASIS.

PRIMARY REFLEX AREA

- Along the Dai Mai from the navel to the lateral edge of the abdomen, including the ASIS

PRIMARY REFLEX POINTS

- ST 25 and ASIS

The reactions for the YWD are unique, principally because the primary reflex points are located within the primary reflex area, the belt line, and the ASIS. The ASIS is the gall bladder reflex point, and ST 25 is the TB reflex point. Moreover, there are secondary reactions as well, also located in the primary area. These are KID 16 and SP 15. We will study the secondary reactions later, but for now, you can think of these two points as additional confirmatory signs. Essentially, diagnosing the YWD belt is easy because all the points are along the belt of the Dai Mai. We can break this area down according to theory into primary points—the ASIS and ST 25, corresponding to GB and TB, and secondary reactions such as KID 16 and SP 15.

The ASIS also appears as a primary area for the YQD pattern. To confirm a YWD reaction, look for both belt line and ASIS reactions, or a clear belt line reaction on its own. ASIS reactions, without belt line involvement, are more suggestive of YQD.

YQD

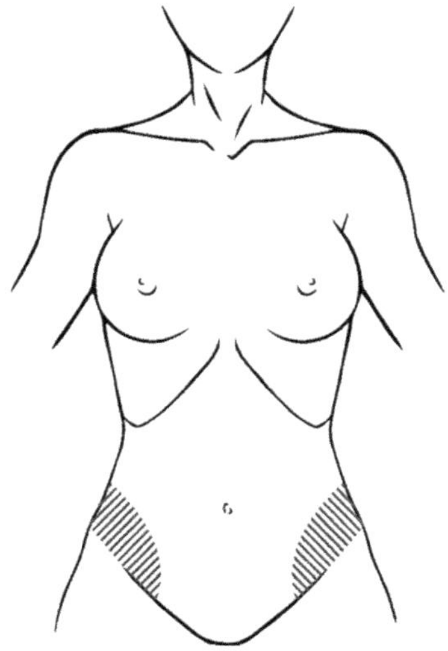

Figure 5-10: YQD primary areas.

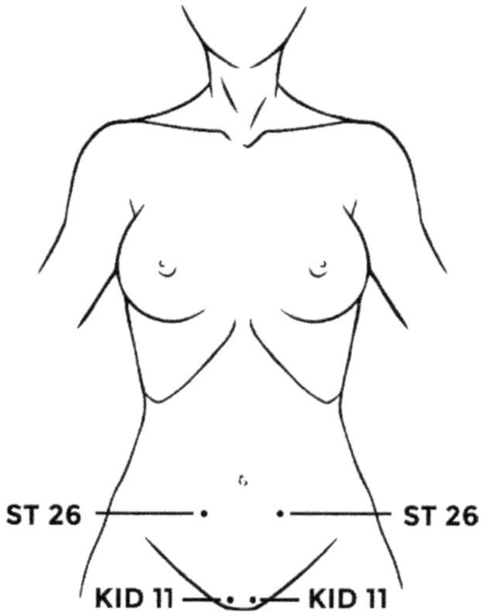

Figure 5-11: YQD primary points.

The reflex area for the YQD is the ASIS. Unlike the midline reflex area for the YQR, its logic isn't immediately obvious. We can offer a few working theories to make sense of this and to help us remember.

One idea is that the spine is anchored in the hips, which may explain why the Asian squat is considered a healthy resting posture that helps reposition the spine. Manaka explored this in another way. Drawing on a 1925 article describing a muscular chain that "suspends" the pelvis from the occiput, he outlined a sequence of linked muscles running up the body: internal oblique to external oblique to serratus anterior to the rhomboids. Seen this way, you can imagine a continuous line of tension running from the ASIS up to the neck, which might explain the diagnostic relationship between the ASIS and the YQD pattern.

These ideas are also useful when thinking about the next pattern, the Cross Syndrome. For example, if the liver (a right-sided organ) is affected, it may distort the right external oblique, which could then affect the left internal oblique and related muscles on the right side.

PRIMARY REFLEX AREA

- ASIS

PRIMARY REFLEX POINTS

- KID 11, ST 26

CROSS SYNDROME

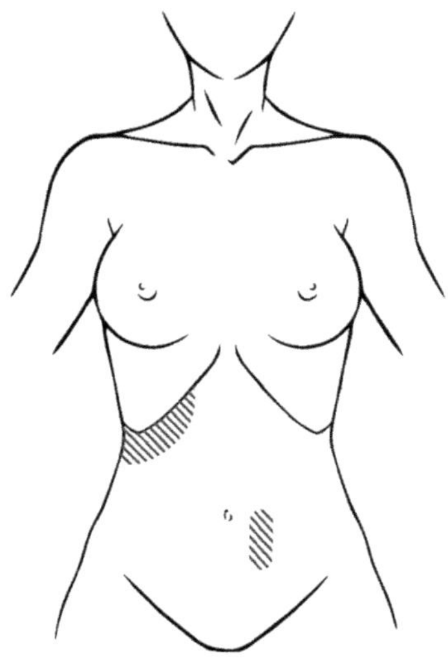

Figure 5-12: URQ and left ST 25–ST 27.

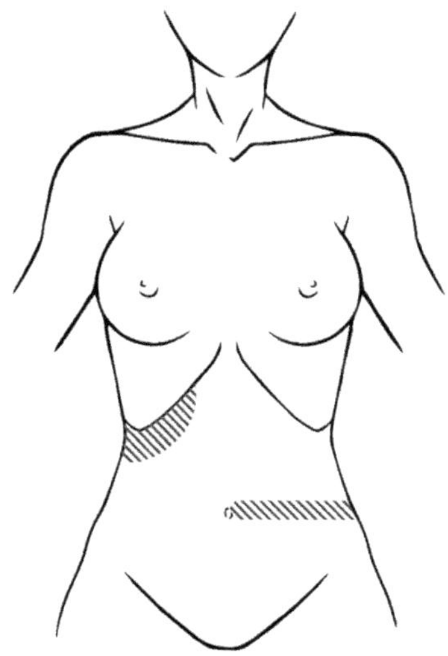

Figure 5-13: URQ and left belt.

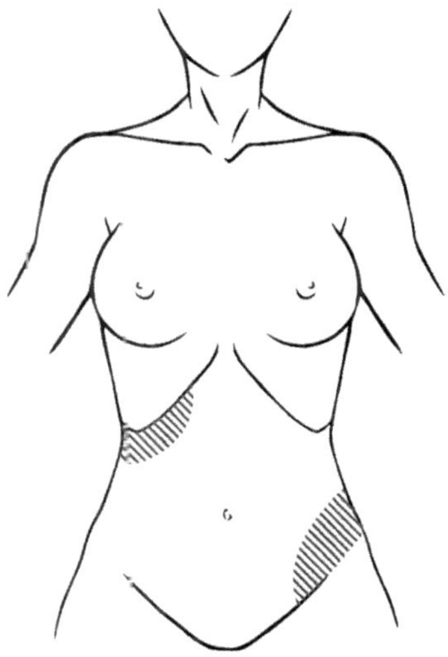

Figure 5-14: URQ and left ASIS.

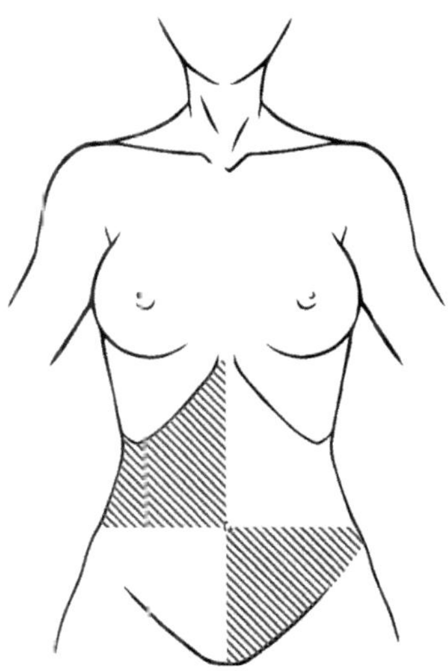

Figure 5-15: Any URQ and LLQ reactions.

The fifth pattern is a combination pattern, which is a mixture of YWC on the patient's right and YWD on the patient's left. In other words, there are reactions in both the upper right quadrant and the lower left quadrant.

PRIMARY REFLEX AREA

- The upper right quadrant (right subcostal area) and the lower left quadrant. The lower left quadrant reactions manifest in one to three areas: ST 25 to ST 27, along the left trajectory of the Dai Mai itself, and at the left ASIS. One, two, or all three of these reactions together, combined with the upper right quadrant reactions, constitute Cross Syndrome (CS).

PRIMARY REFLEX POINTS

- In theory, we would palpate the primary points related to the individual components of this pattern, such as REN 17, P 1, and the mid-axillary line from SP 21 to GB 26. In practice, though, when Cross Syndrome presents with clear reactions in the upper right and lower left quadrants, further point-checking is rarely necessary.

The right subcostal area is consistently tight, while the lower left quadrant may show tenderness at any or all three sites: the left ASIS, the left ST 25–27 region, or along the left belt line.

Finally, when the left ST 25–27 area is hard, lumpy, and painful, it indicates more advanced blood stasis. In contrast, milder reactions in this region—whether at ST 25–27, the belt line, or the ASIS—are more suggestive of a musculoskeletal distortion and a milder degree of blood stasis.

CS is a combination pattern created by Dr Manaka. Later in this book, we will study some contemporary patterns developed by Stephen Birch and Brenda Loew that treat different combinations of Manaka's basic patterns.

A ROUTINE FOR PALPATING THE *HARA*

The previous chapter introduced the idea that palpation is done in two stages: first with light pressure on the primary reflex areas, then with deeper pressure into any reactive areas or points. All the authors of this book palpate slightly differently—there's no single 'correct' way to proceed. Our individual approaches have evolved through clinical practice.

Beginners, however, need a starting point. We recommend a simple, consistent strategy to begin with. As your palpatory sensitivity, observation skills, and understanding develop, you'll naturally begin to adjust your approach.

While Manaka's close colleague Kazuko Itaya palpated very lightly and Manaka used comparatively deeper pressure, both had clear reasons for their approach, based on long clinical experience. What follows is a practical outline, especially useful if you haven't yet trained directly with a Manaka teacher.

We recommend palpating in three rounds. It's important to palpate every patient from the same side, every time. Right-handed people usually palpate standing on the patient's left. This consistency is important when comparing findings from week to week. Do things the same way, each time.

ROUND 1: LIGHT PALPATION OF THE PRIMARY REACTIONS

Begin by making contact with the patient and helping them relax. Explain what you're about to do and get verbal consent. Then, place one hand gently on the upper abdomen and rest your other hand lightly on the lower abdomen. This initial contact helps ground the patient, calms the nervous system, and gives you a first impression of general tone, temperature, and asymmetry—without applying pressure. For example, the upper abdomen might feel tight, the lower abdomen cool or flaccid, or you may notice asymmetry in the rectus abdominis. These initial impressions, gathered without applying pressure, may also contribute to your sense of prognosis. For example, if everything feels firm and toned, it suggests a better prognosis; if the entire abdomen feels weak, flaccid, and lacking in tonus, it is likely that more treatments will be needed.

With the patient relaxed and grounded, begin your first round of active palpation. Use light pressure to examine each of the primary reflex areas:

- **REN MAI**: Palpate lightly from REN 15 to the navel, noting any tension.
- **YWC**: Start at the right subcostal area, with your fingers resting on the ribcage. Press your thumbs gently under the lateral rib cage at about a 45° angle and move medially. Repeat on the left subcostal area, starting laterally and moving medially. Compare both sides.
- **DAI MAI**: Palpate gently from KID 16 to ST 25, SP 15, and the ASIS. Note any left-right differences.
- **LOWER ABDOMEN**: Palpate from the navel to the pubic symphysis along the Ren Mai, then from ST 25 down to ST 27 on each side.

At this stage, simply observe—note tightness, tone, temperature, or tenderness. If anything is particularly tender or reactive with light pressure, remember to return to it later with firmer palpation.

ROUND 2: MEDIUM PRESSURE AND CONFIRMING REACTIONS

Now go back over the same areas with slightly deeper pressure to confirm your findings. This is where jump reactions and pressure pain tend to appear. Use variations such as:

- Cross-fibre palpation on hard or raised areas; for example, across the upper Ren Mai
- Circular or cross-fibre palpation across ST 25–ST 27 or over the ASIS
- Lighter touch for softer, weaker, or cooler regions—especially over the lower Ren Mai, where the abdominal wall may be thinner or overlying internal organs (a lighter touch gathers more information when the area is more deficient)

Take note of where reactions are clearest—this will guide you towards one or more of the five primary patterns.

ROUND 3: DEEPER PALPATION AND PATTERN CONFIRMATION

By now, you should have some clear candidates for the pattern. You will have noticed areas that feel tight or abnormal in some way, and you can now do a third round, slightly deeper, to confirm these. As you apply the deeper pressure to each of the same regions in the same sequence, this is where you more commonly find pressure pain and jump reactions.

Once you've identified the likely pattern(s) based on reflex areas, palpate the primary reflex points associated with them. A pattern is considered valid if there's a reaction in both the primary area and its corresponding points—either unilaterally, bilaterally, or contralaterally. You don't need to palpate reflex points for patterns that didn't show a reaction in the primary area.

Use light cross-fibre or circular palpation as needed to assess the degree of pressure pain or jumpiness. If only one pattern shows a clear set of reactions, you've identified the root pattern to treat. If two or more patterns are active, you'll need to use the secondary reactions as tiebreakers.

CLARIFICATION WITH THE SECONDARY REACTIONS

Sometimes, things don't go the textbook way! Several patterns present simultaneously. The primary areas and primary points all check out positively. Manaka employed various strategies to clarify the pattern identification process, including palpating an additional group of points to confirm one pattern over another. These secondary reactions are covered in detail in Chapter 14.

SYMPTOMS

There's one final way to differentiate between the Eight Extras patterns: symptom presentation. Sometimes, two patterns present with clear primary and secondary reactions, making it difficult to choose between them based on palpation alone. In such cases, symptoms can help tip the balance.

For example, if YQR and YQD both present, and the patient has a cough or shortness of breath, that might support YQR. If they have neck or back pain, we might lean towards YQD. While later volumes will describe treatments for specific symptoms within the MSA model, symptoms are not usually the primary basis for selecting a pattern. That said, they can help us weigh one pattern more heavily than another when palpation alone is inconclusive.

We'll explore this approach further in Chapter 14.

CONCLUSION

We've seen that the *hara* has been used since antiquity to diagnose the condition of the whole body, perhaps because of the "moving qi between the kidneys". Manaka mapped out reaction zones for the Eight Extraordinary Vessels on the *hara* and developed his own reflex points, the Manaka-*mu* points, to help decide what to treat. When we palpate, we can start lightly and then with each pass press more deeply, looking for primary reflex areas, primary reflex points, and, where necessary, secondary reactions. In this chapter, we have described palpation for diagnosis. In the next chapter, we'll see how palpation can also serve as a feedback mechanism—to assess the effectiveness of our treatment strategy and point selection.

SUMMARY

- **Abdominal palpation is central to MSA diagnosis:** it draws on classical theory and Manaka's innovations in mapping the Eight Extraordinary Vessels onto the four quadrants of the abdomen.
- **Manaka mapped diagnostic zones for the Eight Extras:** These include primary reflex areas and corresponding primary reflex points.
- **The primary reflex areas define five core patterns:** Each is associated with one or more of the Eight Extras and is located along specific anatomical landmarks or quadrants.
- **The Manaka-*mu* points are side-specific:** They enable left–right differentiation of meridians, unlike many classical front-*mu* points, which lie on the midline and which Manaka sometimes found to be less responsive.

- **Eight Extras patterns confirmation:** Each pattern is confirmed by finding reactions at both the primary reflex area and its corresponding primary reflex points (the Manaka-*mu* points).
- **Secondary reactions act as tiebreakers:** When two or more patterns coexist, palpating specific points and areas on the limbs, neck, or trunk can help clarify the diagnosis. We'll examine them in more detail in Chapter 14.
- **Symptom presentation can support decision-making:** If palpation does not clearly distinguish between patterns, symptoms can help differentiate pattern selection (see Chapter 14).

WHAT'S NEXT

Once the five basic patterns are clear, the next step is to treat them. In the following chapter, we'll introduce the tools and procedures you need to perform Step 1.

CHAPTER 6

STEP 1 PATTERNS: TOOLKIT AND TREATMENT

INTRODUCTION

In the last chapter, we looked at Manaka's five basic patterns. There are quite a few more abdominal patterns to come, but the beauty of this system is that when we identify a pattern, we don't need to think too much about choosing the treatment. If we identify a YQD pattern, we treat the master and couple points of the YQD pair. If we identify a YQR pattern, we treat the master and couple points of the YQR pair. Moreover, when we move to Step 2, releasing the yang aspect of the body, our treatment options are clearly defined by our choices at Step 1. The pattern and treatment are inextricably linked. Although the theory of MSA may at first feel bewildering, its practice is powerfully simple. This chapter will examine the nuts and bolts of Step 1 treatment: which points do we use, which side do we treat them, and how (and why) do we apply polarity agents.

THE MASTER AND COUPLED POINTS

The Eight Extras are described as reservoirs of energy, absorbing excess flows from the main meridians and filling them when they are empty. They are activated by needling two points simultaneously: the master point and the coupled point. Imagine these two points as two locks at the top and bottom of the door of a safe. Both keys must be inserted and turned at the same time for the door to open. Thus, to unlock Manaka's system, we need to memorise the master and coupled points of each pair.

Table 6.1: Master and coupled points.

PATTERN	MASTER AND COUPLED POINTS
YQR	LU 7 + KID 6
YWC	P 6 + SP 4
YWD	TB 5 + GB 41
YQD	SI 3 + BL 62

POINT LOCATION

At this stage in the book, it should come as no surprise that Dr Manaka's point locations for the master and coupled points differ from the textbook locations we all learned in school. Once again, this comes down to pragmatic considerations in JAAM. In many traditions in JAAM, there is a concept of the 'currently alive' point, first coined in the early twentieth century by Takeshi Sawada, the renowned moxibustion practitioner. For example, in contemporary Meridian Therapy, the alive point is the location that, when stroked gently, elicits the best possible change on the pulse. It might not be so close to its textbook location and can only be located by skilful palpation. Denmai Shudo, a renowned teacher and author, says it takes "effort and ingenuity" to find the alive point and reminds us that the acupuncture points came first, and the point location textbooks came second.[109]

We can draw from Shudo's comment that, despite what is taught in acupuncture colleges, there is no standard of acupuncture point location. The famed Bronze Man models, filled with liquid and covered in wax, were designed to leak when hopeful students needled the correct point location. But most people would agree that this was a learning tool rather than an accurate gold (or bronze) standard of where these points occur in the infinite anatomical variations of the human body.

109 Shudo, D. (1990). *Japanese Classical Acupuncture: Introduction to Meridian Therapy.* Seattle: Eastland Press.

As is often found when looking across different traditions of acupuncture, some Japanese point locations differ from Chinese locations. For example, while LIV 14 is (mostly) on the mammillary line in both traditions, in JAAM it is found below the costal margin, and in TCM it is in the sixth intercostal space. Moreover, different traditions emphasise different attributes when searching for acupuncture point locations. By definition, the Bronze Man locations were fixed; moreover, contemporary Chinese textbooks also describe point locations in exact ways, using proportional measuring and anatomical landmarks. This approach stands in marked contrast to the concept of the alive point. The alive point can be found in different ways. Isaburo Fukaya, another twentieth-century moxibustion pioneer, used strong palpation to define effective moxa points by pressure pain and induration. In Meridian Therapy, the alive point is the one that elicits the best change on the pulse when stroked lightly. **In MSA, it is the pressure pain point that, when treated, gives the most comprehensive change in the palpable reactions on the abdominal wall.**

Manaka's point locations are shown in Figures 6-1–6-9. Using these anatomical descriptions as a starting point, explore the meridian above and below the location with pressure. Use your thumb or index finger to palpate, supporting your hand with fingers and thumb on the area to be treated. Palpate firmly for indurations and pressure pain along the meridian and around the location.

LU 7		
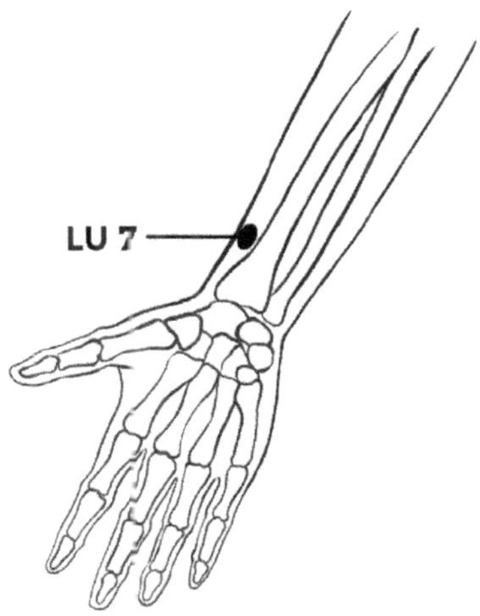		
LOCATION	**FINDING THE POINT**	**COMMENTS**
On the anterior surface of the wrist, LU 7 is located with the palm facing up. The point is proximal to LU 8 on the radius, proximal to the prominence of the radial styloid process.	Place your finger proximal to the styloid process, apply pressure until pressing to the bone, and then slide the fingertip proximally along the surface of the radius until you encounter a small knot or mound that is painful on pressure.	In keeping with all Japanese traditions and older Chinese practices, Manaka's LU 7—unlike its location in modern TCM textbooks—lies on the line connecting LU 9 and LU 5.

Figure 6-1: Finding LU 7.

P 6		
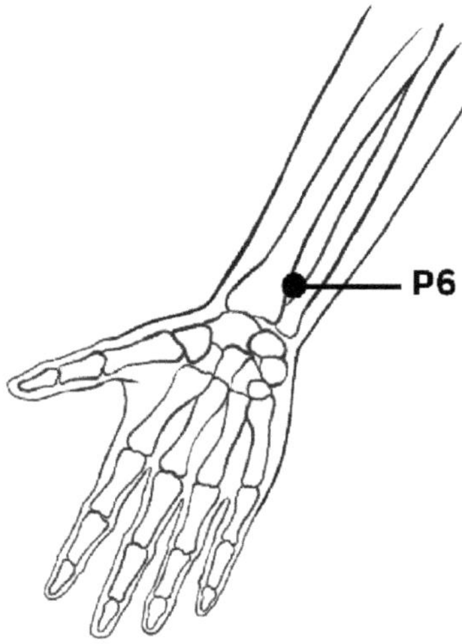 		
LOCATION	**FINDING THE POINT**	**COMMENTS**
On the palmar surface of the wrist, P 6 is located between the tendons of palmaris longus and flexor carpi radialis, most commonly at the proximal edge of the ulnar-radial joint or slightly proximal to that.	To find the point, find the proximal edge of the joint of the radius and ulnar bones, and press to look for pressure pain. If it is not there, move the finger slightly proximal to that and press. Repeat until you find a pressure pain point. It may feel like a hard sheet of tissue, which is more pronounced when the hand is dorsiflexed.	In marked contrast to many contemporary descriptions, Manaka's P 6 is not 2 *cun* above the wrist. It is more distal.

Figure 6-2: Finding P 6.

SI 3

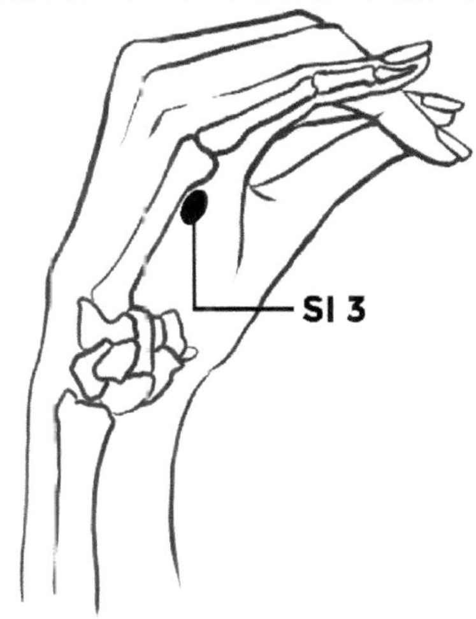

LOCATION	FINDING THE POINT	COMMENTS
On the ulnar border of the hand, in the depression proximal to the head of the fifth metacarpal bone, along the palmar margin of the fifth metacarpal bone.	This point does not often present with obvious pressure pain—this is more common when there are clear symptoms along the small intestine meridian in the shoulder and arm. If no pressure pain is present, palpate for the most tense point, which may even lie a little more proximally, towards SI 4.	This point location is pretty consistent with contemporary locations, except with the proviso that you need to palpate for the most reactive or tense point in the region indicated.

Figure 6-3: Finding SI 3.

TB 5

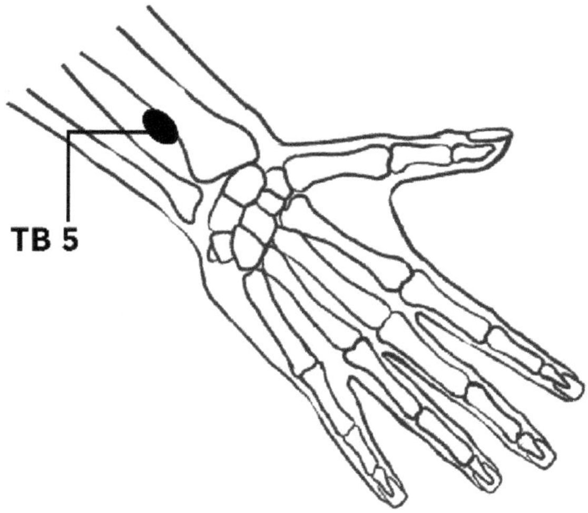

LOCATION	FINDING THE POINT	COMMENTS
With the palm facing down, the point is on the dorsal aspect of the wrist and proximal to the wrist joint. This is a hard, tender point on the ulnar border of the radius.	To locate the point, place your finger in the depression at TB 4, then move it radially along the wrist crease to the next depression. From this position, press down to the surface of the bone and glide your finger proximally along the ulnar margin of the radius. When you encounter a small knot or bump, apply firmer pressure—there should be a distinct pressure pain reaction.	Just like P 6, this point is found more distally than the contemporary location 2 *cun* above the wrist, and more radially, towards the large intestine meridian. Once again, palpation is key.

Figure 6-4: Finding TB 5.

BL 62		
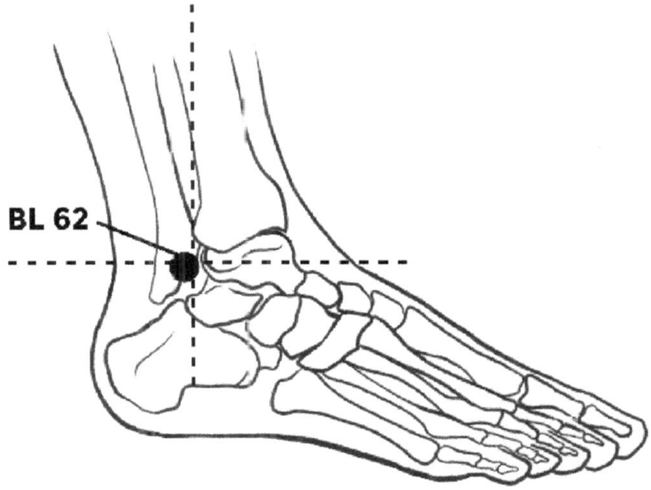		
LOCATION	**FINDING THE POINT**	**COMMENTS**
On the lateral aspect of the ankle, the point is located in the region of the angle formed by the lines from the posterior and inferior margins of the lateral malleolus; if not here, it can be slightly inferior and anterior to that.	Start looking for pressure pain in the region of the posterior–inferior angle. It can be quite distinctive when found. If there is no pressure pain at that angle, palpate a little more anteriorly or inferiorly and continue until pressure pain is found. Inverting the foot medially may make the point more obvious.	This point is more posterior than most contemporary descriptions.

Figure 6-5: Finding BL 62.

KID 6

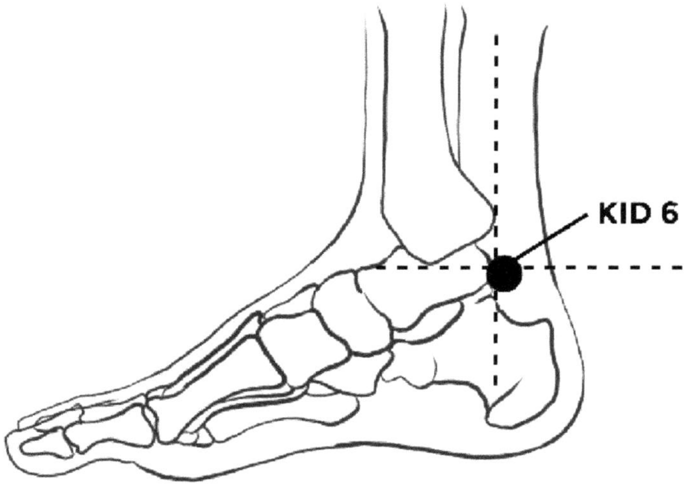

LOCATION	FINDING THE POINT	COMMENTS
On the medial aspect of the ankle, the point is located in the region around the angle formed by the lines from the posterior and inferior margins of the medial malleolus; if not here, it can be slightly inferior and anterior to that.	Start looking for pressure pain in the region of the posterior–inferior angle. It can be quite distinctive when found. If there is no pressure pain at that angle, palpate a little more anteriorly or inferiorly and continue until pressure pain is found. Everting the foot laterally may make the point more obvious.	This point is more posterior than most contemporary descriptions.

Figure 6-6: Finding KID 6.

GB 41

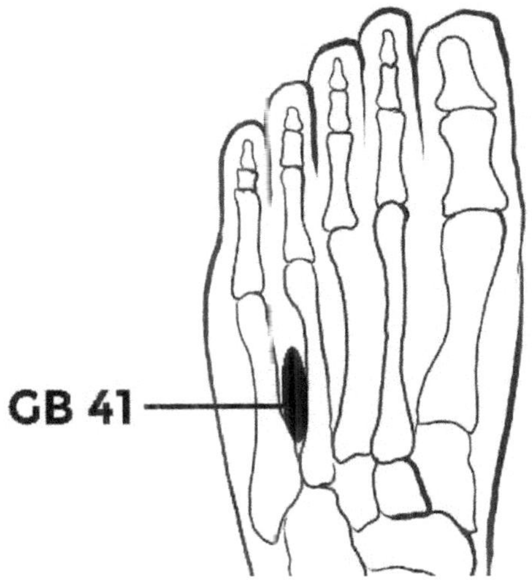

LOCATION	FINDING THE POINT	COMMENTS
On the dorsum of the foot, at the juncture of the 4th and 5th metatarsals, or slightly distal to the juncture along the edge of the 4th or 5th metatarsals.	Start palpating from the juncture of the 4th and 5th metatarsals. As you press, the point should show a clear pressure pain reaction. If there is none, angle your finger to press against the edge of the 4th metatarsal, just distal to the juncture. If no pressure pain is found there, repeat, this time pressing against the edge of the 5th metatarsal slightly distal to the juncture. If there is still no reaction, repeat moving slightly more distally along the margins of the 4th and 5th metatarsals.	Contemporary textbooks emphasise the tendon as a landmark for finding this point; in this system, the juncture of the 4th and 5th metatarsals is the starting point for palpation.

Figure 6-7: Finding GB 41.

SP 4

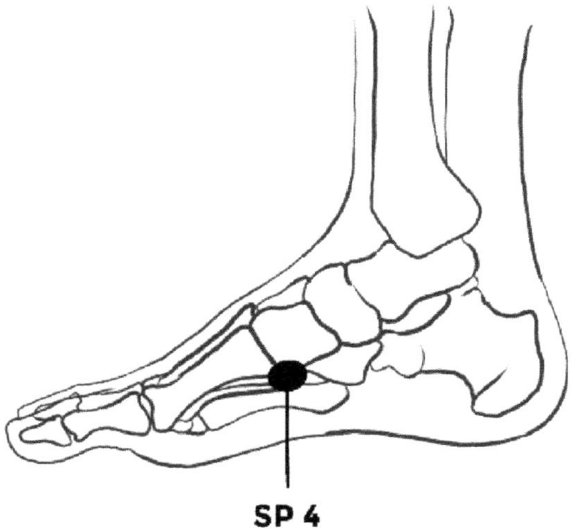

LOCATION	FINDING THE POINT	COMMENTS
On the medial aspect of the foot, slightly proximal or inferior to the base of the 1st metatarsal.	Located as a sensitive knot below the base of the 1st metatarsal bone or slightly more proximal. To find the point, run your finger proximally along the inferior margin of the 1st metatarsal bone. Once at the base of the bone, move just slightly below that and apply pressure. If there is no pressure pain here, move slightly more inferiorly again and press. If the reaction is still not found, press slightly more proximally so that you are below the 1st metatarsal joint.	This point is much more proximal than in contemporary descriptions and can be a little more inferior (towards the sole of the foot). It can usually be recognised by the distinctive hard, painful knot found there.

Figure 6-8: Finding SP 4.

POLARITY AGENTS

We are about to explore the treatment of the master and coupled points. Some renowned Western teachers, such as Dr Dick van Buren and his student Giovanni Maciocia, have suggested creating polarities between the two points by, for example, needling one on the right and the other on the left, according to gender.

Manaka's approach was different. His use of the master and coupled points grew directly out of clinical experience. While treating severe burn injuries during the war, he experimented with ways of moving excessive positive ions from the damaged tissue and observed that polarities applied across certain pairs of points produced striking therapeutic effects. Later, he recognised that these pairs corresponded to the master and coupled points of the Extraordinary Vessels. In this sense, the practice came first and the theoretical framework followed.

As he continued exploring these phenomena, he examined a range of polarity agents already being used in Japan and Germany, such as Cu–Zn and Au–Ag needles and north–south magnetic treatments. He used these mainly as testing tools, helping him understand the behaviour of polarity in the body, rather than as routine clinical treatments. From this work, he eventually developed his own polarity devices—the ion-pumping cords and later the electrostatic adsorber and ion-beam devices. These tools are an integral part of Manaka's Step 1 treatments and sometimes of Step 4. Although they're different in construction, all these tools come in pairs: two metals, two probes, or two clips—one positive, one negative. Here's how Manaka described the origins of his approach, as a wartime doctor treating burn injuries:

> *In the 1940s, I invented a treatment for burns using the ion-pumping technique. With severe, painful burns, excessive numbers of positive potassium ions abound in the area of the burn. The disruption of the cell walls in the damaged area is the source of the potassium ions. Thinking that it would be helpful to move these positive ions to other areas of the body, I experimented with many ways to achieve this goal and found the following useful.*
>
> *With the patient reclined on an insulated table, I attached the negative lead of a Van de Graaff generator to an undamaged part of the body. I then covered the burn with a sterile, thin, metal foil, attaching a metal chain*

> *and a germanium diode with the opposite (positive) end attached distally on the body. I found that this produced excellent results treating burns. It eliminated or greatly reduced the pain of the burns and accelerated the healing process. After these initial experiments and findings, I then refined and developed the method to treat other diseases. I found that ion pumping (I.P.) techniques applied to the eight confluence-*jiaohui *points on the extraordinary vessels were particularly useful; I was able to eliminate the use of the Van de Graaff generator, and I devised systematic treatment methods using these eight points.*[110]

ION-PUMPING CORDS

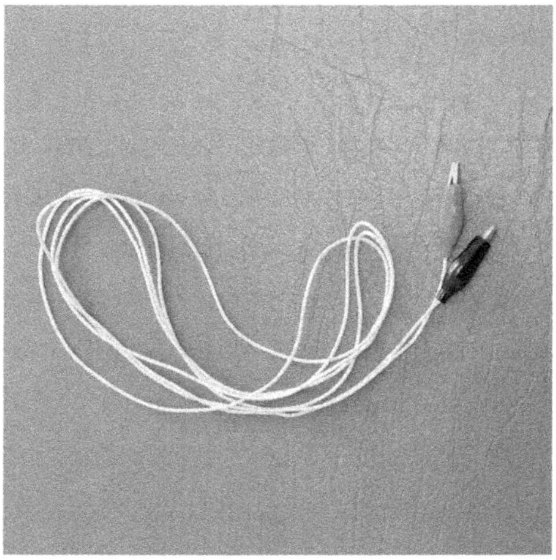

Figure 6-9: Ion-pumping cords.

The ideas for Manaka's ion-pumping cords (IPC) came about through necessity when he was a Japanese army doctor. During the battle for Okinawa, supplies were running low, and he treated many soldiers with burns. He "discovered that applying tin foil to burns not only relieved the pain but also stimulated and seemed to speed the healing process".[111]

---

110 Manaka, Y., Itaya, K., & Birch, S. (1995). *Chasing the Dragon's Tail: The Theory and Practice of Acupuncture in the Work of Yoshio Manaka*. Brookline: Paradigm Publications. p. 120.

111 Matsumoto, K., & Birch, S. (1988). *Hara Diagnosis: Reflections on the Sea*. Brookline: Paradigm Publications. p. 354.

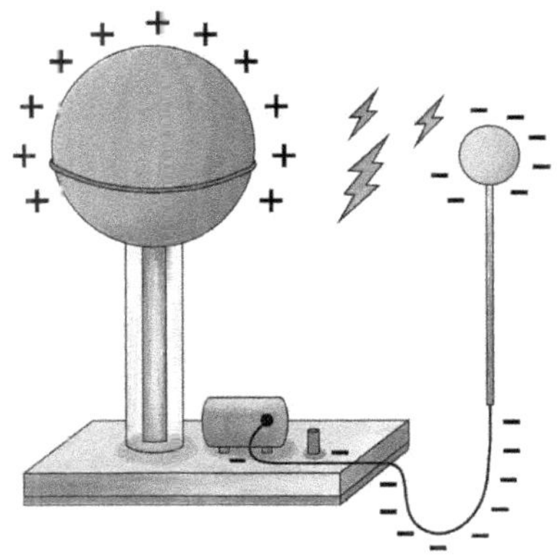

Figure 6-10: Van de Graaf generator, a machine that builds up static electricity to high voltages, which then discharges across its electrodes.

The early burn treatments started with silver foil and a Van de Graaf generator, an electrostatic machine that uses a moving belt to accumulate very high voltages on a hollow metal sphere. In the 1950s, with the invention of diodes, Manaka developed his first ion-pumping cords.

An ion-pumping cord is essentially a length of copper wire with a connecting clip at each end. One clip is red and the other black (positive and negative, respectively). Soldered into the middle of the wire is a diode. Diodes were developed in the 1950s in the new transistor radios that replaced the old valve radios. They only allow electrical current to flow in one direction. Thus, a diode has a positive end and a negative end. If you attach each clip to a pair of acupuncture needles, one needle becomes positive and the other negative.

> *Theoretically, attaching the positive and negative clips of an ion cord to two needles inserted shallowly will create a polarity between the two needles, and electronic and ionic currents will begin to flow inside the body.*[112]

The idea of Manaka's burn treatment theory is that an excess of energy in one area of the body causes a relative deficiency in another. You might remember these as the 'dents and bumps' we explored in Chapter 1. Using polarity devices such as IPC enables us to transfer that energy from one part of the body to another by way of the body's inherent, relative electrical potentials.

---

112 Manaka, Y., Itaya, K., & Birch, S. (1995). *Chasing the Dragon's Tail: The Theory and Practice of Acupuncture in the Work of Yoshio Manaka*. Brookline: Paradigm Publications. p. 121.

Manaka described the treatment of thirty-one patients with second-degree burns in 1965. All of them went from severe pain to no pain within twenty minutes of treatment with IPC. As his work developed in the 1950s, he noticed that certain points were more effective with these treatments than others—these were the eight confluence-*jiaohui* points mentioned above: the master and coupled points of the Eight Extras. This observation greatly influenced the development of his octahedral model.[113]

Manaka researched the properties of the meridians by testing key points with different polarity agents. For example, his tests showed that the Ren and Du vessels do not appear to have a directional flow. He used pairs of needles made from materials with different electrovalences (such as needles made from zinc and copper or gold and silver), the north and south poles of magnets. He even observed that a practitioner's thumb and little finger, when placed on the master and coupled points, could produce a mild polarity effect and alter the reactions at the Manaka-*mu* points. This approach was designed to research meridian behaviour (qi flow, yin–yang relationships, and five-phase correspondences). For treatment, however, he relied on ion-pumping cords applied to the master and coupled points of the Eight Extras.

Table 6.3: Polarity agents.

POSITIVE +	**NEGATIVE -**
Red clip	Black clip
Au (gold)	Ag (silver)
Cu (copper)	Zn (zinc)
N (north)	S (south) magnet poles
Thumb[114]	Little finger

113 Matsumoto, K., & Birch, S. (1988). *Hara Diagnosis: Reflections on the Sea*. Brookline: Paradigm Publications. p. 358.

114 Manaka first described this after attending a Qigong conference in China in the summer of 1986, where he met a Qigong expert using the polarity of pinkie and thumb. Inspired, Manaka began testing the idea and soon incorporated it into his practice. In the early 1990s, the Japanese Acupuncture faculty at the New England School of Acupuncture began experimenting with the same approach—placing the thumb over the red clip and the little finger over the black. We found it effective and began teaching it as a supplement to the regular IPC treatment. Since it felt a bit mysterious and energetic, Stephen Birch dubbed it the '*wuwu* technique'.

[Note: The polarity rules for copper–zinc, gold–silver, and north–south magnet pairs differ from those for ion-pumping cords. They are not interchangeable when used on Extraordinary Vessel points and act on the body in distinct ways.]

Even Manaka acknowledged that the mechanism behind polarity agents was not fully understood. He noted that although electric current flows through a wire from the black clip (negative) to the red clip (positive), the electronic flow—the movement of electrons—actually runs in the opposite direction, from red to black. He extended this idea to the body, hypothesising an internal flow from the site of the black clip to the red, following his clinical logic in burn treatment: placing the black (negative) clip over the burn site (where ionic charge accumulates) and the red (positive) clip near a needle, thereby encouraging ion flow away from the injury. More recently, Stephen Birch, following twentieth-century scholars who translated qi as 'stuff', has described this principle as: inside the body, 'stuff' flows from the black clip to the red. We can summarise Manaka's polarity model as follows: in the wire, stuff flows from the red (positive) probe to the black (negative); in the body, stuff flows from black (negative) to red (positive).

He also developed two more polarity tools that could be applied to the skin without penetrating the skin: the electrostatic adsorbers (EA) and the ion-beam device (IBD). Certainly, for authors Oran Kivity and Paul Movsessian, these non-insertive devices have proved more attractive options than needling with ion-pumping cords. We will discuss these alternatives to IPC in Chapter 17 on fine-tuning treatments. For now, however, in the chapters dealing with Step 1, you should assume that we are needling and using IPC.

GENERAL RULES FOR IPC

There are some general rules for applying IPC, some of which are universal to all polarity agents.

1. The patient should remove all jewellery and piercings, where possible. The reason for this is that we are ion pumping, creating polarities with metals. The more metals there are on the skin, the more different points there will

be in the circuit. If jewellery is retained, especially around the neck and around the wrists or fingers, it might interfere with the efficiency of the treatment, potentially making it less effective.

In some cultures, patients wear a lot of jewellery, so it's worth passing them a bowl in the waiting room so they can get on with the removal process before the session. Sometimes, jewellery won't come off—it's been there too long, or the patient considers it unlucky to remove it. In these cases, work with the items in place and monitor the patient closely.

2. Needle insertion should be shallow, between 2–3mm. We generally use very fine gauge needles with a pipe-head handle, inserted with a guide tube. Manaka used 0.18 gauge needles, but even finer 0.16 gauge needles are an option. We will explore how to do this kind of needling in the clinical section, but for now, the most important consideration is depth. Deep needling, needle manipulation, and acquiring *deqi* sensations are not only unnecessary but also counter-productive for ion pumping. You only need to needle superficially in the upper layers of the skin to create the ionic effects that drive the effectiveness of the IPC. This means that the needle should fall over from its own weight and lie flat on the skin, after being angled with the flow of the meridian.

   As the needle lies flat, there's a second consideration: it should point in the direction of meridian flow or perpendicular to it. For example, if needling LU 7, the needle should point towards the thumb. If needling SI 3, the needle should point towards the shoulder or perpendicularly towards the hand. We should not needle against the flow of the meridian.[115]

3. When the needles are inserted, position the IPC on the wrist or ankle so the clip is stable on the skin. It may be necessary to wind the cord around the wrist, hand, ankle, or foot to allow it to lie in a stable position near the point.

[115] Manaka investigated the properties of angle and direction of needling and found that needling with and against the flow acts like a polarity agent (Chasing the Dragon's Tail, pp. 60–64).

Once stable, clip the cord to the needle. Some practitioners, including Oran Kivity, use micropore tape on the shaft of the needle to anchor it flat to the skin, leaving the handle exposed for the clip of the IPC.

4. The duration of treatment is relatively quick. If it's the patient's first time, retain the clips and needles for five minutes only. If it's a repeat treatment, you can leave them on for a maximum of ten minutes. For sensitive patients, reduce these treatment times (see Chapter 15).

5. While the cords are in place, no other needles should be inserted. This is in part for the same reasons we remove jewellery. We don't want to confuse the circuit of the IPC with extra metals, particularly in the upper quadrant. However, Manaka and his associate Kazuko Itaya also experienced some adverse events when needling other points while the cords were in place. He looked into this and worked out rules for how to do this safely. We will discuss these ideas in Vol. 2, when we explore what to do with stubborn abdominal reactions that have not fully cleared. For now, as a beginner, do not needle any other points while the IPC are on.

   Sometimes there are counterflow qi reactions such as cold feet, red face, headache, dizziness or faintness. To deal with this, one option is to remove the clips immediately. Another is to reverse the polarity of the clips for a few seconds, until the reactions clear. Stephen Birch recommends the following: if there is a counterflow qi reaction on the five basic patterns, reverse the polarity of the clips. We have never observed a counterflow qi reaction in contemporary patterns such as Mixed Yin, Ren Dai, and K3L. If such a reaction occurs, it is advisable to remove the cords rather than attempt to reverse the polarity.

6. A final point to consider about IPCs is maintenance: they can occasionally fail. The soldering at the diode may get damaged, and once that happens, current can no longer flow through the diode. It's therefore a good idea to test them regularly with a circuit tester. Some acupuncture suppliers even sell dedicated IPC-testing devices.

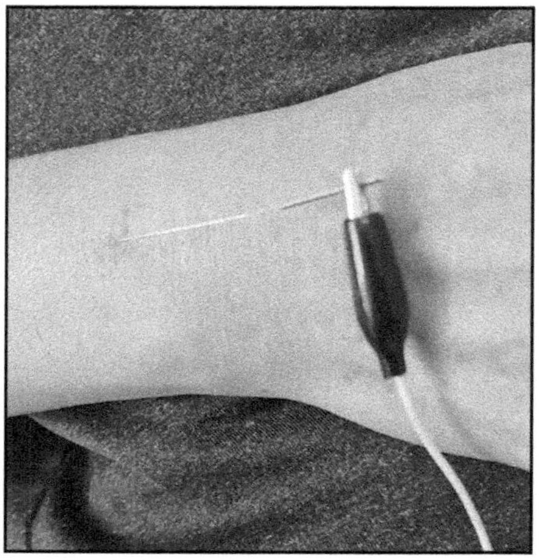

Figure 6-11: Needle and clip.

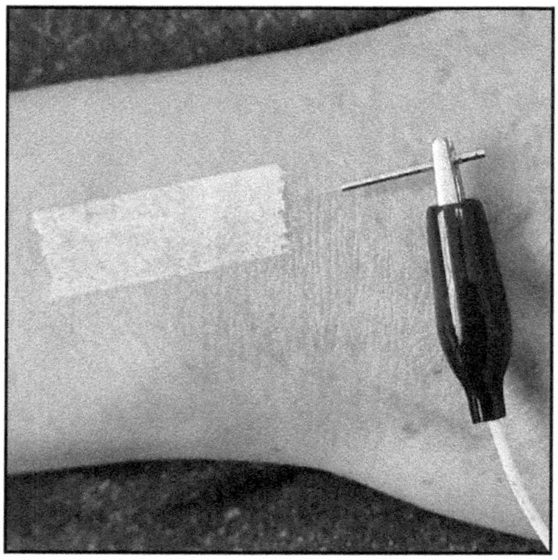

Figure 6-12: Needle and clip taped along the length of the shaft.

PLACING THE RED AND BLACK CLIPS

Let's recap. We've palpated the abdomen and identified a pattern. This has given us our treatment points. We've palpated for the master and coupled points in Manaka's unique locations, and now, finally, we're set to apply the IPC. Which way round do they go?

We can begin to answer this question by looking at the etymology of the character 'wei' of the Yin and Yang Wei Mai (維). The character refers to a rope or binding that, like the rope on a sailing ship, you pull downwards. Thus, these vessels are thought to regulate downward activity and downward movement.

This means that when treating the YWC pair and/or the YWD pair to support the downward action of the Wei Mai, we place the black (negative) clip at the hand and the red (positive) clip at the feet (stuff moves inside the body from the black clip to the red clip).

Manaka pointed out that while the 'qiao' character (蹻) of the Yin and Yang Qiao Mai refers to the heel, etymologically it depicts a heel lifting or kicking upwards. When we run, the heels move upwards. Thus, these vessels appear to regulate upward movement. Consequently, to support this upward action, when treating the YQR or YQD, we place the black (negative) clip on the foot and the red (positive) clip on the hands.

This principle gives us two simple rules.

Table 6.4: Clip placement.

VESSEL	**ARM**	**LEG**
YWC YWD	Black (-)	Red (+)
YQR YQD	Red (+)	Black (-)
CS	Black (-)	Red (+)

After years of fine-tuning the use of the IPC, Manaka found that this placement of the black and red clips of the IPC reduced, almost to zero, the risk of unpleasant counterflow reactions. Thus, he insisted that for the sake of increased safety and efficiency of use, beginners should follow these rules for the placement of black and red clips.

SIDE OF TREATMENT

We have established rules for the direction of flow and placement of clips with the IPC polarity agents, but we also must decide on the side of treatment. These rules are derived from two principles. The first is that for those pairs that include vessels on the midline, such as the YQR and YQD pairs, there is no left or right bias, so treatment should be bilateral. For these two pairs, we therefore treat bilaterally using IPC on both feet and both hands, right hand to right foot and left hand to left foot—no unilateral treatments.

The second principle derives from your palpation findings and relates to the other patterns, such as YWC, YWD, and Cross Syndrome. This principle is that you treat the side with reactions. If the left side is reactive, you treat the left side. If both sides are reactive, you treat both sides. If just the right side is reactive, you treat the right side.

Table 6.5: Side of treatment.

VESSEL	REACTIVE SIDE	TREATMENT SIDE
YWC, YWD	L R L + R	L R Bilateral
YQR, YQD	Both vessels run along the midline, so laterality is not a factor	Bilateral
CS	Left and right	Bilateral

WORKFLOW AND TROUBLESHOOTING

Applying IPC with needles is the standard method. We will discuss the use of alternatives such as IPC with silver spike points (SSP) or applying electrostatic adsorbers (EA) in Chapter 17. If this is the first treatment, retain the needles and IPC for up to five minutes. If this is a repeat treatment, you can keep them on for up to ten minutes.

There are three rules to follow when practising MSA:

1. Palpation
2. Palpation
3. Palpation

This list might seem tongue-in-cheek, but it serves to emphasise an important principle. We palpate to decide the pattern. We palpate to find the treatment points. When the IPC are in place, we palpate again to see how the reactions have changed. If things haven't worked out as expected, we need to troubleshoot to see what might be happening. Manaka provided a straightforward methodology to do this.

POSSIBLE OUTCOMES AFTER ION PUMPING

After applying the IPC, test the results by re-palpating the primary reaction. You may feel a shift immediately and certainly, after thirty seconds, there should be some noticeable change. If this is slow to happen, you can try adding a supplementary polarity technique to accelerate the process. Manaka described the thumb as a positive polarity agent and the little finger as a negative.[116]

To perform this simple technique, hover your thumb (positive) over the red (positive) clip and your little finger (negative) over the black (negative) clip. This adds an extra layer of polarities to the IPC. Relax your posture, arms and fingers and stand like this for 10–20 seconds on each side. Then go back to the *hara* and recheck. At this stage, there are several possible outcomes:

1. The reactions on the abdomen, such as hardness and pressure pain, improve considerably, and you feel satisfied with the changes.
2. There is only minimal change, or one reaction area has not changed at all.
3. There's no change at all.
4. Things feel worse.

---

116 This simple additional polarity of thumb and little finger (Birch's *wuwu* technique) is very effective to accelerate the abdominal changes. Even though you don't touch the clips, you often feel a sense of warmth as you hold your hands over them.

THE BELLY SOFTENS CONSIDERABLY

In this instance, you have achieved the goal of Step 1, and all that remains to do is make sure the polarity device is applied for the required time. For IPC with needles, this means a total of five to ten minutes.

THE REACTIONS CHANGE PARTIALLY

Sometimes there's been a change on the belly, but it's not very much. Instead of the hoped-for reduction of reactions, they've only improved by 10% or so. In these cases, the problem is most likely not your diagnosis of the pattern; it's more likely to be your point location or, sometimes, that a needle fell out.

Stephen Birch has used a salad bowl as an analogy to describe the shape of the acupuncture points. They're bowl-shaped. If you lower a chopstick vertically into the centre of the bowl, you create the maximum change at the point. If you lower it more towards the rim of the bowl, the effect is weaker. If the chopstick is outside the bowl, on the table, it creates no change at all. The more accurate your point location with your needle, SSP, or probe, the more dynamic the change at the *hara*. The less accurate it is, the less dynamic it becomes. The *hara* is a very truthful guide. Even if only one of a pair of points is placed inaccurately, it will let you know.

Let's take the example of Cross Syndrome. Imagine that the left lower quadrant reaction feels better, but the right upper quadrant reaction is only marginally less tight. This means that the point location on one or both points on the right could be at fault. But which point is wrong? Is it P 6, SP 4, or both?

The good news is that it's not always necessary to relocate both points. First, visually inspect the point locations. You may notice that one point looks slightly off from its usual location—if so, remove that needle, repalpate, and reinsert. Or you might notice that the needle has slipped out of the point and simply needs reinserting.

Second, if nothing obvious shows up from your visual inspection, Manaka devised a simple fix: palpate the associated Manaka-*mu* points. In the case of the YWC, these are REN 17 (and P 1) and the mid-axillary line. If one of these *mu* points has become less sensitive, while the other remains jumpy, the one that remains reactive indicates the issue. You should relocate the master or coupled point related to the reactive *mu* point.

For example, if there is reduced pressure pain at REN 17, but the mid-axillary line is still jumpy, then you should relocate SP 4. Conversely, if the mid-axillary line has changed, but REN 17 hasn't, you should relocate P 6. Remove the needle, repalpate for the live point, and reinsert. Often, the correct location is only 1 mm or so away from the original insertion.

As soon as you reinsert the needle, recheck the abdomen. There's usually a clear improvement in the main reactions.

If we take a second example, treating the YQR, we might find that the midline has softened in the upper part but is still reactive more inferiorly. We can check KID 16 and LU 1–LU 2 bilaterally to determine which KID 6 or LU 7 might be misplaced. Just one point of the four will affect the overall reactivity. For example, if the right KID 16 has not softened, remove the needle at the right KID 6, repalpate the point, and reinsert.

This is where the Manaka-*mu* points come into their own. Initially, we used them to confirm a diagnosis. Now, we can use them to fine-tune our treatment. Especially when needling bilaterally, the Manaka-*mu* points will give clear feedback about our point location on the left and right.

THERE'S NO CHANGE AT ALL

No change at all is a somewhat unusual outcome, but not unheard of. The most likely explanations are:

1. All four point locations are off (check the Manaka-*mu* points).
2. There's a fault with the polarity device (use a circuit tester).
3. The patient has a poor prognosis and presents with more pronounced abdominal reactions, suggesting that we should expect slow changes.

The patient is a physically strong person with well-developed abdominal muscles—it is harder to palpate this kind of belly and detect significant changes.

The first possibility implies gross errors in point location. This is exceptionally rare. Once the points are relocated accurately, the abdomen should begin to respond favourably.

In the second case, switch to a functioning IPC unit and recheck the abdomen.

The third explanation is more common. It relates to the patient's ability to change. In some cases, the prognosis indicates that only slow, gradual change can be expected. In a single session, the abdominal wall may *eventually* show only a small shift. However, with repeated treatments, the response tends to build and become more sustained.

Examples include:

- A generally hypotonic abdominal wall
- A patient with a history of chronic illness and significant signs of blood stasis
- Bodybuilders with rock-hard abdominals
- Women in the later stages of pregnancy

THINGS FEEL WORSE

This is an exceptionally rare event. In this case, there are two possibilities:

1. The polarity selection was incorrect (black and red clips wrongly placed).
2. The patient has a unique reaction to standard treatment.

During a busy day, it is possible to err and hook up the points the wrong way. If the reactions seem to increase rather than decrease, the first thing to do is check that the black and red clips are correctly aligned. Particularly with more complicated patterns, it's easy to connect the wrong clip to a needle.

There is a second and very rare possibility—some patients are wired differently!

> *In my practice, this is extremely rare, happening perhaps once every few years. I've reversed the clips from the textbook alignment, and the bad reaction has cleared.*
>
> —Oran Kivity

This is particularly true of the YQD and YQR patterns, which normally bring energy upwards. In some cases, it suits the patient better to redirect the energy in the opposite direction.

Worsened abdominal reactions during IPC treatment can be accompanied by counterflow qi signs, which then become the dominant issue to address. In these cases, the priority shifts to managing the counterflow, especially if the patient shows signs like flushing, restlessness, or visible agitation. This is very rare, and if you follow Manaka's principles about the placement of the red and black clips, you may never see this.

PUTTING IT ALL TOGETHER

Let's run through some examples of these.

EXAMPLE 1

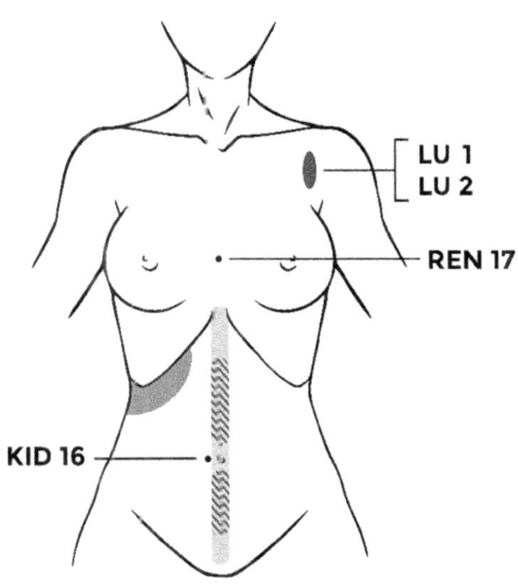

Figure 6-13: YQR is more evident than YWC.

You palpate your first patient of the day, noting reactions along the midline and a little tightness under the right subcostal. So, you are thinking this is either a YQR or YWC pattern. To differentiate, you palpate the primary reflex points, finding no reactions along the Manaka-*mu* for spleen, some tenderness at REN 17, and clear reactions at KID

16 on one side and LU 1 and LU 2 on the other. In this case, the YWC is unconfirmed since there is no reaction on the spleen meridian Manaka-*mu* point (SP 21 to GB 26), while the YQR is conclusively reactive at both the lung and kidney Manaka-*mu* points.

Once you decide this, you know what to do for Step 1! You select KID 6 and LU 7 bilaterally, because this pair includes a midline vessel. Moreover, following Manaka's rules of treatment, you know to put the black clips at the ankles and the red clips at the wrists.

Table 6.6: Weighing between YQR and YWC.

Midline	YQR	Primary area checks out.
Subcostal	YWC	Primary area checks out.
REN 17	YWC	Only one primary point is reactive.
KID 16, LU 1, LU 2	YQR	Almost all primary points are reactive.
		Treatment is bilateral LU 7 (red clip), KID 6 (black clip).

EXAMPLE 2

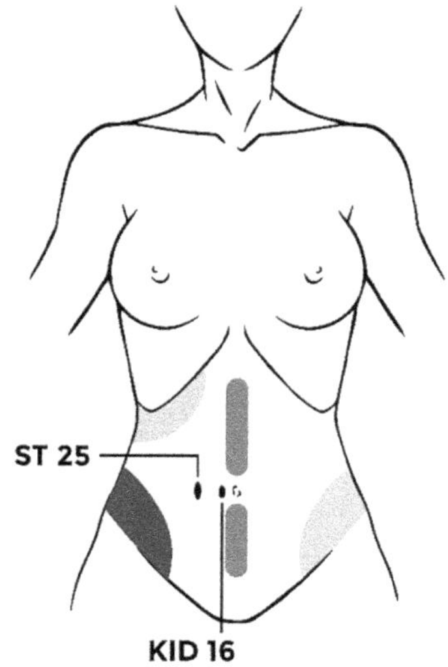

Figure 6-14: YWD with milder CS.

Your next patient has the most significant reactions along the ASIS, more on the right than the left. There's a little tightness under the right subcostal, along the midline, and you notice tightness at KID 16, ST 25 on the right.

The ASIS signs make you think this is a YQD pattern, so you check for the primary reflex points. ST 26 and KID 11 are not reactive. You remember that the ASIS also comes up with YWD, so you check KID 16, which is reactive, but the midline reactions don't check out. KID 16 is tender but the area at LU 1 and LU 2 is not.

The right subcostal and left ASIS could also be Cross Syndrome (CS). You could check the Manaka-*mu* points, but it seems that the right ASIS is much more reactive than the left, so while CS is there, it is not predominant.

What is clear is that the ASIS reactions on the right are tied into the horizontal line tenderness at KID 16, ST 25. YWD is the more predominant pattern here, and as the reactions are on the right, you only treat YWD on the right.

Table 6.7: Weighing between CS, YQD and YWD.

ASIS Both sides, but more on the right	Could be YQD or YWD,	Unclear at this stage
Right subcostal	YWC	Together with the left ASIS, it could be CS, but the ASIS is worse on the right, not the left. You could check out the primary points for YWC to corroborate.
Midline	YQR	Check out the primary points.
KID 16		KID 16 supports a YQR diagnosis, but LU 1 and LU 2 are not reactive.
ASIS	YQD	Could the ASIS relate to YQD? Check out primary points ST 26 KID 11.
YQD	No tenderness at ST 26 KID 11	Primary points do not support YQD.
KID 16, ST 25 (R) ASIS	YWD	This is the most reactive and consistent finding. Right ASIS plus belt reactions on the right.

EXTRA DIFFERENTIATION TOOLS

As you can see from the examples, pattern differentiation can feel complicated. Patterns co-exist. Moreover, some patients are hard to palpate! These include pregnant women, patients who've had extensive abdominal surgery, and sporting types with rock-hard abs. In these cases, default options are available to clarify the diagnosis through alternative means, starting with the secondary reactions. If these do not provide clarity, the approach then shifts to basic theory and symptom differentiation. The use of these two extra layers of differentiation is discussed in Chapter 14.

FINAL THOUGHTS

> *The first and most important step of a root treatment is restoration of harmony on the yin (front) side of the body. The procedures taken in this step are determined by the palpable reactions found on the abdomen and chest.*[117]

In Step 1, we diagnose the condition of the octahedron by palpating the abdomen and chest. We then use the Eight Extraordinary Vessels to alter the octahedral structures of the body. Successful treatment reduces or eliminates the palpable reactions in these regions.

As the first step of four, this diagnosis, pattern recognition, and treatment sets the direction and clears the way for the subsequent steps.

Step 1 requires confirmation through palpation. This palpation method, which is repeatable and verifiable by others, enables the selection of points for patients who might otherwise be difficult to diagnose. Moreover, it can be used for diseases in their beginning stages that have not yet manifested symptoms. It can also be applied when the patient presents with many symptoms or with more than one disease.

SUMMARY

- **Pattern and treatment are inseparable:** Once you identify the pattern, the master and coupled points are already determined.
- **Palpation is essential at every stage:** From diagnosis to point location to confirming treatment effects.

---

[117] Manaka, Y., Itaya, K., & Birch, S. (1995). *Chasing the Dragon's Tail: The Theory and Practice of Acupuncture in the Work of Yoshio Manaka*. Brookline: Paradigm Publications. p. 159.

- **Point location trumps textbook precision:** Use pressure pain and induration, not fixed anatomical distances, to find the 'alive' point.
- **Manaka's IPC technique evolved from treating burns**: It forms the core of Step 1 treatment in MSA.
- **Polarity agents come in pairs**: one positive and one negative. For treatment, we use IPCs. For testing, different metals, opposed magnets, or even the thumb and little finger can create the required polarity.
- **Stuff flows from black (negative) to red (positive)**: Within the body, the IPC polarity creates a directional flow that mirrors Manaka's theory of energetic redistribution (other polarity agents may act differently).
- **Jewellery and additional needles interfere**: Remove metals and don't needle elsewhere during IPC to avoid circuit confusion or adverse reactions.
- **Needles should be shallow and aligned**: No need for *deqi*; depth is minimal, and the angle should follow the meridian flow or lie perpendicular.
- **Correct clip placement reduces counterflow risk**: Wei vessels (YWC, YWD) are black clip at hand, red clip at foot. Qiao vessels (YQR, YQD) are black clip at foot, red clip at hand.
- **Treatment side depends on the vessel**: YQR, YQD and CS are bilateral. YWC and YWD are treated on the reactive side.
- **Use the Manaka-*mu* points to troubleshoot**: They help confirm diagnosis and identify point location errors during treatment.
- **Adverse reactions are rare but real**: Memorise what to do, just in case.

WHAT'S NEXT

MSA has evolved since Manaka's passing. In addition to his five basic patterns, we'll explore contemporary developments, including new ways of using IPC contralaterally, and meet three patients: Christine, David, and Margaret.

CHAPTER 7

EXPANDING STEP 1 OPTIONS: CONTRALATERAL PATTERNS

Before 9/11, I regularly found Cross Syndrome in about one-third of my patients, consistent with Dr Manaka's observations. After 9/11, however, with the country in shock, I began noticing something different: consistent findings on both the Ren and Dai vessels. When I shared this with colleagues, many reported the same thing. Together, we came to recognise a new pattern—the Ren Dai.

—Brenda Loew

CONTEMPORARY ABDOMINAL PATTERNS

This chapter introduces the contemporary patterns developed by Stephen Birch and Brenda Loew. They emerged through repeated clinical use of Dr Manaka's five primary patterns and the realisation that, when two patterns coexisted with equal weight, Manaka's system required you to choose one or the other. Over time, this led to the development of an economical approach—patterns that allow us to treat two or more Extra Vessels at once using fewer needles and cords.

YQR is one of the patterns we see most frequently in clinic. Each of the new patterns in this chapter combines YQR with one of the other primary patterns introduced in Chapter 6. These combinations are known as *mixed* or *contralateral* patterns. Unlike Cross Syndrome (CS), which uses two patterns needled separately on the left and right, each mixed pattern uses a single pair of IPC connected contralaterally across the body, from left to right or right to left. This produces the same treatment effect as a four-needle treatment (two on each side), but milder, with just two needles (one on each side). If we take the YQR as an example, rather than needling LU 7 and KID 6 bilaterally—using four needles and two IPC for the pair of vessels—we can create the same, but slightly milder, effect with just two needles, one on each side.

We now have the option to use, contralaterally, point configurations that were formerly bilateral, achieving similar treatment effects with a lower dose of treatment. Below, we will explore three mixed patterns and their variations.

MIXED YIN PATTERN

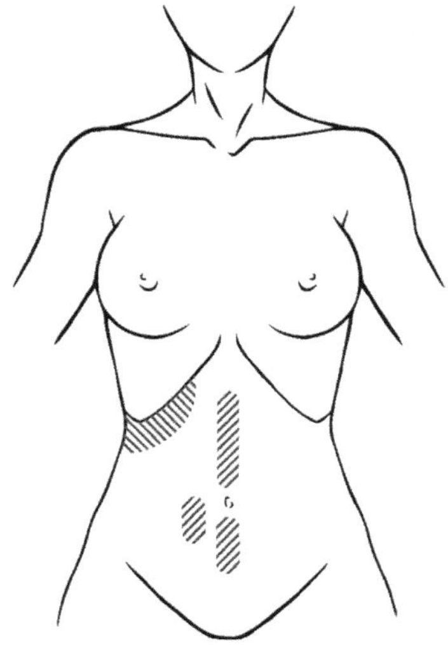

Figure 7-1: Mixed Yin primary areas.

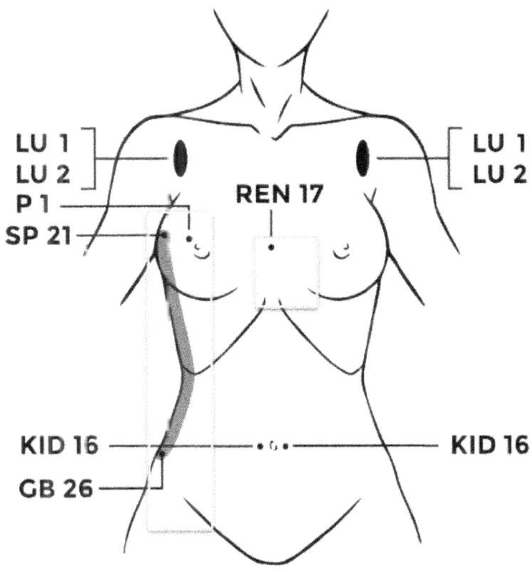

Figure 7-2: Mixed Yin primary points.

This pattern combines YQR with YWC. It developed in response to a commonly occurring clinical observation: a dominant reaction on the right side of the abdomen, specifically from ST 25 to ST 27. While applying one of Manaka's five core patterns sometimes had an effect, it was often insufficient.

In response, Birch began observing consistent accompanying findings. He noted that this right-sided abdominal reaction often appeared alongside right subcostal tightness and midline tightness. After experimenting with treatment using contralateral IPC, he proposed that these findings formed the basis of a distinct diagnostic pattern with reactions at:

- The right subcostal area
- The midline
- Right ST25–ST 27

In the *Nan Jing hara* mapping (Figure 5-1), the ST 25–27 area on the right is associated with the lung reflex. Renowned Japanese acupuncturists Kyoshi Nagano and Kiiko Matsumoto have referred to this same area as the 'immune reflex'.[118] Tenderness in this area is therefore highly significant.

---

118 Matsumoto, K., & Euler, D. (2008). *Kiiko Matsumoto's Clinical Strategies: In the Spirit of Master Nagano*. Vol. 1. Brookline, MA: Kiiko Matsumoto International.

Over time, other associated reactions were noted:

- The left LU 1–LU 2 region tends to be more reactive than the right.
- The right KID 16 is often more reactive than the left.
- Reactions can also appear over the right ASIS.

For a diagnosis of the Mixed Yin pattern, the core findings must include reactions at the right ST 25–27, the right subcostal region and along the midline. There is no equivalent mirrored presentation on the left.

NEEDLING

Unlike previous protocols, this pattern is needled contralaterally. Insert LU 7 on the left and KID 6 on the right. Then insert P 6 on the right and SP 4 on the left.

This approach offers a streamlined economy. Instead of using four needles and two cords to treat YQR bilaterally, as before, plus two more needles and a third cord for YWC, we achieve a similar effect with just four needles and two cords, keeping the overall treatment dose low.

Table 7.1: Mixed Yin clip placement.

POINT	SIDE	COLOUR
LU 7	LEFT	RED
KID 6	RIGHT	BLACK
P 6	RIGHT	BLACK
SP 4	LEFT	RED

THE REDLLL RULE

With Mixed Yin and the other contralateral patterns described below, it might be challenging at first to remember which clip goes where. Although we all memorise things differently, here's a simple mnemonic that might help.

- In this IPC configuration, both red clips are on the left, and both black clips are on the right. So, if you remember that the red clip goes on **LU** 7 on the left, the rest falls into place.
- For English speakers, a handy memory aid is **REDLLL**. The Chinese name for LU 7 is *Lieque*, so this stands for: **RED**, **L**U 7, ***L**ieque*, **L**eft.
- There is one exception to this rule, the final Ren Dai pattern, but all the other patterns follow it.
- If English is not your native language, you can try to come up with another similar mnemonic to hold this important detail in your mind (in Brazil, for example, we developed the VPEL rule: ***V**ermelha*, ***P**ulmão 7*, ***E**squerdo*, ***L**ieque*).

K3L PATTERN

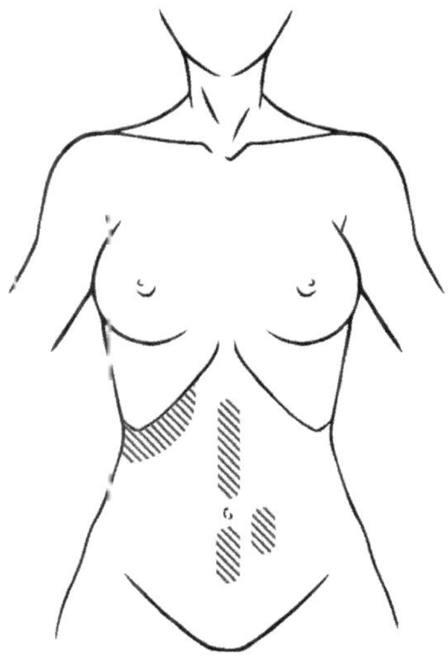

Figure 7-3: K3L primary areas.

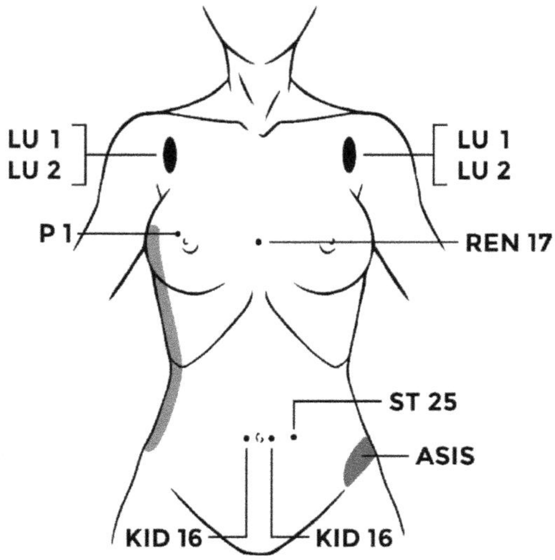

Figure 7-4: K3L primary points.

This pattern combines YQR with CS. Many patients were observed to show both patterns co-presenting, but Manaka's original system required choosing one or the other. The idea was that treating the dominant pattern would improve the other via whole-body effects. But when both patterns kept showing up together, it became a topic of discussion.

In one case involving a patient with severe symptoms, neither pattern alone was enough, so Birch combined them into a single treatment: YQR on one diagonal, and a contralateral treatment using LI 4 and LIV 3 on the other. Birch was inspired by a colleague in Boston who had used IPC on the Four Gates, needling LI 4 and LIV 3 bilaterally. The Four Gates combination is considered to have a strong effect on moving qi and blood. In this instance, LI 4 is needled on the right hand, which is the upper right quadrant, and therefore affects the right subcostal. LIV 3 is needled on the left foot, in the lower left quadrant, therefore it affects the lower left quadrant of the belly. Once again, the contralateral version offered an economy—fewer needles, fewer cords.

The treatment worked well and gradually became a commonly used pattern. Like CS, it may present with reactions in the lower left quadrant, such as left ST 25–ST 27, left belt line reactions or left ASIS reactions.

Like Mixed Yin, this pattern follows the REDLLL rule with contralateral IPC, with black clips on the right and red clips on the left. Birch named it K3L, short for the four meridians needled: **K**idney, **L**arge intestine, **L**ung, and **L**iver—one K, three Ls.

Table 7.2: K3L clip placement.

POINT	SIDE	COLOUR
LU 7	LEFT	RED
KID 6	RIGHT	BLACK
LI 4	RIGHT	BLACK
LIV 3	LEFT	RED

REN DAI PATTERN

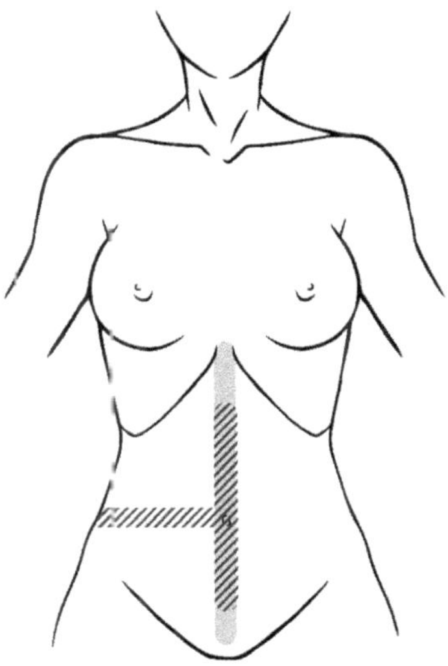

Figure 7-5: Ren Dai (right-belt).

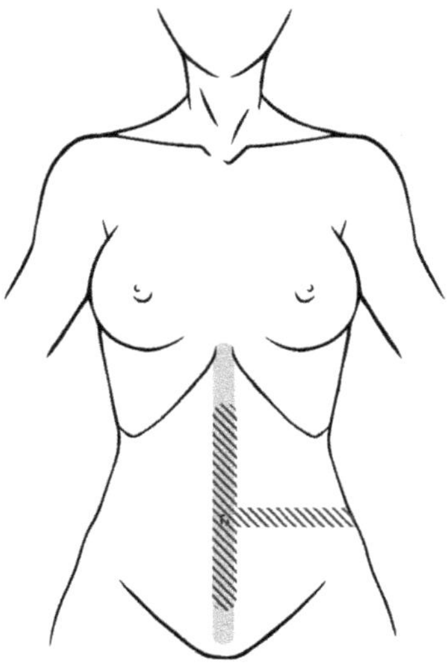

Figure 7-6: Ren Dai (left-belt).

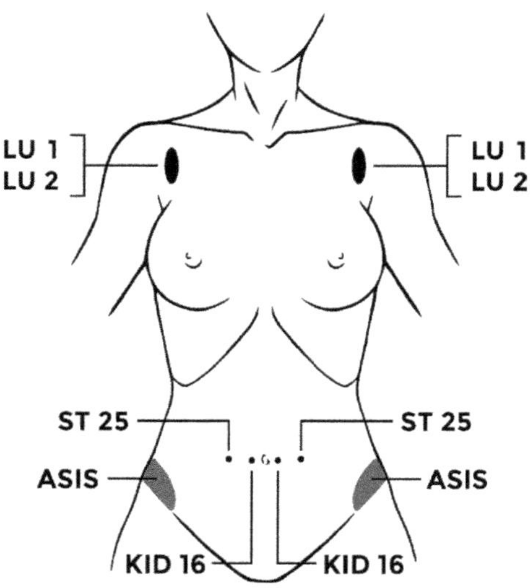

Figure 7-7: Ren Dai primary points.

The Ren Dai pattern, as its name suggests, combines YQR with YWD. As the opening quotation in the chapter shows, Brenda Loew started to observe it on patients in the traumatic aftermath of the 9/11 attacks on the United States. It is characterised by midline tightness, usually above the umbilicus, sometimes with accompanying softness below. At the same time, belt reactions appear, occasionally combined with ASIS reactions.

The Ren Dai pattern has two variations: left-belt and right-belt. These reflect which side of the belt region shows the stronger reaction. Identifying the more reactive side is essential, as it determines whether we select TB 5 on the left or on the right.

Ren Dai (right-belt) manifests with midline reactions on the Ren Mai and horizontal reactions along the Dai Mai from SP 15, ST 25, and KID 16, especially on the right. The ASIS may or may not be reactive. The red clip goes to LU 7 *Lieque* on the left (REDLLL rule), so KID 6 goes on the right. From there, it's the same principle: black clips on the right, red clips on the left. ST 25 is important here. It's the Manaka-*mu* point for the triple burner, so if it's tender on the right, needling TB 5 on the right should release it. If TB 5 goes on the right, G 41 must go on the left.

Table 7.3: Ren Dai (right-belt) clip placement.

REN DAI (RIGHT-BELT)		
POINT	**SIDE**	**COLOUR**
LU 7	LEFT	RED
KID 6	RIGHT	BLACK
TB 5	RIGHT	BLACK
GB 41	LEFT	RED

Ren Dai (left-belt) manifests with midline reactions and horizontal reactions along the Dai Mai from SP 15, ST 25, and KID 16, especially on the left. The ASIS may or may not be reactive.

In this case, the rule for LU 7 on the left no longer applies. Because ST 25 (the front-*mu* of triple burner) is tight on the left, we need to needle TB 5 on the left with the black clip. The cord traverses the body to GB 41 on the right with the red clip. So now, exceptionally, we have to needle LU 7 on the right with the red clip. There's only one place left for KID 6 and the black clip—on the left. Our usual configuration is reversed: the black clips are on the left, and the red clips are on the right.

This is one of those situations where the bilateral Manaka-*mu* points really shine. If you find tightness on Ren Mai and Dai Mai, it's the left–right location of the ST 25 reaction that helps you decide the placement of TB 5 and LU 7. The traditional *mu* point, Ren 7, could not give us this information.

Table 7.4: Ren Dai (left-belt) clip placement.

REN DAI (LEFT-BELT)		
POINT	**SIDE**	**COLOUR**
LU 7	RIGHT	RED
KID 6	LEFT	BLACK
TB 5	LEFT	BLACK
GB 41	RIGHT	RED

REMINDER: THE REDLLL RULE

In Ren Dai (right-belt), *the red clip goes to LU 7 on the left (Red, LU 7,* Lieque, *Left—LLL).*

In Ren Dai (left-belt), *this configuration reverses: black clips on the left, red clips on the right.*

Ren Dai (right-belt) *follows the same clip placement principle as the other contralateral patterns, while* Ren Dai (left-belt) *is the single exception.*

Both patterns are common in clinic: palpation of the belt will determine which variant to use.

DISCUSSION

PRIMARY POINTS

In practice, we rarely need to check the primary points when diagnosing the mixed patterns. Birch generally does not use them for Cross Syndrome (CS), the Mixed Yin pattern, or the K3L pattern. In CS, the combination of upper right quadrant reactions with lower left quadrant reactions is usually so clear that confirmation with the primary points adds nothing. Because the K3L pattern is essentially CS plus YQR, he also seldom checks the primary points for this pattern. The same applies to the Mixed Yin pattern; once those three primary reaction areas appear, the diagnosis is effectively conclusive.

The Ren Dai variations are similarly straightforward. Diagnosis depends on finding midline reactions together with either the left belt or right belt area. If both of these primary zones are present, the pattern is already obvious, and confirmation with the primary points is rarely necessary.

HORIZONTAL AND VERTICAL REACTIONS

In the Mixed Yin and K3L patterns, we also find reactions to the left and right of the navel and at the ASIS. How do we differentiate between these patterns and the Ren Dai?

With the Ren Dai pattern, the reactions are limited to the belt, which includes KID 16, ST 25, and SP 15, often with the ASIS. But for the Mixed Yin and K3L, not only is the right subcostal present, but the reactions to the left or right of the navel lie along the stomach meridian, ST 25–ST 27. In both the K3L and Mixed Yin, KID 16 is often present, as well as SP 15 and the ASIS reactions.

One way to simplify this is to consider that Ren Dai reactions tend to be horizontal, with reactions at points along the belt such as KID 16, ST 25, SP 15, while Mixed Yin and K3L show more vertical patterns along the stomach meridian, from ST 25–ST 27.

IN PRACTICE: STEP 1—STORIES FROM THE CLINIC

In a change from our normal format, this and the subsequent chapters about each of the Four Steps will introduce cases from our practices. As we've covered all the basic patterns, it's time to see them in action. We've decided to present our cases in two ways:

1. You'll meet three patients whose stories unfold in episodes, one for each step, so you can follow their journeys in instalments through the treatment process and see how each step builds on the last.
2. We've included two chapters of longer and more dense, self-contained case studies that you can either read in one sitting or come back to as your understanding deepens. This dual approach is designed to spare you the feeling of ploughing through an endless thicket of case notes, while also giving you real people to follow, root for, and learn from.

Before we dive into the first instalments, let's introduce Christine, David, and Margaret—three patients with very different challenges, each showing in their own way how Manaka's system comes to life in the clinic.

CASE STUDY 1: SCIATIC PAIN

Christine, Female, 56

Occupation: Business consultant

PRESENTING CONDITION

Christine presented with right-sided sciatic pain, with occasional twinges in the left leg. The pain originated at the base of the right buttock and radiated down the stomach meridian above the knee. She experienced some weakness in the legs, especially on the right. The pain disturbed her sleep, waking her frequently and forcing her to move.

RELEVANT HISTORY

- Duration: 2 months
- Advised to exercise, but no improvement
- No scans or diagnostic testing performed
- Avoids medication
- Previous long-term acupuncture treatment for migraines (more than 9 years)
- Migraine treatment was effective; the patient ceased acupuncture 3 years ago after menopause
- Past migraine patterns mostly liver-related (CS, K3L, Mixed Yin)
- Auto accident at 32: head/face trauma, chronic neck and shoulder stiffness, occasional left arm numbness
- Managed previous back issues well with exercise

PALPATION

- Slight tension in the right subcostal region
- Right ASIS, SP 15, ST 25, and KID 16 tight and jumpy
- Bilateral ST 26 stiff/sore, right ST 27 stiff
- Left ASIS tight
- REN above navel stiff; below navel flaccid (age-related pattern)

TREATMENT 1

Diagnosis: Ren Dai pattern. Dominant right-sided Dai Mai reaction. Mixed Yin pattern present but milder.

Step 1: Ren Dai (right-belt) with IPC (10 minutes)

PRACTITIONER NOTE

Christine's presentation suggested a Ren Dai pattern from the start: the dominant right-sided Dai Mai reaction matched her right leg sciatic pain. Abdominal findings showed classic hypotonia below the navel, likely age-related, and tightness around the ASIS and Dai Mai points on the right. The Ren Dai is often selected when leg problems occur on the same side as Dai Mai reactions; in this case, the right leg pain and right-sided Dai Mai findings strongly supported that choice.

CASE STUDY 2: NECK PAIN POST-WEIGHTLIFTING INJURY

David, Male, 39

Occupation: Corporate manager

PRESENTING CONDITION

David reported right lateral neck pain that began after a weightlifting injury 8 years earlier. There was a palpable swelling between GB 9 and GB 10, which occasionally radiated to the right shoulder with intermittent tingling into the face. He experienced a background pain level of 5/10 daily, which increased to over 8/10 under stress.

RELEVANT HISTORY

- High-stress managerial role
- Hypertension (controlled with medication)
- Hernia surgery 2 years ago
- Cholecystectomy 7 years ago

PALPATION

- Very tight along the Dai Mai bilaterally
- ASIS tender on palpation

Diagnosis: YWD

TREATMENT 1

Step 1: YWD with IPC (10 minutes) bilaterally

PRACTITIONER NOTE

David's symptoms appeared on the right, which might suggest right-sided treatment. However, in Manaka's system, palpation findings determine the treatment side. As he was tender along both sides of the Dai Mai, treatment was applied bilaterally.

CASE STUDY 3: HIP DEGENERATION AND CHRONIC PAIN

Margaret, Female, 60

Occupation: Retired

PRESENTING CONDITION

Margaret experienced back and groin pain associated with hip joint degeneration. The pain originated in the right lumbar region and referred into the right groin, with additional sacral discomfort. Her hip pain began 4 years earlier and had worsened over the past 2 months. The pain was constant, severe and deep, and limited her mobility. The pain was relieved by movement, pressure, and heat. She was particularly concerned about coping with an upcoming long-haul flight.

RELEVANT HISTORY

- Lumbar fusion at L4–L5 25 years earlier, leaving severe scarring
- Hip degeneration confirmed by MRI 4 years earlier
- Previous cortisone injections for hip pain (with no lasting improvement)

PALPATION

- Very flaccid below the navel, slightly tight above
- Right ASIS is very sore

TREATMENT 1

Diagnosis: YQR

Step 1: YQR with IPC (15 minutes)

PRACTITIONER NOTE

This abdominal finding commonly indicates a YQR pattern: a midline that feels hollow and weak below the navel but tight and reactive above. It is often accompanied by a corresponding tightness in the lumbar area, and sometimes rounded shoulders in the upper back (see Chapter 14).

[Note: These cases are continued in the Step 2 instalment.]

SUMMARY

- **Mixed patterns expand the Step 1 options:** They allow us to treat the YQR and other Extra Vessels together using fewer needles and cords by connecting the IPC contralaterally.
- **Mixed Yin combines YQR and YWC:** It is diagnosed by right-sided ST 25–27 reactions with accompanying right subcostal and midline tightness.
- **K3L combines YQR and CS:** It appears when upper-right and lower-left quadrant reactions present together, creating a pattern best treated contralaterally.
- **Ren Dai combines YQR and YWD:** It is identified by midline reactions together with left or right belt findings, especially reactions at ST 25, which determine the placement of TB 5 and the resulting cord configuration.
- **Cord placement follows the REDLLL rule:** All contralateral patterns follow this rule except for the left-belt Ren Dai variation, where the configuration reverses.

WHAT'S NEXT

Step 1 releases the yin aspect of the body. In the next chapter, we turn our attention to Step 2 and the yang aspect. We'll look at Manaka's principles for selecting points on the back, and the practical use of *chishin* (retained needling) and *kyutoshin* (moxa on the needle).

CHAPTER 8

STEP 2: PALPATION AND NEEDLING

PROGRESSING FROM STEP 1

Step 1 and Step 2 are of equal importance, together comprising the root treatment, balancing yin and yang. As we have seen, Step 1 involves releasing the yin/anterior aspect. We now move to Step 2, releasing the yang/posterior aspect. What does this mean?

In Dr Manaka's practice, this entailed focusing on the back and, to some extent, on all the yang meridians. In practical terms, we examine the back-*shu* points that relate to the treatment we have just performed. This involves two simple principles of point selection. We treat:

1. The back-*shu* points relating to the meridians of the master and coupled points
2. Tight, reactive pressure pain points (PPP)

For example, if we treat the YWD pair in Step 1, we have used IPC at TB 5 and GB 41. Next, we turn our attention to those points on the back that relate to these two points, namely BL 22 and BL 19, the back-*shu* points of the triple burner and gall bladder, respectively.

As you can see, there's a clear progression from Step 1 to Step 2. Each of the points selected in Step 2 relates to the master and coupled points used in Step 1. Manaka recommended palpating firmly around each related back-*shu* point to find the most reactive point. PPP are the most significant finding and should always be treated, in keeping with the goal of Step 2. When palpating, we look for certain qualities: tightness, hardness of muscle tissue, and reactivity such as pressure pain or jumpiness.

Usually, Manaka used *kyutoshin* (moxa on the needle) technique. If the patient was thin and unsuitable for the deeper needling required, he would use *chishin* (shallow retained needle) and a heat lamp. However, he was both flexible and creative, deploying many different methods to achieve the goals of Step 2. These approaches are listed at the end of this chapter, all of which will be covered in this book series.

Sometimes, Manaka's choice of back-*shu* point was based on other non-theoretical considerations, such as reactivity or needle depth. For example, for the YQR pattern, we would expect to needle BL 13 and BL 23, the back-*shu* points of the lung and kidney. Instead of BL 13, however, Manaka recommended needling BL 25 or a PPP near it. This is because performing *kyutoshin* at BL 13 is a more difficult procedure, as the point is over the lungs and deep needling can cause pneumothorax. A simple, pragmatic equivalent is to needle the back-*shu* point of the lung's paired meridian, the large intestine.

Moreover, Manaka's locations for the back-*shu* points were not textbook, but very much influenced by the realities of reactivity and induration in the general area. For our purposes, we take the region of the upper back from the level of BL 17 and above as being contraindicated for *kyutoshin*; hence, other points like BL 14 (corresponding to P 6 in a YWC pattern) are also contraindicated for this technique. If you do choose to treat points such as BL 13 or BL 14 at Step 2, use *chishin* with a heat lamp.

[Note: For this kind of treatment, we recommend far infrared (FIR) or TDP plate lamps, as the far infrared spectrum they generate most closely replicates the therapeutic effect of moxa.]

STEP 2 FOR THE BASIC FIVE PATTERNS

Table 8.1 lists the default Step 2 back-*shu* choices. In the YQR pattern, BL 25 may be used as a substitute for BL 13, since it corresponds to the large intestine—the paired meridian of the lung.

Table 8.1: Back-*shu* points.

PATTERN	TREATMENT POINTS	LOOK FOR REACTIONS AT
YQR	LU 7, KID 6	BL 23 + BL 25 and/or PPP
YWC	P 6, SP 4	BL 18 or BL 20 and/or other PPP
YQD	BL 62, SI 3	Lateral to BL 27 or BL 28 and/or other PPP
YWD	TB 5, GB41	BL 19 and/or BL 22, BL23 and/ or other PPP
Cross Syndrome	P 6, SP 4 TB 5, GB41	BL 18 or BL 20 + either BL 23, BL 25, or BL 27 and/or other PPP

The YWC pattern frequently corresponds to liver or spleen dysfunction. BL 18 is commonly selected when liver reactivity predominates, while BL 20 relates to spleen pathology and its link to SP 4.

For the YQD pattern, reactions are often found lateral to BL 27 or BL 28; these are described further in the discussion of the inner and outer bladder lines below. Sometimes other PPP are more prominent than the associated back-*shu* points. In these cases, it is good to treat them. For example, in CS you may find reactions at BL 18 or BL 20 as well as PPP in the lower back not on the list above. It's fine to treat these reactive points as part of the goal of Step 2. The main consideration in these cases is not to choose every reaction and overtreat.

STEP 2 FOR MIXED PATTERNS

As with Manaka's original treatments, Step 2 for the contemporary mixed patterns follows the choice of points for Step 1. Once again, theory and palpation combine to give you your treatment points. Steps 1 and 2 together comprise the root treatment.

The Mixed Yin and K3L are variations on a theme: they are both patterns where the liver and kidney need to be addressed together. Hence, the default back-*shu* points are BL 18 and BL 23.

Table 8.2: Step 2 for combination patterns.

PATTERN	TREATMENT POINTS	LOOK FOR REACTIONS AT
Mixed Yin	KID 6, LU 7, SP 4, P 6	BL 18 + BL 23
K3L	KID 6, LU 7, LI 4, LIV 3	BL 18 + BL 23 or BL 27 instead of BL 23
Ren Dai	KID 6, LU 7, TB 5, GB 41	BL 19 or BL 22 and BL 23 or BL 25 or other PPP

In Ren Dai, pressure pain is often found around BL 19 and BL 22, as well as BL 23 and BL 25. In some cases, especially when BL 23 is less reactive, palpation lateral to BL 27, just as in CS, may reveal stronger PPP that can serve as effective substitutes.

When doing Step 2 for YWD, you may find that BL 19 and BL 22 are often too close together for *kyutoshin*, as the combined heat of four needles in such close proximity can be excessive. In that case, choose either BL 19 or BL 22 and add a PPP. On some people, however, BL 19 and the area lateral to BL 22 are far enough apart to use both.

FINDING THE BACK-*SHU* POINTS

> *Those who know how to apply the needle rely on their left hand; those who do not know how to apply the needle rely on the right.*
>
> —*Nan Jing* Chapter 78[119]

As you finish Step 1 and ask your patient to turn over, you will already have an idea of where to treat, based on Tables 8.1 and 8.2. It's important to realise that these point choices are not set in stone; they are a filter to narrow down your options. Thus, when you actually contemplate your patient's back, it's good to start off by looking. Looking reveals raised and sunken areas on the back, which immediately guide your hands when you start palpating. In terms of workflow, it's helpful to have a needle prepared in your dominant hand before you start, and to palpate with your non-dominant hand.

As when palpating the *hara*, start with a light touch, stroking the back and letting its contours guide you to the indurations. For example, for a YWC pattern, if theory suggests that you needle BL 18 or BL 20, try stroking up and down the bladder meridian lightly, and see where the muscle feels most contracted. Once you have an idea of the broad location of the tight band, start with a relatively light cross-fibre palpation. This will allow you to map out the demarcation and shape of the tight band. Finally, palpate deeper across the fibres, looking for the tightest, most reactive point within the tight band. The needle goes here, into the tight band. The back-*shu* points are needled bilaterally. Repeat the process on the other side.

The back-*shu* points are described as on a line 1.5 *cun* lateral to the midline of the spine. In clinical practice, however, the reactions at the back-*shu* points can be more medial or more lateral to the textbook location.

---

119 *Nan Jing* Chapter 78, quoted in Birch, S., & Ida, J. (1998). *Japanese Acupuncture: A Clinical Guide.* Brookline: Paradigm Publications. p. 67.

CROSS-FIBRE PALPATION

As can be seen from the tables above, PPP feature strongly as alternative points to the ones suggested by theory. In JAAM, pragmatism usually trumps theory, and in Step 2, your guide to point selection should always be palpation. In particular, *cross-fibre palpation* is the key to finding effective points.

As the name suggests, this method entails palpating at right angles to the muscle fibres running vertically along the spine. Your fingers should slide back and forth across the bladder line, since only by going across the fibres can you detect the hardest, most reactive points to needle. The point to be treated should lie within a tight band of muscle tissue, as releasing that tightness is the aim of treatment. As you reach the sacrum and buttocks, you may need to change direction and palpate vertically to cross the gluteal fibres.

THE INNER AND OUTER BLADDER LINES

Dr Manaka investigated the flow of the inner and outer bladder meridians along the spine and found that they act like a single wide stream—in other words, the *Huatuo-jiaji* points and both bladder lines function as one meridian. From this and his clinical experience, he suggested that treating BL 23 or BL 52 produces essentially the same effect, and that needling a reactive point anywhere between them can do so as well. He therefore concluded that treating BL 23 means palpating at the level of L2 and selecting the most reactive point—whether closer to the *Huatuo-jiaji* points, on the inner bladder line, or the outer bladder line.

In the interscapular region and from the level of BL 17 to BL 22, the back-*shu* points may feel like hard, stringy knots, and cross-fibre palpation can often provoke jump reactions. Occasionally, this same kind of knot can be felt down to the level of BL 23 or below, but more often, the reactions at the level of BL 23 are like a plate of hard, reactive muscle, and often the lateral edge of that hard area, around BL 52, shows the best reactions.

Manaka found that the reactive points for BL 27 and BL 28 often migrate further laterally, into the middle of the buttocks. They appear along a tight band of muscle running from the side of the sacrum towards the hip joint and the head of the greater trochanter. Because this band lies more horizontally at this level, we adjust our cross-fibre palpation: pressing vertically, along a caudal–cranial line, with firm pressure. We refer to these as the *mid-gluteal* points.[120] They are located on deeper palpation, probably in the piriformis muscle, and typically feel tight, hard, painful, or jumpy.

Interestingly, these ideas about points at the same level having similar effects resonate very much with the theories of Kurakichi Hirata (1901–1945), who pioneered a holographic mapping of the body consisting of horizontal zones. Indeed, Manaka practised his own interpretation of Hirata's work and wrote a book about this approach. Taku Yokoyama, a former student of Manaka, has suggested that these zones are the horizontal influence of the Dai Mai at different levels.[121]

INSERTING A NEEDLE WITH A GUIDE TUBE

In Chapter 3, we looked at some of the key defining features of JAAM. One of these was the use of the *shinkan*, or guide tube, invented in the seventeenth century by Waichi Sugiyama, the 'Father of Japanese Acupuncture.'[122] Given that so many contemporary acupuncturists all over the world now use guide tubes, and that so many needles are sold with disposable guide tubes, Sugiyama is arguably the most influential acupuncturist of all time. Moreover, the use of *shinkan* is one of the key differentiating techniques between Japanese and Chinese needle insertion methods. It has several advantages:

- The guide tube stops the needle from bending during insertion, which makes it possible to use much finer gauges, or even needles made of soft metals such as silver or gold.
- Since we don't need to grasp the shaft with fingers or cotton wool, the needle remains cleaner and more sterile.
- The first few millimetres of insertion (up to 4 mm) can be controlled with great precision, allowing us to advance just 2–3 mm if needed.

---

120 This formal name is often shortened by the irrepressible Birch to the 'mid-butt points'.

121 Kivity, O. (2021). *Hirata Zone Therapy with the Ontake Method: Repurposing the Lost Art of Japanese Dermatome Moxibustion for Contemporary Practice*. London: Sayoshi Books.

122 Birch, S. (1997). *Japanese Acupuncture and Moxibustion: A Brief Overview*. Course handout. Anglo-Dutch Institute for Oriental Medicine.

- The downward pressure of the lip of the guide tube reduces the sensation of insertion, making it less painful for the patient.

The following pages describe procedures for inserting a needle with a guide tube, both for the shallow oblique insertion required for Step 1 ion pumping and Step 2 needling, such as *chishin* retained needling, and *kyutoshin*, which requires a deeper, perpendicular insertion.

POSTURE

Your posture is of great importance to the success of your insertion. In Toyohari-style acupuncture, the instructors emphasise that you stand with the point you are needling directly in front of your *hara*. Your posture should be upright and relaxed, and your arms should form a soft circle. Make sure you feel comfortable and aren't leaning awkwardly to reach the point.

OSHIDE

Both hands play essential roles in the location and needling of points. *Oshide* means left hand. Use the tip of the index finger of your left hand to locate the point. Once the location is clear, form an *oshide* over the point (a ring shape formed by touching the index finger to the thumb).

Cross-fibre palpation can also be used when locating the master and coupled points. Some Japanese practitioners use their thumb to palpate, as this is a strong digit and can exert much force, but we recommend using the index finger, which is more sensitive to the underlying tissue.

The entire left hand, including the palm and remaining fingers, stabilises the area to be treated. The *oshide* itself fixes the point location and serves as an accurate marker for the placement of the guide tube and needle.

It is important to keep the *oshide* stable and relaxed, and to do this, it's good to keep an inner eye on your whole arm and shoulder, making sure it feels soft and open.

SASHIDE

Some guide tubes come with a plastic holding piece for the needle handle, or the needles are fixed with a drop of glue. To release the needle, break the seal or remove the plastic holding piece from the guide tube.

The right hand is referred to as the *sashide*. Hold the needle and guide tube in the *sashide* with your index finger, anchoring the needle handle at the top of the tube. When you've located the point, place the tube into the *oshide* at the correct angle. The guide tube should touch the skin. For more sensitive points, apply more downward pressure with the guide tube. The pressure of the guide tube lip pressing down masks the sensation of the insertion.

Before you start to insert the needle, make sure that the tip is resting lightly on the skin. If you start inserting the needle when the needle tip is halfway up the guide tube, it will shoot along the empty tube like a dart and will definitely cause discomfort when it hits the skin. To bring the tip to the skin gradually, before insertion, tap the side of the guide tube lightly or stroke the handle of the needle gently.

INSERTION

To insert, tap the top of the needle handle lightly several times. You can also vary the part of your finger you use to tap. Using the proximal phalanx produces a lighter force, while using the distal phalanx delivers more force. This allows you to moderate the tap and control the depth of insertion. On sensitive areas, such as points on the hand like SI 3, a single firm tap can work better.

Another variable is the angle of the tapping finger. This can range from vertically above the guide tube, to about 45°, to tapping from the side. At 45°, the edge of the guide tube acts as a brake to the tapping movement.

As with the *oshide*, it is important to keep the *sashide* relaxed and light. If your fingers, arm, or shoulder are stiff when needling, this tension will be transmitted through the needle and increase the risk of causing discomfort during insertion.

A PROGRESSION OF SKILLS

This chapter focuses on *chishin* and *kyutoshin. Kyutoshin* was Manaka's favoured approach. However, with years of practice in different settings, we also find *chishin* very useful. This chapter introduces needling methods as a progression of skills, arranged as an incremental sequence for ease of learning. We begin with *chishin*, commonly used in Step 1 on the hands and feet. We then explore *chishin* on the back, and finally progress to *kyutoshin*, which requires deeper insertion and more advanced skills.

However, although we describe *chishin* on the back before *kyutoshin,* this does not mean it should be the first choice for Step 2. **In practice, Manaka's default Step 2 method was *kyutoshin*.** *Chishin* was reserved only for those who were not suitable for *kyutoshin*—for example, thinner patients with tight spinal muscles.

CHISHIN IN STEP 1

In Step 1, we have seen that the needles are inserted and then the IPC clips are attached. The needle technique is shallow, and since the needle is retained for a few minutes with no manipulation beyond attaching the IPC clip, the needling is a form of *chishin* (retained, shallow needling).

Manaka recommended inserting the needle 2–3 mm. If the needle handle normally protrudes 4 mm from the top of the guide tube, this means that you can't tap the handle so that the top is flush with the top of the guide tube—that's already deeper than he recommends. Just tap until the needle is inserted 2–3 mm and then remove the guide tube. The needle will immediately fall over from its own weight and lie flat on the skin. Make sure that it falls so that it's pointing in the direction of the meridian flow by angling the needle and tube with the flow of the meridian; for example, at TB 5, it should be pointing towards the elbow.

CHISHIN IN STEP 2

Use the steps above to palpate for and needle two pairs of back-*shu* points. Needle downwards, in the direction of the bladder meridian. As above, the needles should fall under their own weight. Retain for about ten minutes. With this kind of shallow needling, you will often see reddening of the skin at the insertion points. A pragmatic rule of thumb is to remove the needles when the reddening starts to dissipate.

KYUTOSHIN: MOXA ON THE NEEDLE TECHNIQUE

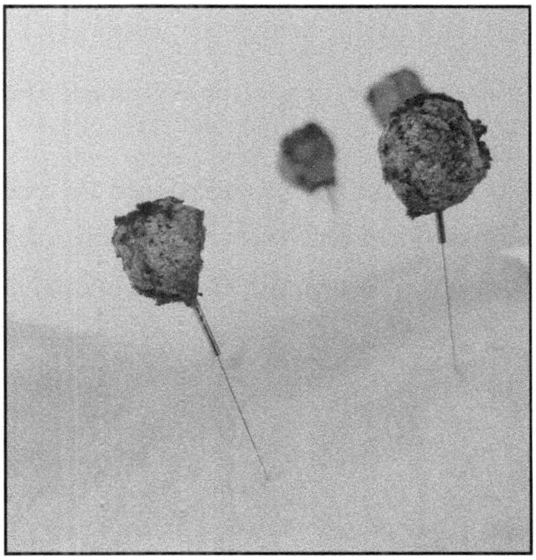

Figure 8-1: *Kyutoshin*—moxa on the handle of the needle.

This is an indirect moxa method in which small balls of moxa are burned on the handle of a needle. In JAAM, a special grade of moxa wool—known as semi-pure moxa—was developed for this purpose. One popular and widely available brand is Wakakusa. It is fluffier and more yellow than the coarser, greener grades.

Less refined moxa does not adhere well to the needle handle, and fragments of hot material can drop onto the patient's skin. With semi-pure moxa, most of the coarse matter has been sifted out, so the rolled ball sticks well to the handle and does not shed particles. If you plan to use this technique, make sure you purchase semi-pure moxa or Wakakusa moxa, made specifically for this purpose.

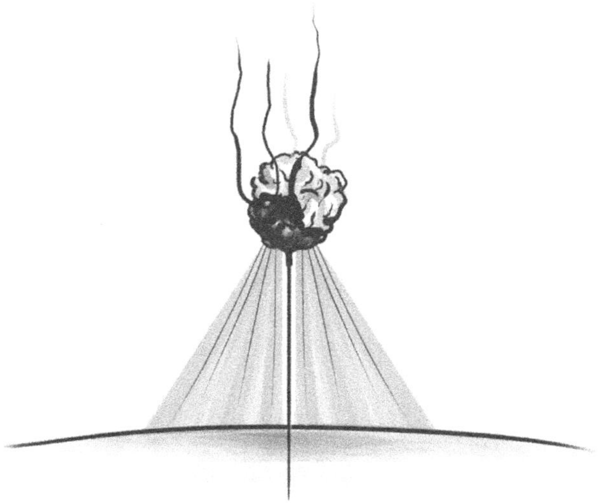

Figure 8-2: The main effect of needle moxa is radiated heat on the skin.

As can be seen in Figure 8-1, a moxa ball is placed onto the needle handle and ignited. The main effect of the moxa is radiant heat on the skin. Although some penetrates through the needle shaft into the tissues, this effect is much less.

WARMING AND MOVING

The purpose of the moxa in *kyutoshin* is to enhance the muscle-relaxing effect of the needle. This is achieved by generating a mild, comfortable warmth around the insertion site, helping the muscles release.

Manaka also believed that these warming and relaxing effects improved blood flow and, over time, could gradually resolve blood stasis. Since blood stasis was a pivotal construct in his system, he used *kyutoshin* with almost every patient at Step 2, regardless of what was done at Step 1. (We will explore Manaka's thoughts on blood stasis and prognosis in later books.)

Although Manaka routinely applied *kyutoshin* at Step 2, the method is versatile and can also be used at Step 4 to treat symptoms (see Chapter 13). In JAAM, *kyutoshin* (moxa on the needle) is understood and used quite differently from the Chinese technique *wenzhen* (warm needle). This difference may stem partly from the influence of Chinese herbalism on Chinese acupuncture, which makes clear distinctions between warming and cooling medicines in ways that JAAM does not. It may also reflect practical considerations about the type of heat each technique generates.

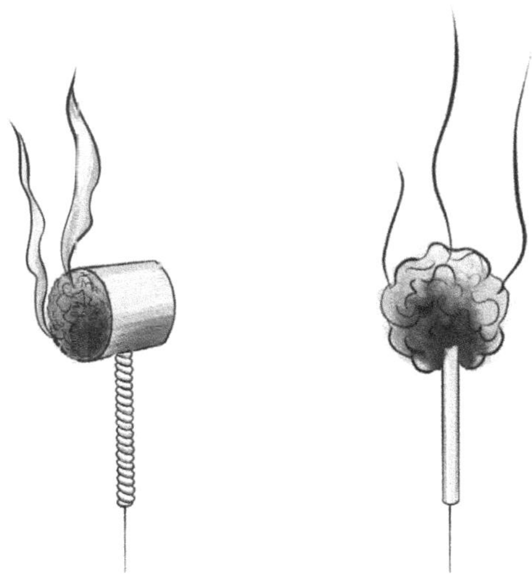

Figure 8-3: *Wenzhen* and *kyutoshin*.

In China, *wenzhen* is applied to add heat to patients considered cold—the needled area must become hot for the technique to be judged effective. By contrast, *kyutoshin* is used to aid muscle relaxation and improve blood circulation, so only mild heat is required. *Wenzhen* involves placing a cut piece of moxa stick on the end of the needle. In contrast, *kyutoshin* uses loosely rolled balls of *semi-pure moxa*, refined to burn at a lower temperature than the tightly compressed moxa in sticks. The needles are also designed differently: solid pipe-handled needles conduct less heat than copper-wound handles.

Table 8.3 compares the *kyutoshin* (needle-moxa) and *wenzhen* (warm needle).

Table 8.3: Comparing needle moxa and warm needle.

JAPANESE *KYUTOSHIN*	**CHINESE *WENZHEN***
Semi-pure moxa burns less intensely at a lower temperature since it is loosely compressed.	The moxa pole segment burns hotter and longer since the moxa is tightly compressed.
Lightly rolled balls burn faster at a lower temperature.	Densely packed stick segments burn longer and hotter.
A solid pipe handle conducts less heat.	A copper-wound handle conducts more heat.
Warm sensation.	Hot sensation.

ACTIONS

In JAAM, *kyutoshin* is considered to be a *mild* treatment that:

- Relaxes the muscles
- Warms mildly
- Stimulates the microcirculation of blood.

TECHNIQUE

LOCATION AND INSERTION

Using cross-fibre palpation as described above, locate the most prominent point within the tight band of muscle. Place your *oshide* on the point and insert the guide tube into the *oshide*, directly over it. Tap the needle in as far as the tube will allow, then advance it to the depth needed so it stands upright and can support the weight of the moxa ball. Do not manipulate the needle to obtain qi sensation.

If you accidentally elicit *deqi*, Manaka advised waiting for the sensation to diminish. If not—or if the patient seems distressed—remove the needle and reinsert 1 mm or so away.

APPLICATION OF MOXA

Roll moxa balls lightly between the palms of both hands. Each ball should be approximately 1–2 cm in diameter. Avoid compressing the moxa as you roll, so the final ball is light and not dense. The denser the ball, the hotter it will burn and the more difficult it can become to get it to bind on the needle handle.

Gently break the ball in two and rejoin the halves on the needle handle, firmly but without squeezing. The ball of moxa should sit centred on the handle. As you press the two halves of the ball together, apply horizontal pressure, neither upward nor downward. Pressing downward may insert the needle more deeply without your noticing; pressing upward may withdraw it so that it no longer stands upright. With practice, applying this horizontal pressure becomes easy.

For safety reasons, remember these two rules:

1. The base of the needle handle should be visible below the ball.
2. The top of the needle handle should not be visible at the top of the ball.

The principles behind these two rules are simple. If the base of the handle is not visible, three risks can occur:

1. The ball is lower on the handle than it should be, which can affect its stability.
2. If the ball is lower down the handle, it is closer to the skin and may feel uncomfortably hot.
3. The needle shaft is sensitive to heat and may warp or bend if heated directly, whereas the thicker handle will not.

We don't want the moxa ball sliding down the shaft like a hula hoop dropping to your feet—it should sit firmly on the handle, like a top hat jammed on your head. To secure it, leave a good portion of the ball above the handle and finish by squeezing the top last. The needle handle should remain hidden within the moxa, with only its base visible below.

To prevent it from slipping downward, leave a substantial portion of the ball above the top of the handle. When you press the two halves together, finish by squeezing the top of the ball last—this secures it firmly to the handle. The top part of the handle should not protrude through the moxa.

The moxa ball should sit 2–3 cm from the skin. Adjust the size of the ball to the needle length and body area. To check it is secure, tap the ball lightly or tap the skin around the needle: it should remain secure as the needle sways. Remove any loose fragments of moxa from the ball or handle that could fall.

Light the ball from the bottom, close to the handle. As moxa burns, it produces a sticky resin; lighting it near the handle ensures the resin binds the ball firmly to the needle. It will typically burn for around two minutes.

PROCEDURAL ISSUES

It is important to explain the procedure, so patients anticipate the warmth of the moxa and know to alert you if it feels too hot. Remind them to stay completely still while the moxa is burning. Minimise conversation during *kyutoshin*, especially anything that might make them move or laugh—it is unnerving to watch four needles with smouldering moxa wobble as a patient guffaws. Restrain your sense of humour!

Kyutoshin demands absolute focus. Keep your eyes on the needles at all times and anticipate accidents. If a ball looks precarious, be ready with an ashtray underneath to catch it, should it fall. Never leave the room while moxa is burning. If you must look away—for example, to write notes—keep glancing back frequently to monitor the needles.

If the heat is too much for the patient, you can use a home-made heat shield: a piece of cardboard with a narrow V-shaped cut. Slide it around the needle so that it sits beneath the moxa. You can remove it when the heat has reduced. Sometimes it may be necessary to remove the needle while the moxa is still burning. Prepare an ashtray and tweezers in advance for this possibility. If removal is required, grasp the needle carefully with tweezers and drop the whole assembly into the ashtray to cool.

To check that the moxa has gone out, hold your palm over the ball to feel for residual heat. Once it is cool, gently pick up the ash ball with your fingers and place it in the ashtray. Take care not to touch the needle handle, as it retains heat.

Alternatively, you can use a moxa spoon or scoop designed with a slit to slide around the needle and lift the ash. Care should be taken not to catch the bottom of the handle of the needle as the hot needle may fall on the skin.

When removing the needles, remember the handles may still be hot. One option is to grasp the shaft, which will already be cool.

SMOKE

A final consideration is that *kyutoshin* generates a lot of smoke. Make sure your treatment room is well ventilated, not just for your patients' sakes but for your own. Oran Kivity recalls that when he first started using the technique in 1997, he developed a smoker's cough until his clinic installed an extractor fan in the treatment room.

TOOLBOX PHRASES

Much of what we do in acupuncture is unfamiliar to patients. With its abdominal palpation, unusual polarity devices, and rapid changes in pressure pain, MSA can seem more unfamiliar than many other approaches. Naturally, these things spark curiosity and questions, so it helps to have ready-made explanations.

No technique in this book needs more introduction than *kyutoshin*. This is where *toolbox phrases* come in: a simple, reassuring, pre-planned explanation of what you're about to do.

You need to find your own way of gently and reassuringly explaining that you're planning to insert needles into their back, place balls of a herb on the needles, and set them alight. There's very little that can go wrong, and if anything feels uncomfortable, you'll be right there to take care of it.

Work out what you need to say; practise saying it to friends until it comes out smoothly and naturally. It's as important to get that right as it is to light the moxa cone from the bottom.

CLINICAL APPLICATIONS

Manaka used *kyutoshin* in Step 2 on the related back-*shu* points, which are usually tight and reactive. He applied it as a simple "muscle-relaxant" treatment, taking advantage of its mild and comfortable stimulation. *Kyutoshin* is also effective for musculoskeletal problems, especially on the back, knees, and shoulders, and it can be used as a Step 4 treatment (see Chapter 13).

With extremely tight back muscles (as in acute spasms and pain), *kyutoshin* may be challenging to apply. In such cases, distal points on the legs can be used to relieve the tension. Palpate BL 40, BL 55, BL 56, BL 57, and BL 58 for reactions; if one of these is very tight or sore, it may be used as the Step 2 treatment.

With very thin patients, beginners often struggle to adjust needle depth, moxa size, and ball placement safely. In such cases, *chishin* with a heat lamp is the simpler and safer option. Far infrared (FIR) and TDP lamps are recommended, as they best emulate the warmth of moxa.

DOSAGE

We will discuss dosage extensively in Chapter 15 and how to lower the dose of *kyutoshin* to accommodate the needs of sensitive patients. For typical patients, Manaka recommended two pairs of points, with two balls on each. This can be increased to a maximum of three pairs of points, with two balls on each.

The skin should turn a pinkish red. If it becomes very red or the patient cannot tolerate the heat, protect the skin by placing a piece of card around the needle or by sliding two fingers alongside the shaft to cover the skin for a few seconds.

CONTRAINDICATIONS

For acute low-back problems, Manaka recommended using distal leg points rather than local points. When there is inflammation and strong pressure pain, local needling can aggravate the condition, and many patients will also find it difficult to lie prone and remain still.

NEEDLE SIZES

As we have seen in Chapter 3, there is a preference in JAAM for less stimulation. Particularly with the invention of the guide tube, it is possible to use much finer needles. Japanese needle sizes are referred to differently from Chinese needle gauges.

Table 8.4: Needle sizes.

NEEDLE DIAMETER (MM)	0.12	0.14	0.16	0.18	0.20	0.22	0.25	0.30	0.35
CHINESE GAUGE	#44	#42	#40	#38	#36	#34	#32	#30	#28
JAPANESE GAUGE	00	0	1	2	3	4	5	8	10

In MSA, we use fine needles for three primary purposes: shallow needling for ion pumping, shallow retained needling for symptom relief (*chishin*), and *kyutoshin* at Step 2 or 4. The length and gauge vary by function.

Table 8.5: Needle size by function.

METHOD	GAUGE	COMMENT
Ion pumping	**30–40 mm No. 1 or No. 2** *(Chinese 1–1.5", 0.16–0.18 mm)*	The finer the needle, the more easily it will fall out. Micropore tape may be required.
Chishin	**30–40 mm 00 to No. 2** *(Chinese 1–1.5", 0.12–0.18 mm)*	Select according to patient sensitivity. If they don't like needles, use 00 or 0; for most patients, you can use No. 1 or No. 2.
Kyutoshin	**40 mm No. 3** *(Chinese 1.5", 0.20 mm)*	The needle must carry the weight of the moxa, so it needs to be slightly thicker.

NEEDLE DEPTHS AND ANGLES OF INSERTION

CHISHIN

Insertion is generally very shallow, as little as 1 mm, and no more than 4 mm, about the length of the handle protruding from the guide tube, so that the needle falls over from its own weight. The insertion is oblique or transverse.

KYUTOSHIN

The insertion is perpendicular and deeper into the muscle tissue, so the needle can stand upright and support the weight of moxa on the handle. Table 8.6 provides safe needling depths for *kyutoshin*.

Table 8.6: Needle selection for *kyutoshin*.

AREA	NEEDLE LENGTH AND GAUGE	DEPTH OF INSERTION
BL 18–BL 20	**40 mm No. 3** *(Chinese 1.5", 0.20 mm)*	Around 1 cm
BL 21–BL 23	As above	Up to 1.5 cm
BL 25	As above	Slightly less deep, as the muscle bands at BL 25 are more medial
Sacral area (lateral to BL 27, BL 28)	As above	Around 1.5 cm
Buttocks	**40 mm or longer No. 3** *(Chinese 1.5"+, 0.20 mm)*	May require a longer needle, depending on body size

CONTEMPORARY MANAKA: ONTAKE

A full description of Ontake is beyond the scope of this chapter, but it can be a handy tool for Step 2. Because it is such an effective contemporary moxibustion method, we introduce it briefly here. For more details, see *Moxa in Motion with the Ontake Method,* which includes a full chapter on the use of Ontake with MSA.[123]

DEFINITIONS

Ontake is a short tube of bamboo, filled with moxa wool. When lit, the mouth and sides of the bamboo become warm, allowing it to be applied as a dynamic pressing and rolling tool. When combined with Manaka's theory of meridian frequencies, it can be

123 Kivity, O. (2020). *Moxa in Motion with the Ontake Method: Rhythmic Moxibustion Methods from Japan for Mind-Body Healing*. London: Sayoshi Books.

applied to the skin rhythmically at specific frequencies of beats per minute, according to the meridian affected. This meridian frequency moxibustion brings about rapid changes in muscle tightness and relieves pain fast.

Applied on the back, it can easily achieve the goal of Step 2, without needles. Particularly for patients who are averse to needles, it offers a comfortable alternative to *chishin* and *kyutoshin* at Step 2.

OTHER OPTIONS FOR STEP 2

This chapter has introduced *chishin* and *kyutoshin* for Step 2, but as the goals of Step 2 are so broad, to release reactions on the yang aspect of the body, there are many other methods to achieve them. The *Manaka Made Simple* book series will cover all the techniques presented in Table 8.7, which shows the breadth of approaches Manaka used for this purpose. The historical methods reflect his use of shallow needling, moxa, and percussive tools, while the contemporary methods highlight newer innovations such as Ontake.

Table 8.7: Options for Step 2.

HISTORICAL MANAKA	*Kyutoshin* (moxa on the needle)	This was what Manaka did routinely for Step 2. Needles are inserted perpendicularly, and moxa is burnt on the handle of the needle.
	Chishin needling	Shallowly inserted retained needle.
	Chishin needling with heat lamp	Used when the patient is thin and unsuitable for the relatively deeper insertion required for *kyutoshin*. Far infrared (FIR) and TDP lamps are recommended, as they best emulate the warmth of moxa.
	Needling yang meridian points	Manaka listed several points on the yang meridians that frequently get congested and suggested palpating and needling these in sequence (known as Manaka's reactive points).
	Stretch moxa	Stretching the yang meridians while burning moxa on reactive points.
	Okyu, chinetsukyu, choseikyu	Small-cone moxibustion, large-cone moxibustion, and platform moxa to release tender, tight points.
	Kyukonshin	Shallow needling combined with small-cone moxibustion.
	Manaka's wooden needle and hammer	A percussive tapping instrument, often applied with a metronome.

CONTEMPORARY MANAKA	Ontake	A heated piece of bamboo, often applied with a metronome. Ontake can be applied to the whole back for Step 2, or it can release Manaka's reactive points.

IN PRACTICE: STEP 2—STORIES FROM THE CLINIC

In this section, we return to our three patients—Christine, David, and Margaret—to follow their progress into Step 2 treatment. To save you flipping back and forth, we'll begin each instalment with a short recap of their Step 1 presentation and treatment, before discussing how their cases unfolded with Step 2.

CASE STUDY 1: SCIATIC PAIN

Christine, Female, 56

- **Chief complaint:** Right-sided sciatic pain, disturbed sleep
- **Notes:** History of migraines and old car accident injury; age-related abdominal hypotonia
- **Diagnosis:** Ren Dai (right-belt) (dominant right-sided Dai Mai reaction, Mixed Yin milder)

Step 1: Ren Dai (right-belt) with IPC (10 minutes)
Step 2: *Chishin* with an infrared lamp (FIR) on BL 23, BL 26, and lateral to BL 27 (mid-gluteal point)

PRACTITIONER NOTE

With a Ren Dai pattern, we look for pressure pain around BL 19, BL 22, BL 23, BL 25, or other PPP. Palpation lateral to the inner bladder line revealed tenderness at the mid-gluteal point in the piriformis muscle. This point typically feels tight, hard, painful, or jumpy.

CASE STUDY 2: NECK PAIN POST-WEIGHTLIFTING INJURY

David, Male, 39

- **Chief complaint:** Chronic right lateral neck pain with swelling between GB 9 and GB 10, radiating at times to the right shoulder and face
- **Notes:** Old weightlifting injury (8 years earlier); background pain rated 5/10 daily, rising to 8+/10 under stress
- **Diagnosis:** YWD

Step 1: YWD with IPC (10 minutes)
Step 2: BL 19, BL 22 with infrared (FIR) lamp

PRACTITIONER NOTE

In this clinic, moxa was not permitted. Step 2, therefore, followed the textbook approach for point selection, with a heat lamp used in place of *kyutoshin*. This is the standard alternative whenever *kyutoshin* is unsuitable.

CASE STUDY 3: HIP DEGENERATION AND CHRONIC PAIN

Margaret, Female, 60

- **Chief complaint:** Chronic right lumbar and groin pain with hip joint degeneration; constant deep pain disturbing sleep and mobility
- **Notes:** History of lumbar fusion (L4–L5) with severe scarring; multiple cortisone injections with no relief; pain relieved by movement, pressure, and heat
- **Diagnosis:** YQR

Step 1: YQR with IPC (15 minutes)
Step 2: *Kyutoshin*—2 balls on GB 30, GB 31, GB 26

PRACTITIONER NOTE

This was an atypical Step 2 treatment. Normally, BL 23 and BL 25 would be used. In later sessions, BL 25 was indeed selected, but on this occasion, the practitioner addressed the most reactive yang meridian, the gall bladder. In some ways, this overlapped with Step 4, as the needling targeted the area of greatest pain.

[Note: These cases are continued in the Step 3 instalment.]

SUMMARY

- **Step 2 complements Step 1:** Together, they form the root treatment.
- **Focus:** Releasing the yang/posterior aspect via the back-*shu* points.
- **Point selection:** Back-*shu* points related to Step 1's master and coupled points, plus pressure pain points (PPP) found by cross-fibre palpation.
- **Principal method:** *Kyutoshin* (moxa on the handle of the needle).
- **Alternative method:** *Chishin* with a heat lamp when *kyutoshin* is unsuitable.
- **Contemporary option:** Ontake provides a needle-free Step 2 treatment, especially for sensitive or needle-averse patients.

- **Dosage:** Usually two pairs of points with two moxa balls each; increase to a maximum of three pairs if needed.
- **Contraindications:** Acute local inflammation, severe sensitivity, or inability to lie prone.
- **Flexibility:** Other historical and contemporary methods (cone moxa, reactive point needling, Ontake, etc.) may also achieve Step 2 goals.

WHAT'S NEXT

Steps 1 and 2 form the root treatment. In the next chapter, we'll turn to Step 3—structural adjustment with Sotai, a gentle bodywork method that Manaka adapted by combining it with *okyu*.

CHAPTER 9

STEP 3: SOTAI

The objective in step three is to adjust any remaining imbalances of the muscular and skeletal structures. These physical components not only support the body's structure, but also make all physical movement possible. Balance is of great importance for health. Structural adjustment is a very effective method of treating pain in the muscles, tendons, and joints. Some exercises, usually Sotai, *are performed during step three.*

—Yoshio Manaka[124]

Sotai is a popular method of neuromuscular re-education developed by the Japanese doctor Keizo Hashimoto in the 1970s. Sotai uses gentle movements and focused breathing to unwind muscular tension patterns to promote healing in the whole body.

The objective of this method is to help the body restore and maintain its natural structural balance. Hashimoto developed a model of treatment for this purpose using breath and movement. He maintained that Sotai was not just a system of exercises or a method of therapy; it was part of a deeper, broader principle that embraced all of life, a natural result of right living. Improvement and maintenance become the responsibility of each individual.

---

124 Manaka, Y., Itaya, K., & Birch, S. (1995). *Chasing the Dragon's Tail: The Theory and Practice of Acupuncture in the Work of Yoshio Manaka*. Brookline: Paradigm Publications. p. 195

Dr Manaka was constantly assimilating new methods. He had heard of Dr Hashimoto and arranged to study his approach. In typical fashion, once he had the basic concepts, he was tempted to adapt and develop Hashimoto's ideas in his own way. Not content simply to practise orthodox Sotai, he decided to integrate it with his own ideas about Traditional East Asian Medicine (TEAM).

In the *Ling Shu*, the Fire Needle (*fazhen*) was often used to treat the sinew channels. In this case, Manaka's big idea was to develop the notion that Sotai works primarily on the soft tissue. He developed methods to perform Sotai while simultaneously applying Fire Needle. By combining these two modalities, movement and heat, he created something different and unique—a bodywork method that also uses heat. As Fire Needle is a relatively extreme treatment, he also adapted this approach by applying small-cone moxibustion instead. Sotai with moxa is an augmented Sotai—to our knowledge, the first ever combined moxibustion/bodywork method.

It's worth noting that we do not perform Sotai on every patient. Step 3 is reserved for cases where clear structural asymmetries are observed, such as differences in shoulder or pelvic girdle height, leg-length discrepancies, or curvature of the spine. At this stage in treatment, however, it is important to check for these asymmetries, as they can signal the need for deeper physical examination (see below).

It is also not necessary to combine Sotai with moxa every time. Some presentations respond well to Sotai alone, while others, particularly those involving blood stasis, benefit more from the addition of moxa. In short, Sotai offers a range of options: from no intervention, to Sotai alone, to Sotai with moxa.

In this chapter, we will look at the general principles of Sotai and learn how to apply one of the most useful stretches, called Prone Leg Flexion, without moxa. We will then repeat the exercise with Manaka's variation with moxa. For full details on how to apply moxa, go to Chapter 13.

Prone Leg Flexion is one of many Sotai exercises taught in contemporary Manaka classes by the authors. Subsequent books in the series will cover them all.

PRINCIPLES OF SOTAI

To become free of pain, one must move away from pain towards comfort.

—Keizo Hashimoto[125]

Taiso (体操) means 'exercise' in Japanese. Sotai is the same two characters reversed: *So* (操) meaning 'to work or manipulate' (as in a puppet), and *Tai* (体) meaning 'body'. Sotai, therefore, means 'manipulation or movement for restoring or maintaining health'. It combines breathing and movement, within the natural limits of the patient's range of motion, to induce muscular relaxation. Crucially, the corrective movement is performed in the direction away from the discomfort and pain.

This procedure not only treats structural imbalances but can also address many other conditions. Tight muscles impair qi flow. Distortion in the body's musculature can also affect the internal organs and vice versa. For example, tightness over the mid-thoracic back on the right is often associated with the liver, and tightness on the left is associated with the spleen. When excessive, this unilateral tightness can lead to scoliosis.

Weak lungs can cause tightness in the pectoral muscles, pulling the shoulders forward and down. This slumped position can create tightness in the shoulders, as well as in the interscapular area posteriorly. These ideas tie in perfectly with Manaka's octahedral thinking, where the qi flowing over one facet of the octahedron affects the flow of qi in the other seven facets. It also dovetails nicely with the concepts of regulation and dents and bumps explored in Chapter 1.

Thus, structural adjustment, the third step of Manaka's Four Step protocol, is closely tied to the root treatment. It is particularly useful for the treatment of musculoskeletal problems, especially when structural imbalances impede function.

---

[125] Hashimoto, K., & Kawakami, Y. (1983). *Sotai: Balance and Health Through Natural Movement.* Tokyo: Japan Publications Inc. p. 211.

Table 9.1: Visual signs of structural and functional disorders.

MERIDIAN SYSTEM	STRUCTURAL MANIFESTATION
Lung	Tightness in the pectorals and upper torso; rounding of the upper back and shoulders; tightness in the interscapular region
Liver	Upper right and lower left abdominal tension (Cross Syndrome); right shoulder with left lower back/leg involvement; stiffness and swelling around BL 17–20 on the right
Spleen	Swelling and raising in the left interscapular area; tightness and swelling from BL 17–20 on the left
Kidney	Tightness in the lower back with softening of the lower abdomen

THEORY

> *If the body is imbalanced or distorted for some reason, the centre of gravity will shift slightly, so as to lie off the centre of mass. Thus, someone who has a slightly curved spine, one shoulder higher than the other, or the hips and pelvis slightly tilted in an abdominal gait, will have a centre of gravity that is off-centre. These distortions may lead to disorders and diseases. The Japanese therapeutic exercise system,* Sotai, *devised by Keizo Hashimoto, is based on this perception.*[126]

> *Every freely movable joint in the body has its own characteristic range of motion, and its movements can be classified into "octants" or eight kinds of motion... These octants are anteflexion and dorsiflexion, right and left lateral flexion, right and left axial rotation, and contraction and extension by compressing or pulling on the joint.*[127]

---

126 Matsumoto, K., & Birch, S. (1988). *Hara Diagnosis: Reflections on the Sea*. Brookline: Paradigm Publications. p. 187.

127 Hashimoto, K., & Kawakami, Y. (1983). *Sotai: Balance and Health Through Natural Movement.* Tokyo: Japan Publications Inc. p. 165.

According to Dr Hashimoto, a movement never takes place in one segment only (i.e. a single joint or body region). It is not separate from the rest of the body. It spreads out as a chain, starting from one link and moving to the adjoining one, and finally covering the whole body. In this way, the distortions usually begin at the feet and then, in a chain, move from one side to the next, distorting the joints and muscles. For example, right foot distortion will manifest into the left ankle, then the right knee, then the left hip, and so on, with the body always moving away from pain, looking for its preferred position—the position of holding without pain.

As interpreted by Manaka, Sotai aims to correct left–right imbalances and adjust the octahedral structure of the body created by the Eight Extraordinary Vessels.

PRONE LEG FLEXION WITHOUT MOXA

When a movement is painful, it is just like a red light ahead. It is a warning signal to stop further movement because if continued, it could cause more complications. All one needs to do is back the movement up, and this will cure the problem.[128]

OVERVIEW

Let's start this section with a general introduction to Prone Leg Flexion (PLF), one of the most useful Sotai structural adjustments. You may notice one of the holding patterns listed above relating to the lung, liver, spleen, or kidney. In such cases, you can proceed with the first, investigative step, which is called *doshin*.

The patient lies face down, and the practitioner stands at their feet, lifting the patient's feet from the ankles to test their range of motion and leg flexion. With some people, it's easy to bring their ankles to their buttocks, but with others, there's a lack of flexion, and the ankles don't want to go that far. Most commonly, one leg is more flexible than the other.

[128] Ibid. p. 166.

Let's imagine that as you flex your patient's legs, the left side is more relaxed, and the right is more tense. Manaka suggested starting the exercise on the healthier (more flexible) left side and performing it twice, then moving to the less healthy (restricted) right side and performing it once.

The sequence starts with moving the leg passively towards the resistance (passive flexion), then moving it passively away from the resistance (passive extension). At the end of that extension, you ask the patient to actively extend for a count of three while you apply resistance, then relax. These passive and active movements are combined with focused breathing.

PRACTITIONER

As with so many aspects of JAAM, the emphasis is on being relaxed yourself. Sotai cannot be performed with strength—you need to be relaxed and gentle. As with needling, this means adopting good posture in relation to the part of the body you're treating, usually with your *hara* positioned directly in front of it so you're grounded and centred. Keep your arms and wrists loose. If they are stiff, you won't be able to assess the patient's mobility accurately; instead, you may end up forcing the ankle towards the buttocks rather than gently guiding it to assess resistance.

You'll need to develop a set of toolbox phrases to explain this procedure, just as you did for *kyutoshin*. The patient must understand their role. In the first part of the exercise, they are passive, allowing you to flex and extend the leg. In the second part, they actively extend the leg, so they need guidance on how much force to apply. Some patients are very tentative, while others think you want them to kick you across the room. To keep the movement slow and controlled, try resting your hand lightly on the leg and asking them to 'follow your hand'. At the final stage, encourage them to 'meet your resistance', using just enough force to lift the knee off the table without straining.

DEFINING *DOSHIN*

Before starting Sotai, you need to get a baseline reading to know what you're treating and how it will change. This assessment procedure is called *doshin*:

- Note any asymmetries between the left and right sides.
- Check the general structural imbalance.
- Find restricted ranges of motion.

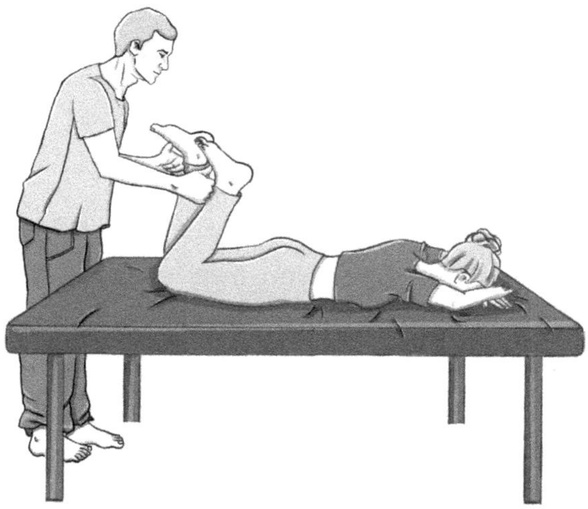

Figure 9-1: Doshin—testing range of motion.

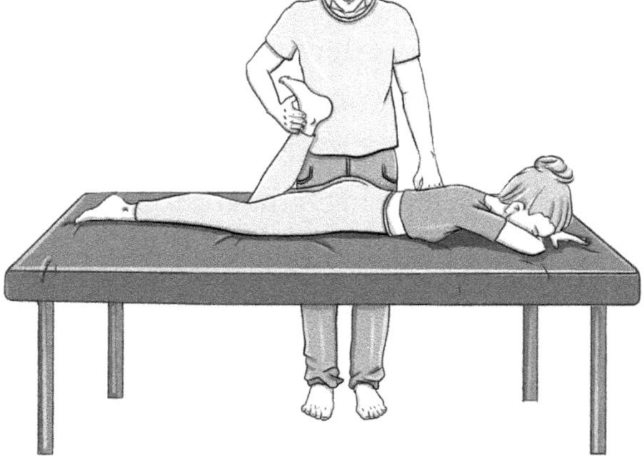

Figure 9-2: Passive stretch to the point of resistance.

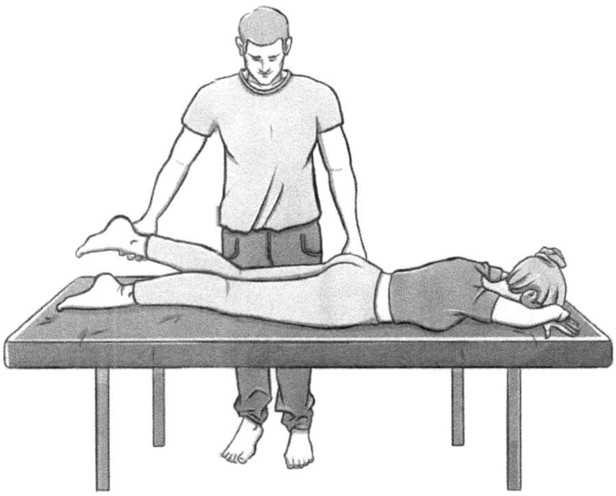

Figure 9-3: The patient pushes against resistance.

STEP-BY-STEP PROCEDURE

For this exercise, the patient lies face down, with their feet level with the edge of the treatment table. Stand at their feet and place your hands around the ST 41 area.

1. ***Doshin*:** With the patient lying prone, lift both legs from the ankles to assess the range of motion in Prone Leg Flexion. Compare how easily each leg flexes towards the buttocks, noting which side feels more restricted. At the same time, observe asymmetries in the paraspinal musculature—for example, one side appearing tighter, raised, or more swollen than the other, as we noted earlier with liver–spleen imbalances.
2. **Begin on the flexible side:** In Manaka's system, the exercise is first performed on the more flexible side. After two repetitions there, move to the restricted side for one repetition.
3. **Breathing and movement:** Ask the patient to inhale as you flex the leg towards the buttocks, bringing it to the point of restriction. Then ask them to exhale as you slowly extend the leg away from the restriction. Your script is *"Breathe in"* as you flex towards resistance, then *"Breathe out"* as you extend slowly towards the horizontal.

Make sure the leg feels supported, with your hand above the ankle. Just before full extension, ask the patient to push lightly against your hand while you resist. Cue them to keep exhaling as they press for a count of three, then release: *"Press gently—one, two, three... relax."* If they run out of breath, they can hold it during the count and exhale again on release.

4. **Reassess:** Recheck mobility. Working the looser side first often increases flexibility on the tighter side, reducing left–right asymmetries.
5. **Repeat:** Perform the sequence twice on the flexible side and once on the restricted side, checking after each cycle. The goal is to increase the range of motion on both sides and, ideally, equalise them.

OTHER POINTS

- Unlike osteopathy or chiropractic, power and speed are not required.
- Keep all movements light and comfortable; avoid anything that feels tiring or painful.
- If the point of resistance produces pain in the lower back, hip, or knee, do not use this exercise.
- There is no fixed rhythm or pace—the priority is to follow the patient's breath.

PRONE LEG FLEXION WITH MOXA

Manaka modified Hashimoto's protocol by adding direct moxa. The *Ling Shu* describes how the Fire Needle can treat the *jinjing* (sinew channels) and help the muscles relax. Manaka exploited the properties of direct moxa for the same objective, using small moxa cones over stiff muscles.

Once you are familiar with PLF without moxa and feel comfortable with your *doshin* and basic treatment sequence, you can graduate to Manaka's first variation. This involves applying a small moxa cone around the BL 18 area on the same side while the patient pushes against your resistance.

OVERVIEW

Once again, let's look at the sequence in broad strokes, then in detailed steps. It works like this. In addition to the *doshin* above, you're going to identify a PPP around BL 18 on the same side as the leg you're treating. Once identified, place a small cone of moxa on it (to learn how to apply moxa, see Chapter 13).

There are several things to consider here. The Sotai sequence is exactly as above, but now, instead of simply counting to three, you light the moxa at the same time as you ask the patient to push against your resistance. Your command to relax comes at the same time as you extinguish the moxa. Ideally, the patient will feel a tiny gnat's bite of sensation from the heat of the cone just as you say, "Relax".

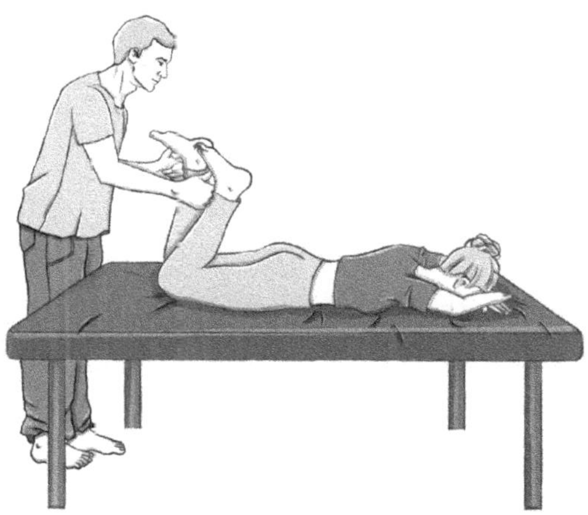

Figure 9-4: Doshin—testing range of motion.

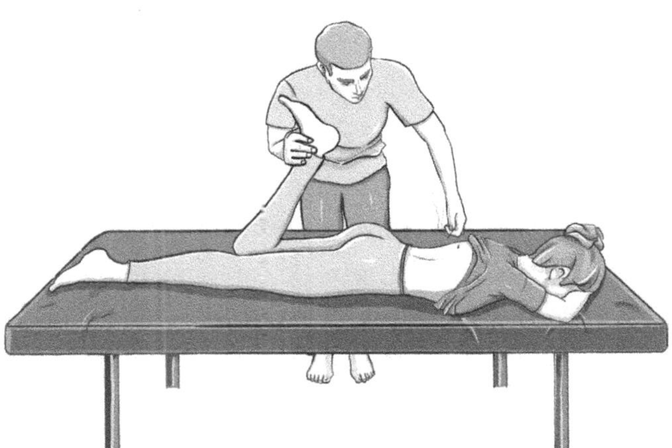

Figure 9-5: Use a longer rice grain of moxa and light on reaching the point of resistance.

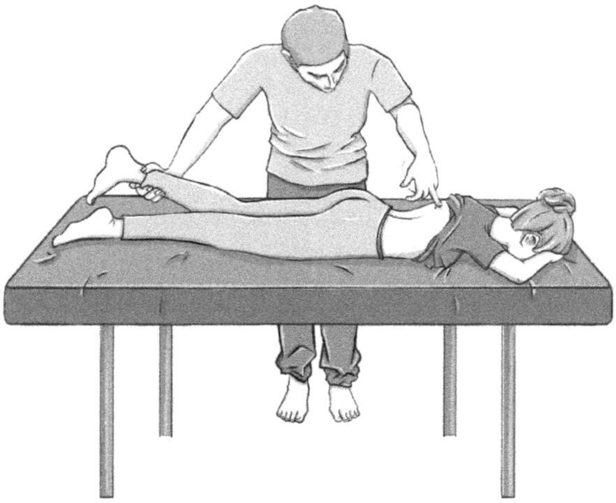

Figure 9-6: Say "Relax" as you extinguish the moxa.

STEP-BY-STEP PROCEDURE

1. ***Doshin*:** With the patient lying prone, lift both legs from the ankles to assess the range of motion in Prone Leg Flexion. Compare how easily each leg flexes towards the buttocks, noting which side feels more restricted. At the same time, observe asymmetries in the paraspinal musculature—for example, one side appearing tighter, raised, or more swollen than the other, as we noted earlier with liver–spleen imbalances. Identify a PPP around BL 18 on the same side as the leg you will treat.
2. **Begin on the flexible side:** In Manaka's system, the exercise is first performed on the more flexible side. Roll a small cone of moxa (about 2–4 mm, depending on your dexterity) and place it on the most reactive PPP near BL 18 on the side of the leg you're treating. Perform the exercise twice on the flexible side, then move to the restricted side for one repetition.

    Breathing, movement, and moxa: Ask the patient to inhale as you flex the leg towards the buttocks, bringing it to the point of restriction. Then ask them to exhale as you slowly extend the leg away from the restriction. Your script is *"Breathe in"* as you flex towards resistance, then *"Breathe out"* as you extend slowly towards the horizontal.

Make sure the leg feels supported, with your hand above the ankle. Light the cone of moxa. Just before full extension, ask the patient to push lightly against your hand while you resist. Cue them to keep exhaling as they press for a count of three, or until they feel the heat of the cone. Say: *"Press gently—one, two, three... relax,"* extinguishing the moxa at the exact moment you give the cue to relax.

It's much easier to light a long cone of moxa when you've just reached the point of resistance than to light a smaller cone as you're moving the leg or when the patient is pushing against your resistance.

3. **Reassess:** Recheck mobility. Working the looser side first often increases flexibility on the tighter side, reducing left–right asymmetries. The addition of direct moxa typically enhances this effect, particularly when the paraspinal muscles are stubbornly tight.
4. **Repeat:** Perform the sequence twice on the flexible side and once on the restricted side, checking after each cycle. The goal is to increase the range of motion on both sides and, ideally, equalise them.

AETIOLOGY

> *As a child, I always turned my head away from the page when writing, instead of looking at it directly. This eventually turned out to be because I had better vision in one eye than the other, so I was compensating by turning my best eye to the page. Even when I got glasses, it took a long time to correct that instinctive tilt of the head when writing.*
>
> —Oran Kivity

Structural imbalances may arise from many causes, including:

- Organ disease; for example, liver problems leading to right hypochondriac tension
- Old injuries and scars
- Favouring one hand or foot

- Activities or sports that over-emphasise one side (e.g. golf, using a mouse, working in a supermarket checkout)
- Biased muscle tone in the neck from unbalanced vision
- Hearing with compensatory postural adjustments leading to muscular and skeletal structural changes
- Right–left differences in the bite of teeth
- Imbalances due to footwear, such as high heels
- Extended use of one limb or part of the body; for example, students carrying heavy books or laptops on one side only
- Changes due to ageing

Aetiology may also include poor dietary and lifestyle habits (such as repeated exposure to cold without adequate clothing), congenital abnormalities of the skeleton, structural abnormalities from injury or disease, and poor posture, both habitual and occupational.

BALANCING THE WHOLE

Not all stiffness is pathological. Sometimes when postural muscles tighten on one side of the back, the stiffness is compensating for weakness or lack of tone on the other side, often linked to internal problems. While Hashimoto emphasised working on the stiff side, Manaka modified the method to begin on the more flexible side. This approach avoids destabilising useful compensations and often restores balance more smoothly. The key is not to correct stiffness unthinkingly but to understand its function—whether it's pathological or compensatory—and adapt Step 3 accordingly.

Step 3 should be adapted to the needs of each patient. For many, it will not be necessary at all. For some, it can be applied as a mild stimulation without moxa, while for others it can be increased in strength, either alone or in combination with moxa.

For sensitive patients, Sotai alone is often sufficient. Adding *okyu* can enhance the effect, especially when the back muscles are tight and resistant. In cases of blood stasis, combining Sotai with moxa usually produces the most effective release. For robust patients, this combined method can be remarkably powerful in correcting long-held structural imbalances.

PLF is the first of several Sotai routines that Manaka adapted and arguably the most useful. It releases the whole bladder meridian; in other words, all the posterior muscle chains from the neck to the ankles.

Since the bladder meridian links the back-*shu* points to the whole body and the organs, applying PLF may have many more profound effects on the overall health of the body and symptoms.

Step 3 can be invaluable in augmenting the root treatment. Stubborn abdominal reactions will start to change when you add structural adjustment to Steps 1 and 2, which in turn can help improve the overall health of the patient.

Manaka also proposed variations, even for this simple PLF, notably using his wooden needle and hammer, which we will look at in subsequent books.

IN PRACTICE: STEP 3—STORIES FROM THE CLINIC

We return to our three patients—Christine, David, and Margaret—to follow their progress into Step 3 treatment. Once again, each instalment begins with a short recap of their Step 1 and 2 presentations and treatments, before showing how their cases unfolded at Step 3.

These cases are real, not constructed for teaching purposes. And tellingly, only one of them was treated with Sotai. As Stephen Birch observes, he uses Sotai in only about one in ten patients. That ratio itself is instructive: Step 3 is an option, not a requirement.

CASE STUDY 1: SCIATIC PAIN

Christine, Female, 56

- **Chief complaint:** Right-sided sciatic pain, disturbed sleep
- **Notes:** History of migraines and old auto-accident injury; age-related abdominal hypotonia
- **Diagnosis:** Ren Dai (right-belt) (dominant right-sided Dai Mai reaction; Mixed Yin milder)

Step 1: Ren Dai (right-belt) with IPC (10 minutes)
Step 2: *Chishin* with infrared (FIR) lamp on BL 23, BL 26, and lateral to BL 27 (mid-gluteal point)
Step 3: None

PRACTITIONER NOTE

If Step 3 had been considered for Christine, PLF with moxa would have been the most likely choice. Her sciatic pain and history suggested blood stagnation, which would lead us to select Sotai with moxa rather than Sotai alone.

CASE STUDY 2: NECK PAIN POST-WEIGHTLIFTING INJURY

David, Male, 39

- **Chief complaint:** Chronic right lateral neck pain with swelling between GB 9 and GB 10, radiating at times to the right shoulder and face
- **Notes:** Old weightlifting injury (8 years earlier); background pain rated 5/10 daily, rising to 8+/10 under stress
- **Diagnosis:** YWD

Step 1: YWD with IPC (10 minutes)
Step 2: BL 19, BL 22 with infrared (FIR) lamp.
Step 3: N/A

PRACTITIONER NOTE

No Step 3 treatment was applied in David's case.

CASE STUDY 3: HIP DEGENERATION AND CHRONIC PAIN

Margaret, Female, 60

- **Chief complaint:** Chronic right lumbar and groin pain with hip joint degeneration; constant deep pain disturbing sleep and mobility
- **Notes:** History of lumbar fusion (L4–L5) with severe scarring; multiple cortisone injections with no relief; pain relieved by movement, pressure, and heat
- **Diagnosis:** YQR

Step 1: YQR with IPC (15 minutes)
Step 2: *Kyutoshin*—2 balls on GB 30, GB 31, GB 26
Step 3: Sotai—Prone Leg Flexion (PLF) and Waist Rotation (this Sotai for the waist will be covered in Vol. 2)

PRACTITIONER NOTE

PLF is commonly used for back and hip pain, as it releases the whole posterior chain. Sotai routines can also be combined: there is no rule limiting you to one. The second, Waist Rotation, involves sitting the patient upright and rotating the torso away from the restricted side against resistance. This Sotai will be covered in Vol. 2.

[Note: These cases are continued in the Step 4 instalment.]

SUMMARY

- **Purpose of Step 3:** Structural adjustment is the third step in Manaka's Four Step protocol. It targets musculoskeletal imbalances that impede function and may reinforce abdominal reactions.
- **Sotai basics:** Sotai is a gentle 'stretch and resist' therapy combining movement with breath, always moving *away* from pain. Manaka integrated Sotai into TEAM and further adapted it by combining it with *okyu* (direct moxa), creating what may have been the first moxibustion–bodywork method.
- **Indications:** Step 3 is not for every patient. It is reserved for clear structural asymmetries (e.g. uneven shoulders or pelvis, leg-length discrepancies, spinal curvature).
- **Spectrum of application:** Step 3 ranges from no intervention at all, to mild Sotai without moxa for sensitive patients, to Sotai with *okyu* for robust patients with long-held imbalances or signs of blood stasis.
- **Prone Leg Flexion (PLF):** A core Sotai exercise releasing the entire posterior chain. Can be performed without moxa or with Manaka's variation using *okyu* at BL 18.
- **Clinical nuance:** Sometimes stiffness is compensatory. Beginning on the flexible side avoids destabilising useful adaptations and often balances tone more effectively.
- **Case lessons:** In practice, Sotai is used selectively—Stephen Birch reports using it in roughly one in ten patients. Only Margaret received Step 3 but Sotai might well have been used on the other two patients had there been evidence of structural imbalance.

WHAT'S NEXT

After Steps 1–3 comes symptom relief. In the next chapter, we'll see how Manaka used ear and hand microsystems in Step 4, applying 'takeaway' needles such as press spheres, press tacks, and intradermals to relieve symptoms and extend treatment beyond the clinic.

CHAPTER 10

STEP 4: BRANCH TREATMENT WITH ISOPHASAL SYSTEMS AND JAPANESE TAKEAWAY NEEDLES

We've now arrived at the final stage of Manaka's Four Step protocol. By this point, patients may still have a list of symptoms from A to Z they hope you can relieve. As practitioners, we all bring our own favourite methods for tackling problems from amenorrhoea to zinc deficiency—and it can feel tempting to reach straight for them here in Step 4.

Dr Manaka, however, approached this stage with caution. His choice of symptomatic treatments was guided not only by his medical knowledge but also by his sense of the patient's circumstances, his assessment of prognosis, and—crucially—his understanding of dosage. Too strong a dose risks undoing the balance achieved in the earlier steps. This is such an important issue that we've dedicated an entire chapter to it (see Chapter 15). We may not have Manaka's decades of experience, but we can follow his principles: always tailor the treatment to the individual.

Steps 1–3, done well, provide a gentle yet effective foundation that allows the body's regulatory systems to help the body heal itself. Step 4 builds on this foundation—not by overwhelming the body with symptom relief, but by adding carefully chosen branch treatments that match both the dosage of the earlier steps and the underlying pathology. For example, *okyu* can support the immune system, ease inflammation, and improve circulation; shallow needling may soften tense muscles better than strong stimulation; and when blood stasis is more pronounced, cupping or even bloodletting may be appropriate.

For this reason, we encourage you to prioritise Manaka's Step 4 methods over your own. They are often surprisingly effective. If they don't bring the results you want within the expected timeframe, you can always return to your familiar repertoire of branch techniques.

In this chapter, we'll explore Manaka's unique approach to pain relief. We'll see how he used *isophasal* points across *micro-acupuncture* systems such as the hand and ear, and how he integrated these into one coherent clinical method.

In this chapter, we will cover:

- Isophasal systems
- Takeaway needles
- Mapping the body on the hand
- Mapping the body on the ear
- Clinical procedures
- Diverging contemporary approaches

In Part 2, we will look at moxibustion, another powerful way to address the branch.

HOLOGRAPHIC METAPHORS AND ISOPHASAL SOLUTIONS

> *Holography is the study of three-dimensional images created using light waves that interfere with each other. The image created is called a "hologram".*[129]

In Chasing the Dragon's Tail, Manaka explored contemporary holographic theories and how they might relate to acupuncture and TEAM. For example, he discussed the physicist David Bohm's theories that in order to explain observed facts, it could be useful to envision the universe as a hologram:

[129] Manaka, Y., Itaya, K., & Birch, S. (1995). *Chasing the Dragon's Tail: The Theory and Practice of Acupuncture in the Work of Yoshio Manaka*. Brookline: Paradigm Publications. p. xviii.

> *Most of what is, is not perceivable or measurable; it is hidden or enfolded in space. The perceivable and measurable world, the world that our senses detect, is like the ripples on an ocean where everything beneath this surface is hidden from us, and all parts are derived from this ocean.*[130]

Manaka thought this model, where all parts of the whole contain images of the whole, could be a helpful tool to develop a framework and language for understanding important aspects of acupuncture and East Asian medicine.

Bohm explained that his theory of the "hidden or implicate order" gives us a way of describing hidden or enfolded structures in the body, such as those described in the medical theories of China.[131]

One of the fundamental ideas of Chinese thought is that humans occupy the physical space between heaven and earth. Chinese medicine assumes a unity between each organism and its environment, between inner and outer; this philosophy of unity is described as Heaven, Earth, and Humanity in Harmony.[132]

It is from these ideas that we can begin to understand holographic theory: the idea that every small part of the body contains the information of the whole. A hologram can be understood as "a three-dimensional image of a given object which contains the information of the object in itself and in every part of itself".[133]

This holographic metaphor can be a valuable tool for understanding the various micro-acupuncture systems that have been developed, assuming that each part of the body is a connected microcosm of the whole. The auricular micro-acupuncture system is a well-known example of this kind of small part–whole body correspondence system.

---

130 Ibid. p. xix.

131 Ibid. p. xix.

132 McCann, H., & Ross, H. (2015). *Practical Atlas of Tung's Acupuncture*. Germany: Verlag Muller & Steinicke. p. 17.

133 Dale, R. (1999). 'The Systems, Holograms and Theory of Micro-Acupuncture', *American Journal of Acupuncture*, 27(3–4). pp. 207–242.

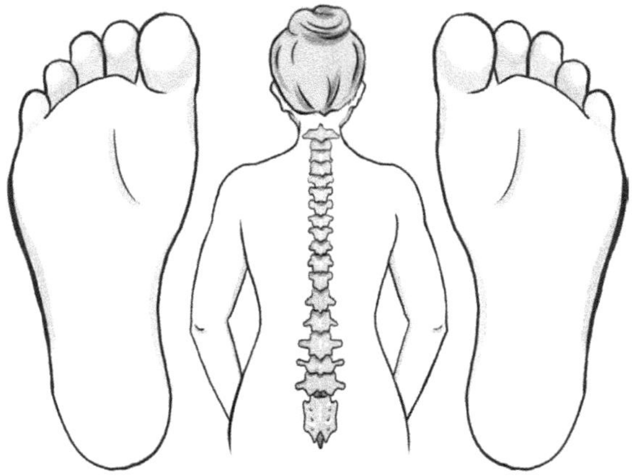

Figure 10-1: Reflexology is the best-known body correspondence system of all: your feet reflect your body.

Perhaps the best-known body correspondence system of all is reflexology, in which the feet are said to reflect the entire body. In Asia, reflexology salons are found in every mall and high street, with practitioners claiming—sometimes more accurately than others—to diagnose problems by identifying painful points on the feet. In the mapping in Figure 10-1, the toes reflect the upper body, the heels the lower body, and the two medial surfaces of the feet, when placed together, reflect the midline and spine.

> *How can we understand the various simple and complex systems of reflexology?... As we have already suggested, if we consider the theories of the holographic paradigm, where all aspects of the whole reflect or contain all other parts of the whole, as descriptive of part of the signal system, we can begin to see how such systems may work. These reflex points and areas are able to receive and send very specific information to specific areas of the body.*[134]

Less well-known to the public are the body correspondence systems taught in every acupuncture school. We observe the tongue daily. Its tip corresponds to the upper burner, the middle to the digestive organs of the middle burner, and the root to the elimination organs of the lower burner. Once again, the trinity of Heaven, Humanity, and Earth is reflected in the three burners.

---

134 Manaka, Y., Itaya, K., & Birch, S. (1995). *Chasing the Dragon's Tail: The Theory and Practice of Acupuncture in the Work of Yoshio Manaka*. Brookline: Paradigm Publications. p. 34.

Another microsystem, accessed through palpation, is the pulse. It is taken in three positions—upper, middle, and lower—often seen to correspond to the upper, middle, and lower parts of the body.

Two other familiar yet unsung body correspondence systems are the front-*mu* point and back-*shu* point groupings. Unlike the ear, which is a miniaturised acupuncture reflection of the body, the back-*shu* points operate on a one-to-one scale. The upper points reflect and treat the upper body; the middle points, the middle body; and the lower points, the lower body. Anatomically, they are said to represent the organ-meridian systems and can be used both diagnostically and therapeutically.[135] The back-*shu* points can be thought of as a conceptual bridge between traditional acupuncture ideas and more modern body correspondence mappings.[136]

Some microsystem correspondences, such as the tongue, are diagnostic or therapeutic, while others are used only for treatment.

The first micro-acupuncture system to be fully popularised was that of the ear, developed by Paul Nogier in the 1950s. The ear is said to contain a miniaturised system of acupuncture points that can treat the whole body. It is worth mentioning, however, that an earlier twentieth-century pioneer of body correspondence mappings in the field of acupuncture was Kurakichi Hirata in Japan, who created an entire system of Hirata Zones in the 1930s, which he treated with a heated needle, some twenty years before Nogier.[137]

Further investigations have led to the discovery and development of many different systems. The list is extraordinary; diagnosis and treatment mappings have been developed on the scalp, face, nose, philtrum, lips, hands, fingers, wrists and ankles, and feet. Each one asserts the same principle of correspondence between macro-anatomy and the topography of the microsystems.

---

135 Dale, R. (1999). 'The Systems, Holograms and Theory of Micro-Acupuncture', *American Journal of Acupuncture*, 27(3–4). pp. 207–242.

136 Hecker, H., Steveling, A., & Peuker, E. (2005). *Microsystems Acupuncture: The Complete Guide: Ear–Scalp–Mouth–Hand*. Stuttgart: Thieme. p. xiv.

137 Kivity, O. (2021). *Hirata Zone Therapy with the Ontake Method: Repurposing the Lost Art of Japanese Dermatome Moxibustion for Contemporary Practice*. London: Sayoshi Books.

DR MANAKA'S ISOPHASAL TREATMENTS

> *We have already suggested that the mechanism behind these microsystems may be holographic; if so, perhaps there is some relationship between the holographic paradigm and isophasality.*[138]

While studying these correspondence systems—both modern and traditional, such as the Five Phases—Manaka coined a novel term to capture the apparent relationships between different parts of the body.

Borrowing once again from modern physics, he used the term *isophasal* to describe these correspondences. For example, the wood points on the twelve meridians are isophasal with one another and with the liver meridian and organ; the liver point in the ear is isophasal with the meridian and organ; and the neck point in the ear is isophasal with both the corresponding point in foot reflexology and the neck itself.

Manaka's new language embraces both traditional and modern correspondence systems and places them within the larger X-signal system explanations that draw on the holographic metaphor. In *Chasing the Dragon's Tail*, he attempted to establish these isophasal connections through his testing methods. As potential components of the X-signal system, they remain somewhat inexplicable (the *X* of the X-signal). Still, they can be described and tested in ways that enable practical applications.

Manaka found three body correspondence systems especially useful: ear acupuncture, Korean hand acupuncture, and Hirata's zone or dermatome mapping system. As Hirata Zone Therapy lies beyond the scope of this book, in this chapter we will focus on the remaining two—the hand and the ear micro-acupuncture systems—and how Manaka applied them in treatment.

When one point alone did not achieve the desired result, Manaka discovered that combining similar points from different systems could be more effective. When treating

---

[138] Manaka, Y., Itaya, K., & Birch, S. (1995). *Chasing the Dragon's Tail: The Theory and Practice of Acupuncture in the Work of Yoshio Manaka*. Brookline: Paradigm Publications. pp. xxxii, 19, 24, 35, 91.

hip pain, for example, he often found it helpful to apply an intradermal needle not only to a reactive point on the hip, but also to a reactive point on the ear corresponding to the hip and a reactive point on the hand system corresponding to the hip. These points have the same 'resonance,' 'signature,' or 'phase'—what he called *isophasal*.

> *Treating three points in an isophasal relationship addresses both the general condition and local disorders, especially acute pain.*[139]

Although Manaka specifically described this type of isophasal three-point treatment using the body–ear–hand, the use of any one of these correspondence systems on its own—such as Chinese ear acupuncture or Korean hand acupuncture—also constitutes a treatment that exploits isophasal relationships.

Thus, he could use up to three needles, selecting a local point, a point on the ear, and one on the hand. Moreover, he used a specialised kind of retained needle, the *hinaishin* or intradermal needle. This needle is taped to the skin and left in place for several days at a time, a non-edible Japanese takeaway, thus inspiring the name of this chapter.

During his clinic visits to Japan in 1986 and 1988, Stephen Birch observed that Manaka used intradermals exclusively, because they were highly effective and because Manaka believed they were tolerated much better than the other two types. When you're leaving a needle in place for a week, how it is tolerated, safety concerns, and dosage are all critical considerations. The old-style *empishin* or press tack needles have significant health risks associated with them, which we will discuss below, and Manaka stated unequivocally that they should never be used on the ears.

It is, however, more than thirty-five years since Dr Manaka's death in 1989, and needle technology has changed. In particular, press tacks are now made in much smaller gauges and lengths than ever before, so they are tolerated better than those available to Manaka. This development allows us to reassess his previous reliance on intradermals. For this reason, as teachers, our approaches have all diverged. Hence, the function of this chapter is to show the theory behind Manaka's approach and allow the authors to describe their individual preferences and choices in their practices.

---

139 Ibid. p. 180.

Manaka's system has been used in the West for almost forty years and has evolved to include not just intradermal needles but other kinds of treatment tools that are taped on the skin, including:

- Press spheres (*ryu*): These have been available for decades.
- Press tacks (*empishin*): The type from Seirin in Figure 10-3 has been available since the early 2000s. Its design eliminates the risks associated with the old-style press tack needles and offers significant control over the dose of stimulation (see below).

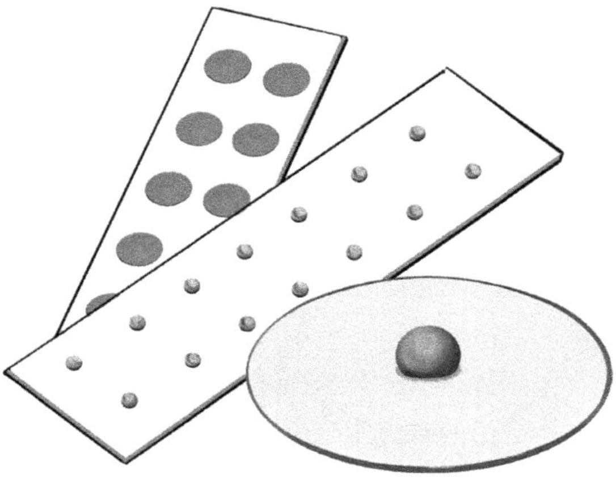

Figure 10-2: Press spheres (ryu).

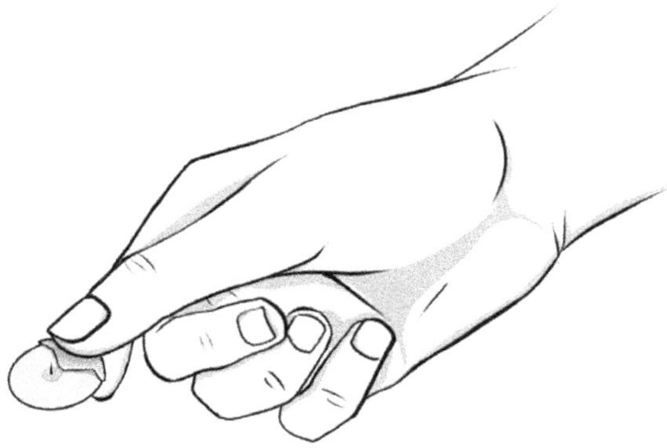

Figure 10-3: Press tacks (empishin)—now available in much smaller sizes than in Manaka's day.

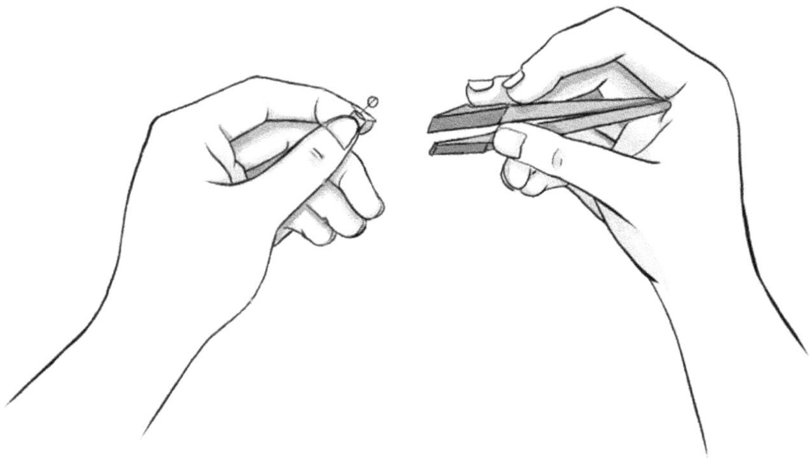

Figure 10-4: Intradermals (hinaishin)—Manaka's first choice when treating isophasally.

GENERAL PROCEDURE FOR PAIN RELIEF

Using Manaka's isophasal approach is straightforward. In addition to changes in pressure pain at the treatment points, it's helpful to have a second feedback mechanism. For pain relief, use reduction in pain and/or improved mobility as your measure.

Before locating a treatment point—local or isophasal—begin with a range of motion (ROM) test. For example, with shoulder pain, ask the patient to abduct the arm and note the range. You can also ask them to rate their pain on a 0–10 scale.

- **Unilateral symptoms**: Search on the symptomatic side.
- **Bilateral symptoms**: Choose the most sensitive points, regardless of side.
- **Multiple systems**: Your prescription may involve contralateral points.

For unilateral symptoms, search the system—such as the ear—on the same side as the symptom. For bilateral symptoms, examine both sides and use the most sensitive points, whichever side they are on. If you are using more than one isophasal system, your prescription may include contralateral points; for example, one on the left ear and one on the right hand.

When searching, begin with a visual inspection of the relevant microsystem. For example, in the case of back pain, examine the lumbar region on the ear. Effective reflex points often show discolouration, dryness, or swelling. In the ear, the cartilage is usually more rigid, and the area is tender when squeezed between thumb and finger, even before you start to search more specifically for reactive points.

Next, palpate the area with a blunt probe or the rounded end of a *teishin* (a ball-tipped probe used for contact needling in JAAM: see Figure 3-1). Look for a pressure pain response. The small surface area of the probe tip is better for eliciting a response than your fingertip.

When you think you have found it, press it with the *teishin* or a blunt probe. Then, test the same movement again. There should be a significant improvement in pain and mobility. If there is no change, try another.

Just like the live points we've discussed in previous chapters, the effective point may not correspond precisely with the mapping location, and there may be several candidate pressure pain points. Test each for effect.

Once you've identified a point with a clear impact on pain or range of motion, insert one of the three types of takeaway device: *ryu*, *hinaishin*, or *empishin*. A further improvement should follow insertion. In the next section, we'll look in detail at each of these three types and how to apply them effectively.

PRESS SPHERES, PRESS TACKS, AND INTRADERMALS

PRESS SPHERES: *RYU*

Ryu are generally used for branch treatment and can easily be applied to microsystem points to relieve pain; for example, placing one on the lumbar point of the ear to ease back pain. They can also be used to support root treatment; for instance, if someone is being treated for kidney meridian problems, *ryu* may be left at BL 23.

APPLICATION

Ryu are simple to use. Firstly, locate a tender point and check that pressing on it brings relief; for example, an improved range of motion. If so, tape the *ryu* onto that point.

Traditionally, tweezers are used to handle the plaster, but you can also use a *teishin*. Attach the adhesive part of the *ryu* to the tapered tail of a *teishin*, then use the other rounded head to press, test, and confirm the point. This pressure may leave an indentation. Once you're sure of the point, flip the *teishin* and apply the *ryu* precisely on the indentation.

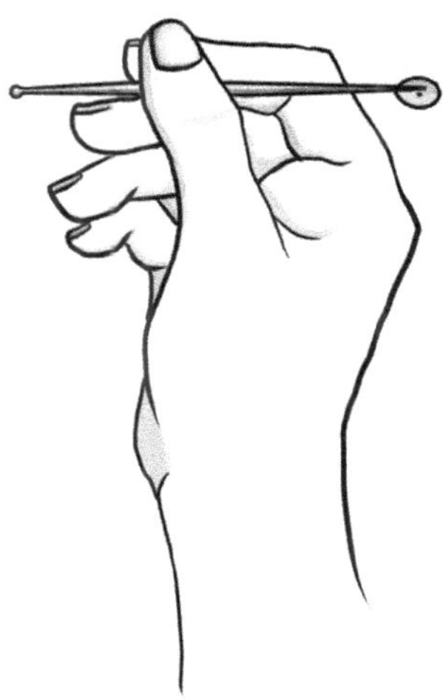

Figure 10-5: Ryu on the sharp end of a teishin.

EAR SEEDS AND DIFFERENT METALS

Some readers may wonder whether ear seeds can be substituted for *ryu*. Superficially, they appear similar, but there are significant differences. Seeds such as vaccaria or mustard exert pressure like *ryu*, but they also have a chemical, vesicatory action that is quite different.

By contrast, steel press spheres (in particular, gold-plated or silver-plated press spheres) are designed to be hypoallergenic, which is the opposite intention to using plant seeds with irritant qualities like mustard. This hypoallergenic quality is important because skin reactions overstimulate the point and surrounding area, risking overtreatment. In

Japanese thinking, the goal is to control dosage precisely, not provoke an uncontrolled reaction—quite the reverse of the rationale for mustard seeds. Moreover, press spheres may exert electrical effects, as we saw with ion pumping, and so are likely "talking" to the X-signal regulatory system.

These electrical effects raise another issue. Gold-plated press spheres (*ryu*) are commonly used because gold tends to cause fewer skin reactions than other metals. However, there is a crucial rule to observe: if you retain gold *ryu* on a patient, you should not combine it with other retained tools made of different metals, such as silver-plated or stainless steel *ryu,* or *empishin* or *hinaishin*.

Combining metals is used intentionally in JAAM—for example, on the master and coupled points of the Eight Extras—but done in a controlled way. Retaining takeaway needles made of different metals without that intention may create unexpected polarities and undesirable reactions. This principle was first noted by Manaka, and it has been strongly reinforced by Stephen Birch, who says simply, "Do not do this!"

For these reasons, as well as concerns about dosage, we recommend avoiding traditional ear seeds and sticking to the three treatment tools outlined here.

TOLERATION AND REACTIONS

Ryu are usually well tolerated, but patients should be firmly advised to remove them after four days. A small minority may find one, two, or all of the points uncomfortable. In such cases, they should be removed immediately. Reactions can include a bruised sensation in the ear or local skin irritation from the plaster or the sphere. This irritation delivers a higher dose of treatment than planned. It may cause a worsening of symptoms or new symptoms such as stiff shoulders, headaches, or fatigue. For more on the complex issue of dosage, see Chapter 15.

Particularly on the ear, the constant pressure of the ball may cause a small indentation sore. While the risk is low, infection is possible—especially in immunocompromised patients. Infections of the ear that penetrate to the cartilage are difficult to treat, as the cartilage has poor blood circulation and antibiotics do not reach it effectively.

In some acupuncture traditions, patients are advised to press on the takeaways for extra stimulation. We strongly recommend against this. Both for reasons of safety and dosage, patients should never press on any of the tools we use: *ryu* (press spheres), *empishin* (press tacks), or *hinaishin* (intradermals).

Finally, in humid weather, the ball and tape can oxidise. After extended wear, the glue breaks down into a slimy residue, and the whole assembly begins to look unhygienic. This is especially common among patients who ignore your instructions (see the Golden Rules below) and return weeks later with their *ryu* still in place.

PRESS TACKS: *EMPISHIN*

An *empishin* (press tack) is a tiny needle, resembling a miniature drawing pin, that is inserted vertically and taped in place on the body (see Figure 10-3). *Empishin* come in various sizes and can be applied almost anywhere. They are particularly useful for pain control, especially on local points; for example, to treat elbow pain, apply one to the most painful pressure point on the elbow.

In Manaka's time, the technology for manufacturing *empishin* was relatively undeveloped and the needles were longer. Although some Japanese practitioners did use *empishin* on the ear, Manaka advised against it, warning that piercing the cartilage risks infection. The older, longer types fall into this category, and we strongly recommend they not be used on the ear.

Today, however, the new Pyonex press tacks from Seirin—unavailable in Manaka's time—offer a safer alternative. The smallest sizes, orange and yellow (0.3 and 0.6 mm), are so fine and short they can be used on the ear without risk of penetrating the cartilage. The longer sizes (0.9, 1.2, and 1.5 mm) remain unsuitable for the ear but can be applied almost anywhere else on the body, except the soles of the feet.

The procedures described in this chapter refer specifically to the new Pyonex press tacks, not other brands or types.

APPLICATION

Firstly, look for a pressure pain reaction and mark the point with a pen. It's better to mark the location with two small dots of ink on either side, rather than directly on the point, since ink is not sterile. Alternatively, you can indent the point with the blunt end of a *teishin*. Once marked, wipe the area with alcohol.

The new generation of Pyonex press tacks comes with a convenient paper tab for handling during insertion, which means you can hold it easily in your fingers and insert it without tweezers. When placing the needle, keep your wrist and shoulders relaxed. Aim for fast insertion with firm pressure and loose wrists—this combination keeps discomfort to a minimum.

TOLERATION AND REACTIONS

The needle side of the *empishin* faces downward, while the reverse side, which contains the plastic sphere that forms the handle, creates a slight bulge under the plaster. Because of this protruding shape, care must be taken with the choice of site. If they are placed on areas like the hands, they are more likely to be knocked or pulled off, for example, when patients put their hands in their pockets.

Needling a point with an *empishin* delivers a stronger dose of treatment than the acupressure provided by a *ryu*. Reactions are rare and may include local soreness or slight skin irritation from the plaster. If a patient experiences a sharp, pricking sensation, the *empishin* should be removed immediately. The same Golden Rules apply, and it is your duty of care to ensure patients understand them and feel confident about removing the needles themselves.

For Manaka's isophasal treatments, use a single *empishin* on the ear and the local point. Treat the hand with the appropriate tool if necessary (see the discussion on diverse contemporary approaches at the end of this chapter).

INTRADERMAL NEEDLES: *HINAISHIN*

Hinaishin (intradermal needles) were invented in the 1950s by the renowned Japanese acupuncturist Kobei Akabane. Intradermals (ID) may be used in various ways: to reinforce a root treatment or to balance left and right meridians, as Akabane did. In this chapter, they are used to relieve specific conditions by providing continuous stimulation of acupuncture points over a period of days.

Hinaishin differ from regular needles in several ways. They are usually 3 mm or 6 mm long and are designed with a ring-shaped handle that prevents them from penetrating deeper into the body. They are taped in place and retained for up to one week (see Figure 10-4).

Hinaishin are available from a wide range of manufacturers, though not always in the two sizes above.

GENERAL

- The insertion is transverse and very shallow. *Hinaishin* lie approximately between the skin and the superficial fascia.
- There should be no awareness of the needle.
- The dosage is minimal, but the signal continues over an extended time.

EQUIPMENT

Hinaishin require a few extra pieces of ancillary equipment. In addition to your standard alcohol wipes, marking pen, or *teishin*, you will need:

- Flat-headed tweezers
- Blunt-headed scissors
- Micropore tape, both white and skin-toned
- Headband lamp (optional)

Most cosmetic tweezers are designed for plucking eyebrow hairs, but for holding the end of an intradermal, it's worth selecting flat-headed tweezers that have a large grasping surface at the tip.

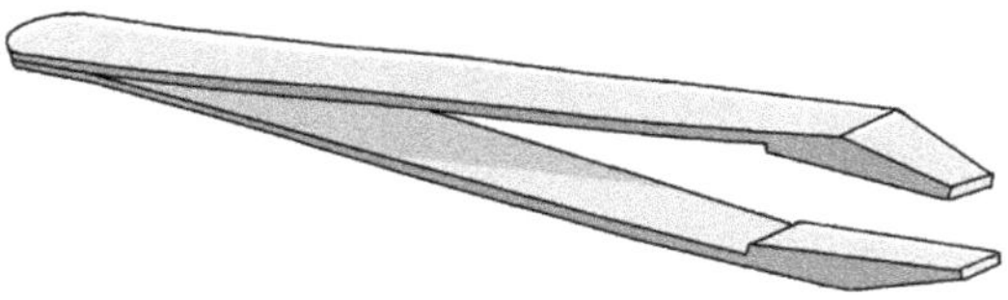

Figure 10-6: Flat-headed tweezers with a large grasping surface at the tip.

Cosmetic shops also provide blunt-headed scissors that are suitable for trimming ear or nostril hair. They can be useful for cutting dressings without the risk of scratching the skin.

Use hypoallergenic micropore tape. In modern times, it seems that an increasing number of patients have sensitive skin. They may react more to the micropore than the needle. It's also worth having a selection of tape colours. White micropore is cheaper and can be used on areas that are hidden, but if the point is visible, it's better to use the more expensive skin-toned tape. You can use a narrow-width micropore for the ear and a wider one for use on the body.

For younger practitioners with excellent eyesight, a headband torch is not necessary. However, as the authors are of a certain age, we believe this can be a valuable addition to the toolkit, particularly when working on the ear or performing small-cone moxibustion. Extra light helps!

APPLICATION

6 MM NEEDLES

Choosing the correct needle length is essential for both safety and comfort. MSA uses two sizes of intradermal needles: long (6 mm) and short (3 mm).

6 mm needles are used only in three specific areas:

1. The midpoints of the thighs and upper arms in larger patients
2. The spine from T8 downwards
3. The posterior torso, including the bladder meridian points in the interscapular area

In short: the back, the spine below T8, and the upper arms and legs.

3 MM NEEDLES

If you memorise those three areas above, it's easy to remember that everywhere else on the body, you use 3 mm needles. They are suitable for:

- Limbs, especially around joints
- The anterior torso
- The spine from T7 upwards
- The neck, hands, feet, ears, and face
- Isophasal points

DIRECTION OF NEEDLING

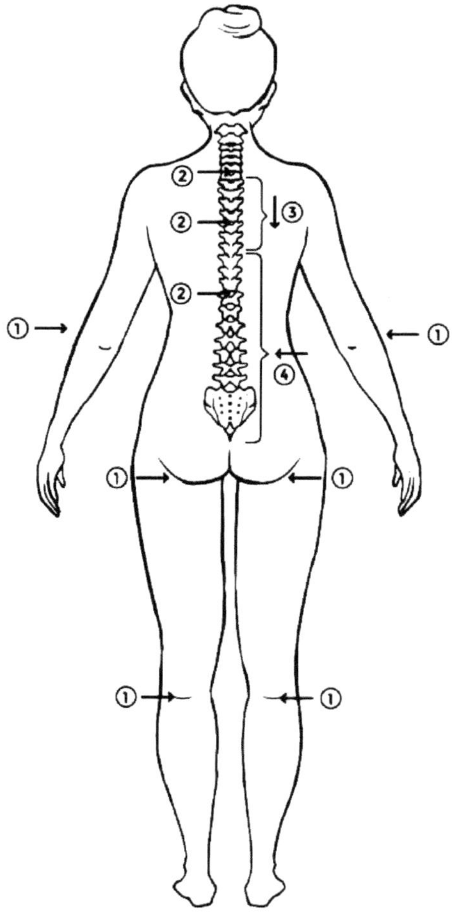

Figure 10-7: Needle direction (see key below).

1. Near joints (e.g. ST 34, LI 11), creases, and flexures (e.g. ST 25, ST 21 or creases on the neck): needle along the crease or flexure, i.e. perpendicular to the meridian.
2. Intervertebral spaces and torso: needle horizontally.
3. Back-*shu* points above BL 17 (T7): needle downwards, to accommodate the lateral movement of the shoulder blades.
4. Back-*shu* points below BL 17 (T7): needle horizontally.

Manaka conducted experiments demonstrating that the direction of needling is of supreme importance.[140] With intradermals, the correct direction is crucial for both efficacy and comfort. His recommendation was **never to needle against the flow of the meridian**. Intradermals are inserted in the direction of the meridian, with the following exceptions based on anatomical considerations:

- Near joints (e.g. ST 34, LI 11), creases, and flexures (e.g. ST 25, ST 21): needle along the crease or flexure (i.e. perpendicular to the meridian). Needling longitudinally across a joint would result in pain on flexion and extension.
- Intervertebral spaces and torso: needle horizontally.
- Back-*shu* points above BL 17 (T7): needle downwards, to accommodate the lateral movement of the shoulder blades.
- Back-*shu* points below BL 17 (T7): needle horizontally.
- Chest and abdomen: needle horizontally towards the midline.
- Ear:
    - Anterior ear—needle upwards.
    - Posterior ear—needle downwards.
    - Concha (inner aspect)—needle in whichever direction is comfortable and can be taped.

DEPTH

Insert the needle subcutaneously so that it lies almost flat to the skin, with the body of the needle within the dermis (hence, 'intradermal'). Insert only one-third to one-half of the needle's length, about 1–3 mm at most. Never insert all the way to the handle, as over-insertion is much more likely to cause discomfort.

140 Ibid. pp. xxxv, 21, 375–389.

INSERTION

Swab the area with alcohol before insertion. Peel back the packaging just enough to expose the handle of the intradermal—like peeling a banana to reveal just the tip. Keeping the needle semi-wrapped reduces the risk of dropping it. Some brands supply the needle embedded in soft cork, which further improves stability when opening the packet.

Using tweezers, grasp the needle by the rounded end at right angles to the tweezers. This makes insertion easier and more controlled.

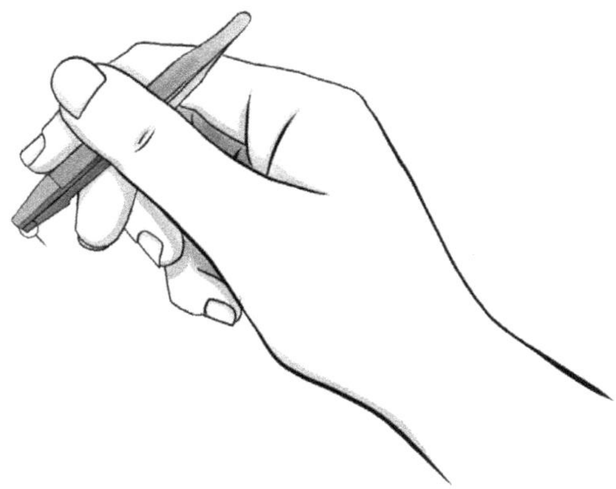

Figure 10-8: Using tweezers, grasp the needle by the rounded end at right angles to the tweezers. This makes insertion easier and more controlled. The needle can point towards you or away from you, depending on the point to be treated.

Place the needle over the point. Unlike conventional fine needles, intradermals are not pushed into the skin. Instead, the skin is pulled onto the needle. There are two methods:

1. With a finger of the other hand, pull the skin away from the point. Angle the needle very slightly into the skin. Gently release the skin, allowing it to move back onto the tip of the needle. You may then need to guide the needle a little deeper to the correct depth.
2. Alternatively, place a finger behind the needle and pull the skin backwards onto its tip. Once the needle has penetrated, adjust the depth as before. This method is especially useful when the skin is flaccid, as in elderly patients.

The needle is inserted transversely so that it lies between the superficial and deep fascia.

DEPTH CHECK

On body and hand points, test the depth by applying gentle pressure to the handle. As the handle depresses, the tip of the needle should rise slightly under the skin. If you can see the skin lift, the depth is correct. If not, the needle is too deep and should be withdrawn and re-angled.

THE EAR

The needle must never be inserted into the cartilage. After insertion, check visually: if the handle stands upright from the skin, it may be too deep. The handle should lie almost flat, and when touched gently, should feel mobile. If it feels immovable, it is likely in the cartilage.

DROPPED NEEDLES

It is inevitable that at some point, an intradermal will fall from your tweezers. Paul Movsessian suggests keeping a small magnet handy that you can pass over the space to retrieve it. Some practitioners magnetise their tweezers, but this creates two problems:

1. The needle clings to the tweezers, making it harder to release.
2. A magnetised needle adds an extra layer of stimulation, which complicates dosage and interactions.

For these reasons, we do not recommend magnetised tweezers.

SECURING THE NEEDLE

Once you are satisfied with the location and depth of the intradermal, you need to secure it in place. Prepare two pieces of micropore tape: one small and one slightly larger. It's best to cut these to size before locating the point or beginning insertion. You can also round the corners with scissors to prevent them from catching on clothing or peeling off during the few days they are in place. Tape one end of each piece to the tape dispenser or any smooth surface nearby, so they are ready to hand.

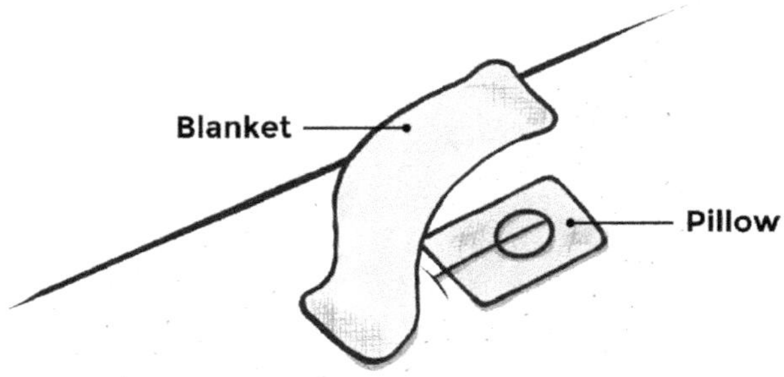

Figure 10-9: The needle resembles a stick figure with its head on a pillow.

Using tweezers, take the smaller piece of tape and slide it under the handle of the intradermal until the end is almost touching the point of insertion. As the head of the needle resembles the head of a horizontal stick figure, imagine this base layer of tape as the mattress, with the needle's head resting on the pillow.

Next, our needle needs a blanket. Take the larger piece of tape and place it over the needle, covering the stick figure's head. As you apply it, make sure the tape first covers the skin just beyond the tip end of the needle, then press it gently back over the handle end. This prevents the tape from accidentally pushing the needle deeper into the skin.

When placing the larger tape, stretch the surrounding skin with your thumb and index finger as you apply it. This helps maintain adhesion as the patient moves. On the body and hand points, this step is important; in the ear, it is not necessary.

Confirm that the needle feels comfortable by pressing gently. If there is discomfort, check that the tape is not tugging on a hair follicle.

REMOVAL

The intradermal is now sandwiched between two pieces of tape. Later in the week, removal is simple: the patient lifts one corner and the whole assembly comes away. Over time, the two pieces of tape adhere to each other, locking the needle handle between them. When the top piece is peeled off, it pulls the lower tape and the needle out together.

Advise patients to dispose of the needle safely, in accordance with the laws and regulations of your country.

FEEDBACK

When an intradermal is inserted into a pressure pain point, the pressure pain often reduces. Counterintuitively, it is fine for practitioners to palpate over the inserted needle, although the Golden Rule for patients still applies—they should never press on takeaway needles themselves. After insertion:

- **Affected area**: Mobility or pain should improve; this is your clinical test of whether the treatment is effective.
- **Site of the intradermal**: Pressure pain may also reduce. For musculoskeletal pain, this isn't essential, since ROM changes and pain relief at the affected area provide a reliable feedback mechanism. However, this local change becomes more important in non-pain conditions, as discussed below.

If pain or ROM does not improve, relocate the intradermal or if the improvement is only slight, add another. This assessment should always be done before the needle is taped in place.

BEYOND MUSCULOSKELETAL PAIN

Manaka mainly used intradermals for musculoskeletal pain, where pain or restricted movement can be demonstrated and tested. In these cases, the feedback is immediate and reliable.

However, this system can also be applied to other conditions such as asthma, chronic digestive problems, or cough. For example, with gastric issues, you might consider the stomach point on the ear. With these kinds of conditions, movement testing is not possible, and immediate changes may not be easy for patients to perceive or report. In such cases, rely instead on the local reaction at the point and your broader clinical reasoning.

TOLERATION AND REACTIONS

Intradermals are usually well tolerated and can remain in place for up to a week. The most common problem is that the tape can catch on clothing—pockets, sleeves, trousers (pants), or socks—and the tape edge may get peeled back. Occasionally, if an intradermal is inserted incorrectly, it can cause a sharp or pricking sensation. Patients should be advised to remove it immediately if this occurs.

INDICATIONS

Intradermals are an integral part of Manaka's isophasal system, where they are used together or combined with other tools to create balanced treatments. They can also be used independently for a local branch treatment, especially for chronic problems or pain in specific areas. Table 10.1 outlines some common clinical indications and suggested approaches for local treatment. The isophasal area on the ear or hand can be added for additional effect.

Table 10.1: Indications for intradermals.

INDICATION	PROCEDURE
Tight tender points	Treat the most reactive area.
Traumas and acute injuries	Treat around the edge of a contusion or break to speed healing.
Lumbar pain	Check *josen* (*shiqizhuixia*, M-BW-25) below L5 and treat if reactive. Korean hand points may also be effective (see below).
Upper limb pain	Treat the wrist on the yang side for carpal tunnel syndrome or RSI.
Repetitive strain injury (RSI)	Treat the most reactive points around the joint.
Bursitis of the shoulder	Palpate along the small intestine meridian; if it feels thick and puffy, check BL 27 (back-*shu* of SI) and treat if reactive.
Knee pain	Around the head of the greater trochanter and either SP 10 or ST 34
Reinforcing a treatment	Suitable for chronic cases where you want to target a specific meridian or organ system. Treat reactive back-*shu* points corresponding to the affected system (e.g. BL 20 for spleen and digestive problems). Leaving intradermals in place for a few days helps reinforce weekly treatments.

CONTRAINDICATIONS

While intradermals are generally safe, there are situations where their use can create unnecessary risk and should be avoided. The most critical contraindication is a compromised immune system: if a patient's immunity is weak, retaining needles of this kind may not be appropriate. Patients can also be remarkably stoic in the face of reactions and may misinterpret instructions, sometimes leaving needles in place even when they are uncomfortable.

Contraindications include:

- Compromised immune system
- Circulatory disorders, such as diabetes—if used at all, limit treatment to the torso and avoid the limbs
- Infectious diseases (e.g. hepatitis B, C, HIV) in immunocompromised patients

DOSAGE: AN INTRODUCTION

Acupuncture, like any medicine, requires us to estimate the patient's reactivity and tailor the dose individually. With herbs or pharmaceuticals, age and weight help guide dosage. In acupuncture, we need to consider two main factors: the sensitivity or robustness of the patient, and the kind of stimulation we apply (e.g. strong or gentle needling). Balancing these allows us to calibrate the tools and techniques to the patient's strength.

For a complete discussion of dosage, see Chapter 15. For now, to keep all the information about takeaway needles in one place, here are some basic guidelines. In brief: *ryu* are the mildest, Pyonex *empishin* are stronger, and *hinaishin* are stronger still.

In order of increasing strength: *ryu* → *empishin* → *hinaishin*.

Table 10.2: Takeaway needles and dosage.

DOSAGE	JAPANESE TAKEAWAY TOOL
Lowest	*Ryu* (provided no skin irritation) 0.3 mm *empishin*
Medium-weak	0.6 mm *empishin*
Medium-strong	0.9 mm *empishin*
Highest	*Hinaishin*

When needling on the body of a sensitive patient, always begin with the lowest dose, such as a *ryu* or a 0.3 mm *empishin*. If this is well tolerated but does not produce results, increase to a 0.6 mm *empishin* at the next visit. If that still proves insufficient, move up to a 0.9 mm *empishin* or an intradermal needle. For sensitive patients treated on the ear, however, stick to the lowest dose.

Sometimes, on a first visit, it may not be easy to judge the correct dose. In these cases, start with a medium–weak option such as a 0.6 mm *empishin*. If it is well tolerated after the session but fails to bring improvement, consider moving to an intradermal at the subsequent treatment.

With more robust patients, where dosage is less of a concern, you can begin with an intradermal needle immediately.

REACTIONS

As we will see in Chapter 15, some patients may return reporting reactions to overtreatment. In these situations, it helps to explain what has happened: your treatment was on the right track, but the dose was too strong. This time, you will reduce the dosage. Explaining this to patients can be very reassuring.

You may choose to lower the dose across all Four Steps of the system. Still, for takeaways specifically, it is best to step down to a milder tool such as a *ryu* or a 0.3 mm *empishin* to see if this can resolve the problem without further overtreatment reactions.

COMMON GUIDANCE FOR ALL TAKEAWAYS

NEEDLING ALONG A MERIDIAN

This final point about dosage applies to all Japanese takeaway tools. It concerns needling along a single meridian stream, such as the left large intestine meridian. Manaka recommended using no more than one takeaway on a single meridian stream; for example, you would not leave takeaways at both LI 4 and LI 11.

When treating the back, rather than leaving intradermals bilaterally on pairs of points (as we do with *chishin* or *kyutoshin*), a simple workaround is to place intradermals contralaterally at BL 18 and BL 23. This rule may have come from his own clinical experience and may relate to avoiding overstimulation of a single meridian flow, which could trigger imbalances.

TOOLBOX PHRASES AND GOLDEN RULES

When you treat patients with any kind of takeaway, clear aftercare instructions are essential. Preparing and rehearsing a few simple *toolbox phrases* allows you to deliver this information quickly, consistently, and with confidence.

Here are four Golden Rules every patient should hear before leaving the clinic:

1. "These needles should stay in for no longer than one week [this may vary—see note below]. Please remove them earlier if they feel uncomfortable."
2. "You should not be aware of the needles. If you feel a sharp or pricking sensation, take them out straight away."
3. "Dispose of the used needles safely and responsibly, in accordance with local regulations."
4. "Never press on the takeaway with your fingers."

Sensitive patients may be more prone to reactions. For these cases, reduce the dosage by using fewer points or recommending shorter retention times. Retention is also influenced by climate: in low-humidity countries, up to one week is safe; in Asia, four days is a better ceiling; and during hot summer months, limit retention to three days. Shortening the retention period is a reliable way to regulate dosage and avoid infection.

Because takeaway needles are retained between visits, they raise legitimate safety concerns. Patients must dispose of their own needles—even though these are tiny—and should be advised to do so responsibly, in line with the laws and regulations of your country of practice. Printing a simple *Guidelines to Takeaways* leaflet is recommended, combining the Golden Rules with clear instructions on removal and safe disposal.

ISOPHASAL MAPPINGS

Dr Manaka's isophasal treatment principle combines local treatment with auricular and Korean hand micro-acupuncture systems. To perform it, you don't need to be an expert in either approach—only to memorise the basic mapping of the musculoskeletal system on the ear and the hand.

This section aims to familiarise you with these two microsystems so that you can quickly locate the areas where the *live points* are most likely to be found.

AURICULAR THERAPY

The role of auricular therapy in Manaka's Step 4 is paramount. He always prioritised the ear over the hand in isophasal treatments. Ear points were treated first, body points second, and hand points added only if the ear–body combination was insufficient. In practice, the ear was his primary starting place.

Given the proliferation of Chinese and Western auricular mappings, for this book, we need a practical working model. For Step 4, our goal is simply to locate the musculoskeletal regions on the ear so we can apply our takeaways effectively. To keep things simple, we use a musculoskeletal layout based on the Chinese model as presented in *Acupuncture: A Comprehensive Text.*[141] Although this differs slightly from the mappings in *Chasing the Dragon's Tail*, it aligns with Manaka's clinical usage and is easy to apply with palpation and range-of-movement testing.

[141] Shanghai College of Traditional Medicine. (1985). *Acupuncture: A Comprehensive Text.* Seattle: Eastland Press.

The following section explores the anatomy of the ear and its relationship to the musculoskeletal system.

ANATOMY OF THE AURICLE

Finding points on the ear depends on recognising its principal anatomical landmarks. Figure 10–9 and Table 10.3 introduce the features used in auricular practice—the helix, antihelix, scapha, concha, triangular fossa, tragus and antitragus. Understanding these structures makes it much easier to map specific body regions onto the auricle.

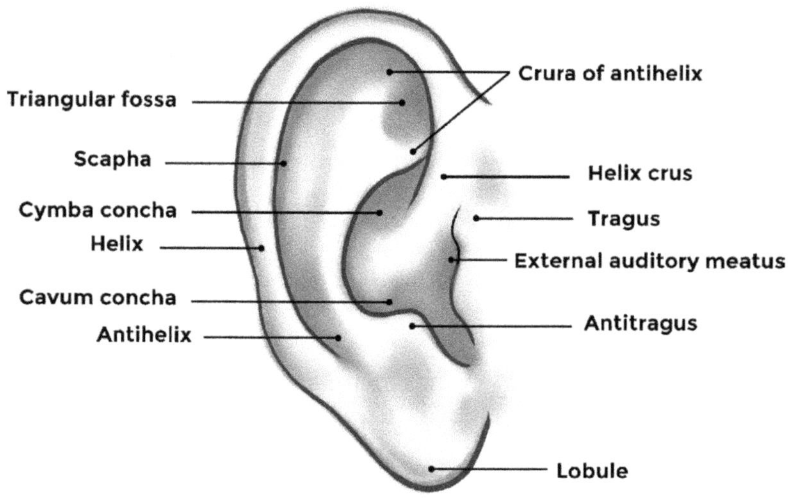

Figure 10-10: Anatomy of the ear.

Table 10.3: Anatomy of the ear.

STRUCTURE	DESCRIPTION
Helix	The inverted rim of the ear, which forms its outer edge, is shaped like a question mark without a dot.
Helix crus	*Crus* means 'root' (plural *crura*). The root of the helix divides the concave depression around the external auditory meatus (earhole) into two areas.
Cymba concha	The upper concavity above the helix crus.
Cavum concha	The lower concavity below the helix crus.
Antihelix	A semi-circular ridge curving around the auditory meatus, branching into two parts at the top of the ear: the superior antihelix crus and the inferior antihelix crus.
Triangular fossa	A triangular valley at the top of the ear, formed by the ridges of the superior and inferior antihelix crura.
Tragus	A triangular flap of cartilage projecting anteriorly over the auditory meatus. Directly above it is the supratragic notch.
Antitragus	A small, rounded cartilaginous prominence opposite the tragus, forming the lower boundary of the concha and contributing to the intertragic notch.
Scapha	The long, narrow groove between the helix and antihelix, curving around the upper two-thirds of the ear like a shallow channel.
Lobule	The soft, fleshy lower part of the ear, forming the rounded lower margin of the auricle.

With these landmarks in place, we can now locate the major musculoskeletal regions on the auricle.

MAPPING THE MUSCULOSKELETAL SYSTEM

In the inverted-foetus model used in Chinese auriculotherapy, the ear reflects the body upside down. The elements of this model that are relevant for Step 4 are:

- The antihelix mirrors the spine, with its lower, middle and upper portions corresponding broadly to the cervical, thoracic and lumbar regions.
- The scapha corresponds to the upper limb, beginning with the shoulder near the cervical antihelix and extending in an arc toward the fingers near the helix root.
- The superior and inferior antihelix crura reflect the lower limb, with the hip, knee and ankle arranged along the triangular fossa and the branching crura.
- The lobule corresponds to the face region.
- *Shenmen* is located in the triangular fossa.
- The reflexes for the internal organs are found within the cymba concha and cavum concha.

A Comprehensive Text provides anatomical locations for the musculoskeletal correspondences, but these are guides, not gospel. They tell you where to begin, but palpation always trumps geometry. In practice, we identify the relevant anatomical zone (for example, the scapha for shoulder pain) and palpate within it to find the most reactive, tender, or relevant point for this patient at this moment—the alive point. The best point is simply the one that improves pain, range of motion, or both—not necessarily the one that sits exactly where the map suggests.

SPINAL SEGMENTS

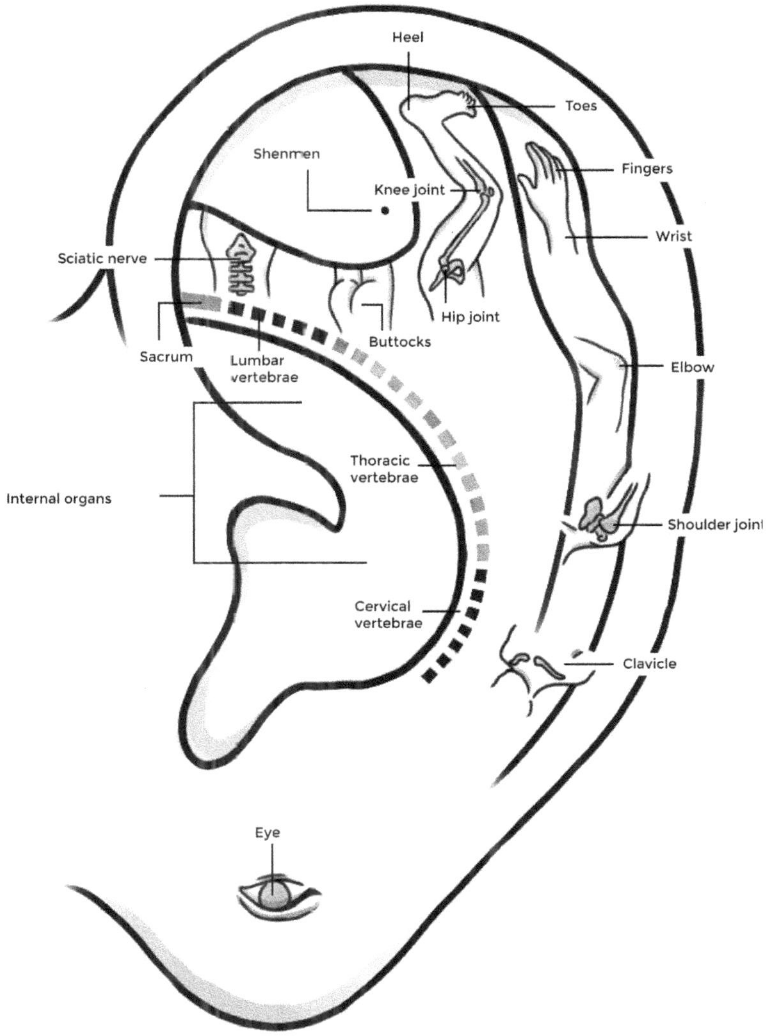

Figure 10-11: Spinal segments.

The spine can be mapped on the antihelix. Palpating inferiorly to superiorly, we often find a series of palpable notches on the antihelix, which correspond to the divisions of spinal vertebrae.

- The first notch is the junction of the antihelix with the antitragus. This corresponds to the Atlas joint.
- The second notch corresponds with C7–T1.
- The third notch corresponds to T12–L1.

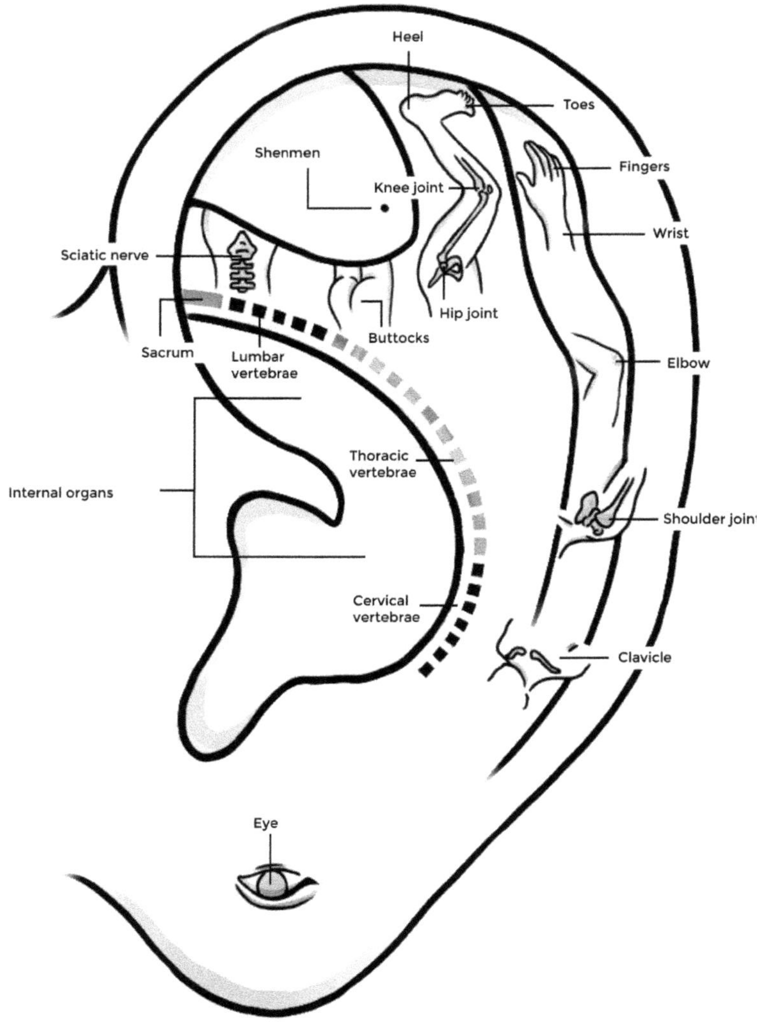

Figure 10-12: The musculoskeletal system of the ear.

UPPER LIMB

The arm lies along the scapha, with the shoulder beginning near the cervical portion of the antihelix. From there, it continues in a parallel arc through the scapha to the fingers, located near the superior antihelix crus.[142]

---

[142] Ibid.

LOWER LIMB

The lower limb is represented on the inferior and superior antihelix crura, following the curve of the triangular fossa. It begins with the sciatic zone on the flat surface of the inferior crus, adjacent to the hip area within the triangular fossa. The buttock area lies just posterior to this. Moving superiorly, the hip joint reflex is found posterior to the triangular fossa, just superior to *shenmen*, followed by the knee. The ankle and toes point posteriorly, roughly level with the finger points in the scapha.[143]

OTHER POINTS

The focus of this chapter is the mapping of the musculoskeletal system on the auricle, as this is all we need for the takeaways at Step 4. Auricular therapy, however, is not limited to musculoskeletal correlations. *Shenmen*, located slightly superior to the apex of the triangular fossa, is widely used to modulate stress, pain and inflammation and can be added whenever these factors influence the patient's presentation.[144]

Points relating to the eyes lie on the lobule, while regions corresponding to the gastrointestinal and other internal organs are found in the cymba and cavum conchae. These additional points lie outside the scope of this chapter, but can be incorporated easily once the basic landmarks presented here are familiar.

LOCATING AURICULAR POINTS

This is all you need to apply takeaways for pain relief. Points can be located in several ways. Manaka himself did not rely heavily on visual signs; instead, he focused on palpation and probing. His method was to compress the cartilage of the ear at the

143 Ibid.

144 The location of *shenmen* on the auricle varies between traditions. In this text, we use the NADA (National Acupuncture Detoxification Association) location, with *shenmen* sitting within the triangular fossa but slightly superior. Other auricular mapping systems place it more centrally or inferiorly.

relevant location between the thumb and index finger; if he found stiffness or tenderness, he would then use a probe to identify the most sensitive spot in that region. At times, he also used an electrodermal device of his own design, the Hibiki 7, which doubled as a point stimulator and was particularly useful with chronic pain patients.

By contrast, contemporary auriculotherapy practitioners often place more emphasis on visual inspection. Changes in skin texture, colour, or the appearance of blemishes in the relevant zone can all serve as useful guides to point location. In practice, the most reliable approach is to combine these methods: observe the ear for visual signs, palpate with even pressure using a blunt probe, and confirm reactivity by testing for effectiveness before applying treatment.

TREATMENT

Insert a 3 mm intradermal needle and secure it in place with tape. For sensitive patients, use a gentler stimulus such as a press sphere or 0.3 mm or 0.6 mm press tack needle.

SAFETY CONSIDERATIONS

Safety is a primary concern in auricular treatments. Two areas require particular attention: protecting the ear cartilage from infection, and managing the risks associated with retained needles.

CARTILAGE SAFETY

The cartilage of the ear has relatively poor blood circulation, which makes infections here especially difficult to treat. Manaka repeatedly warned of the dangers of piercing or irritating the cartilage. The safest technique is to use intradermal needles, which slide in transversely and do not penetrate it.

Historically, press tack needles were too long for safe use on the ear, but modern Seirin versions—orange (0.3 mm) and yellow (0.6 mm)—are sufficiently fine and short to avoid this problem. Press spheres are extremely easy to apply and well tolerated, but care must be taken not to leave them in place too long, as they can cause indentation sores.

AURICULAR NEEDLE RETENTION TIMES

Any retained needle carries the risk of being lost or unnoticed if it falls out. For this reason, the British Acupuncture Council strongly discourages their use. The main risks are missing or lost needles and the potential for infection. Practical precautions can reduce these risks, and these are outlined in the section on empishin.

Retention time must also be managed carefully. In low-humidity climates, an intradermal or press tack needle can generally be left in place for up to one week in adults. In humid climates, such as in Asia, a four-day ceiling is safer, and in hot summer months, it is best to limit retention to three days. Where patients are sensitive or at risk of overtreatment, reducing the retention period is an effective way of regulating dosage.

KORYO SOOJI CHIM (KOREAN HAND ACUPUNCTURE)

Koryo Sooji Chim is a micro-acupuncture system of the hand, developed by the Korean practitioner Tae Woo Yoo. He charted the whole body onto the hands and fingers and also mapped the meridian system and its key acupuncture points. While Dr Manaka did not adopt the system in its full detail, he incorporated a simplified version into his Step 4 symptom control regime. He particularly valued the use of intradermals on the hands, especially on the dorsal surface, as a practical method for pain treatment.

To understand this mapping visually, place your right hand, palm down, on a flat surface. Curl all five digits so your hand stands on its fingers, then extend your middle finger so it points forward. With a little imagination, your hand now resembles a long-necked quadruped—like a small anteater snuffling the ground. The middle finger becomes the head, neck, and chest (moving proximally), the index finger is the left front leg, and the fourth finger is the right front leg. Meanwhile, the thumb and little finger become the left and right hind legs.

If you now lift your hand, the palmar surface represents the yin aspect of the body and the dorsal surface the yang. With another stretch of imagination, you can see how the hand maps onto your own anatomy: head, neck, and chest at the middle finger; left arm at the index finger; right arm at the ring finger; and left and right legs at the thumb and little finger.

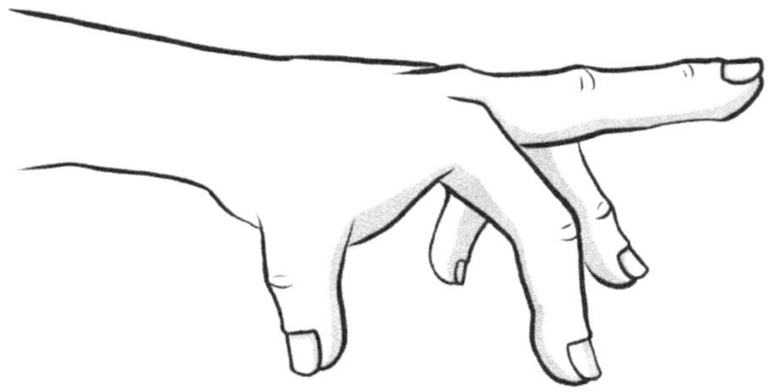

Figure 10-12: Your hand resembles a long-necked quadruped.

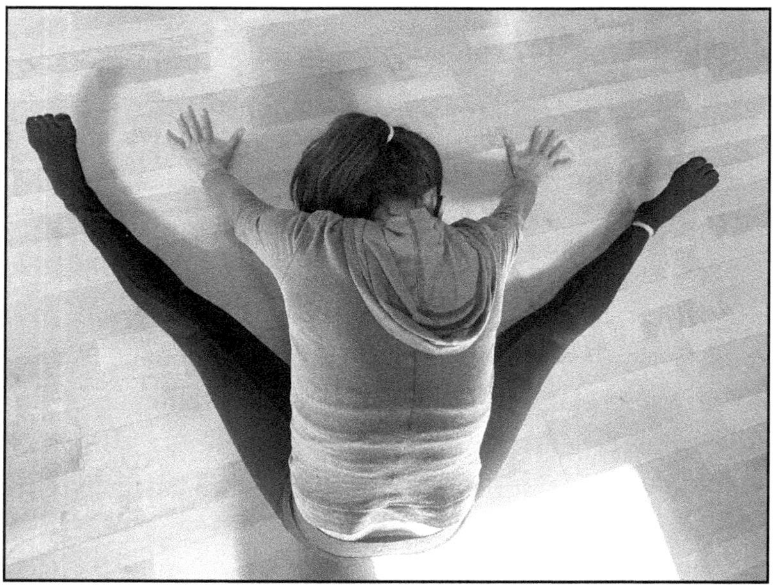

Figure 10-13: The Five Star yoga position mirrors the five fingers in the hand mapping.

What about the left hand? With the dorsal aspect of the hands facing you, place one hand on top of the other. In this position, the lateral aspect of the left hand (little finger, ring finger, and half the middle finger) and the medial aspect of the right hand (thumb, index finger, and half the middle finger) represent the left side of the body. The lateral aspect of the right hand (little finger, ring finger, and half the middle finger) and the medial aspect of the left hand (thumb, index finger, and half the middle finger) represent the right side of the body.

In this mapping:

- The middle finger represents the head and face, as well as the anterior and posterior neck, chest and upper back.
- The index and ring fingers correspond to the upper limbs, while the little finger and thumb represent the lower limbs.
- The metacarpo-phalangeal joints correspond to the shoulders and hips, and the first phalangeal joints to the elbows and knees.
- The second phalangeal joints map to the wrists and ankles.
- The distal phalanges map to the hands and feet.

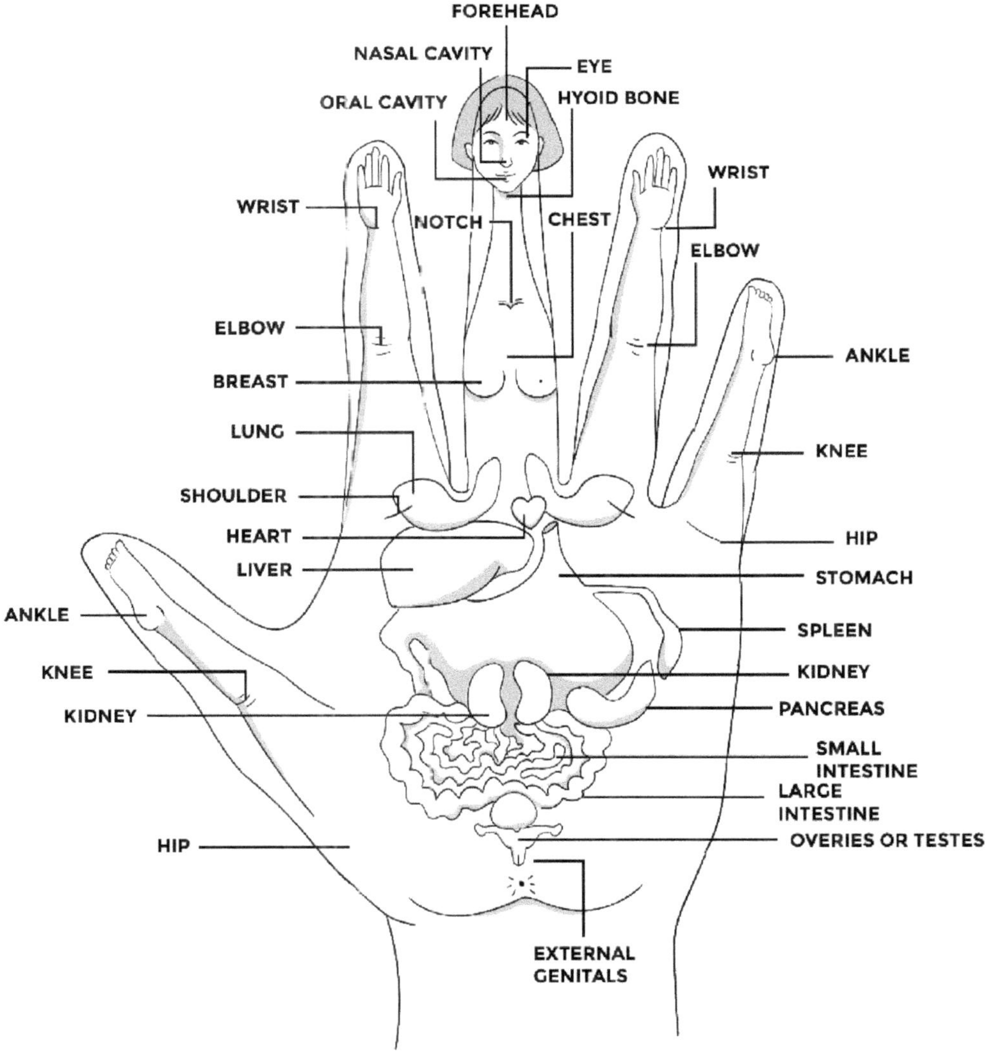

Figure 10-14: Korean hand acupuncture mapping (palmar surface).

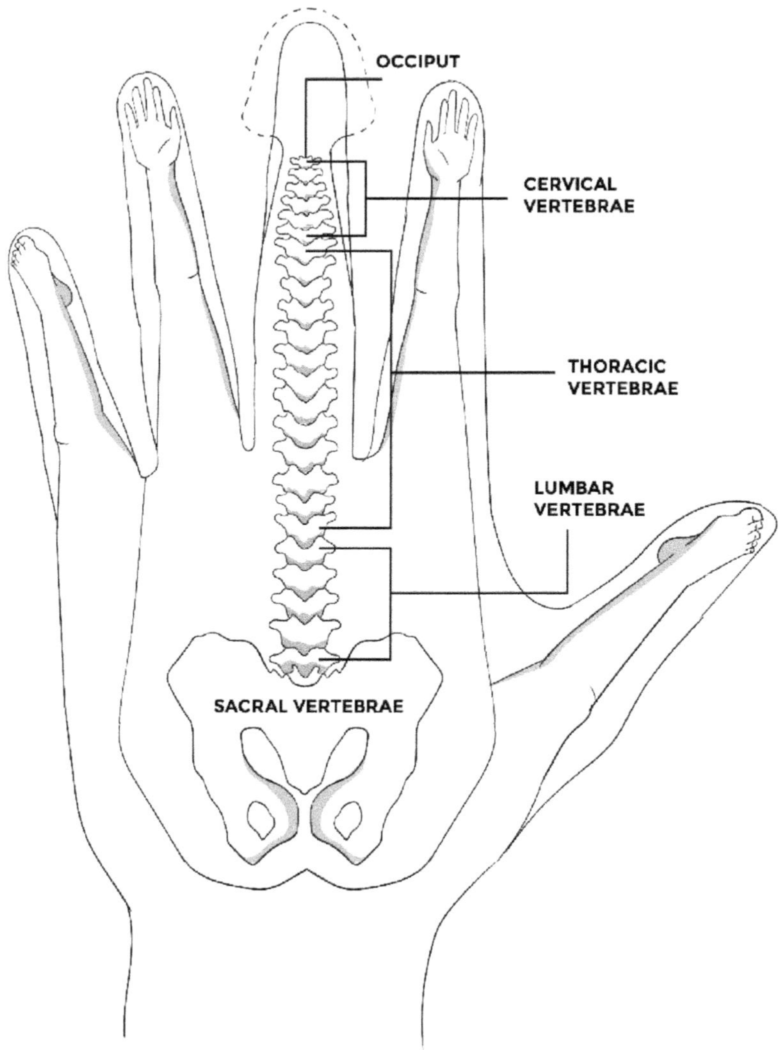

Figure 10-15: Korean hand acupuncture mapping (dorsal surface).

FINDING POINTS

Let's imagine you have pain in your left knee. You'll need to examine your left little finger, around the first interphalangeal joint. Using the same procedures discussed above, look for swelling or discolouration, and use a *teishin* to find pressure pain reactions. It's best to use the reactive point on the hand on the same side as the symptoms. If a greater dosage is needed, you can also treat the related side on the opposite hand.

Tae Woo Yoo would often roll a pen over the relevant region to identify an area of pain before probing with a tool to find the precise point. Manaka, by contrast, did not use a rolling pen but probed repeatedly and quickly with equal pressure until he defined the painful spot. Neither of them relied on visual inspection, beginning instead with palpation. However, Oran Kivity finds a preliminary visual inspection helpful and recommends combining it with palpation for a more complete assessment.

TREATMENT

Use a 3 mm intradermal needle or press spheres. Press spheres are retained better, but their effect is less intense. Press tacks can also be used on the dorsum of the hand for back and hip pain.

Practitioners of Dr Tan's Balance Method may note that the well-known extra points *Ling Ku*, *Da Bai*, and *Zhong Bai* for back sprain, located on the hand, fall within the same region of this mapping. Perhaps this is not a coincidence, but a case of parallel insights.

DIVERSE CONTEMPORARY APPROACHES

You can think of the clinical procedures described above as a kind of baseline, but the reality is that all of us will interpret and practise these procedures differently. Below are some contemporary approaches from our panel of authors.

BRENDA LOEW

Due to their ease of application and rapid effect, I rely primarily on press needles (*empishin*) for Step 4 symptomatic pain relief. Contemporary Seirin Pyonex press needles are comfortable and safe, a significant advance over the original *empishin* available in Manaka's time, and I believe he would have strongly approved.

I usually use the smallest gauge (orange 0.3 mm), which has a good effect on pressure pain points, and rarely apply more than two. Patients are advised to keep the area clean, and while showering is fine, I remind them not to rub or stimulate the needles. Since it's easy for them to forget the needles are in place, I suggest marking a calendar or setting a phone reminder to remove the press needles by the fourth or fifth day, or sooner if there is any discomfort.

I do use the new Pyonex press needle on the ear for Step 4 pain relief. I rarely use *ryu* there, as I worry they might fall into the ear canal. I almost always use *ryu* in paediatric Shonishin, particularly on DU 12 and possibly on ear *shenmen.*

As a standalone practice, I have taught Korean Hand Therapy (KHT) in settings ranging from a hospital trauma centre to homeless youth outreach programmes. Patients learn to massage the hand microsystem for immediate pain relief, and many are amazed at the instantaneous results. In my Step 4 practice, I often teach patients KHT self-massage, particularly for pain and may teach acupressure for non-pain conditions such as nocturia, insomnia, digestive complaints, stress, or anxiety. I may also introduce qigong scalp tapping and low abdominal breathing for autonomic calming. Step 4, for me, frequently includes lifestyle counselling, qigong, breathing, diet, and supplements in addition to Manaka's isophasal treatments.

MARIAN FIXLER

I regularly use *hinaishin* (intradermals), *empishin* (press tacks), and *ryu* (press spheres). If time allows, I prefer 3 mm intradermals in the ear. Unlike Pyonex press tacks, they do not have a plastic 'nipple', so they are better tolerated, especially for patients who like to sleep on that side. I also use Pyonex press tacks (orange 0.3 mm and yellow 0.6 mm), and part of my choice depends on how easy or difficult it will be for the patient to remove the needle themselves—press tacks are easier.

I often use intradermals or press tacks in the ear to reinforce a treatment. For musculoskeletal problems, I assess pain levels and range of movement, looking for a reduction in pain or an improvement in mobility. I also use these devices for low back pain, sciatica, plantar fasciitis (heel point), knee pain, and hip pain, selecting the inner or outer hip point on the ear. Sometimes I combine this with local treatment, but often I prefer to work through balancing methods on other meridians, or with moxa, especially Ontake warm bamboo.

At the end of a treatment, I use press tacks or intradermals on body and ear points as takeaways. On the leg, I tend to favour intradermals, as the direction of the needle can make treatment more effective if placed with the meridian flow. For example, I use SP 6 for dysmenorrhoea and sometimes for fertility in the first half of the cycle. If there is pressure pain on the spleen meridian, I may also use a point near SP 8, leaving a 6 mm intradermal there to help release the groin area.

If I know I won't be seeing a patient when they are likely to need treatment—for instance, before their period—I provide them with press tacks and instructions so they can apply them themselves at the right time.

I mainly use *ryu* press spheres with children as part of Shonishin, most often on GV 12 and occasionally on other points, depending on age and sensitivity. I have also used *ryu* on the hand as takeaways, so patients know where to press after the *ryu* falls out, continuing treatment through acupressure.

ORAN KIVITY

Perhaps because my eyesight has declined over time, or perhaps because I like to save time in clinic, I tend not to use intradermals so much. Instead, I rely on a combination of *empishin* and *ryu*.

For pain, I always begin with a range-of-motion test, then treat locally with a 0.3 or 0.6 mm *empishin*. If the result is good, I may stop there; if not, I'll add a *ryu* or a 0.3 mm *empishin* to the corresponding ear point. I have been consistently impressed with the hand correspondence system, which can be surprisingly effective for conditions outside the musculoskeletal system, such as a sore throat. For this, I place a *ryu* on a tender spot on the palmar side of the third finger and secure it with a loop of micropore tape.

When treating points on the dorsum of the hand for shoulder or hip pain, for example, I use *empishin* and once again rely on lavish amounts of wide micropore tape to keep them in place. Hand points are notoriously difficult to retain, but the micropore extends their lifespan considerably.

For patients, this is often the most exciting part of the treatment. More than once, I've been asked, "Why didn't you start with this?" Patients may be open to talk of root treatment and body balancing, but ultimately they want results—and Manaka's isophasal methods deliver them.

PAUL MOVSESSIAN

Clinically, I choose from a variety of metals when applying Step 4 intradermals or *ryu*, always taking into account the patient's symptoms, constitution, and dosage tolerance. It is essential not to use two different metals on the same body at the same time, as this can create polarity effects and unwanted reactions.

For sensitive patients, such as those with fibromyalgia or chronic fatigue syndrome, *ryu* are often more appropriate than insertive needles. I also prefer *ryu* with immunocompromised patients. Some patients ask if they should press on the takeaways to restimulate the point; I explain that this is unnecessary, as the natural movements of the body gradually build the dosage until it reaches its maximum.

When applying takeaways, I rarely aim for 100% pain relief. Instead, I look for around 75% improvement. This leaves room for the treatment to continue working while avoiding the risk of overdosing. Patients also need to understand that even if they feel better, they are still in the healing stage and should avoid resuming full activity too soon, or they risk undoing the relief.

One of my most common isophasal combinations for back pain or gynaecological issues includes local, hand, and ear points. For example, I place a 6 mm intradermal at *josen* (*shiqizhuixia*, M-BW-25), needled at right angles to the spine, then treat the leg and loin area on the hand with another 6 mm intradermal pointing proximally. Finally, I add a 3 mm intradermal angled inferiorly, either on the antihelix spine region or on the posterior of the ear, depending on which gives the best relief. Although the hand is not an easy place to retain needles—daily friction often dislodges them—I find the 6 mm size holds better than the 3 mm, and a generous pillow of micropore tape helps them stay in place.

Although Manaka generally relied on Chinese-style mappings and pressure pain for point location, I have found that these methods do not always work. In those cases, I turn to Nogier's somatic model with its three phases—mesoderm, endoderm, and ectoderm—relating to acute, chronic, and degenerative conditions.

STEPHEN BIRCH

In my practice of MSA, I found that intradermals could be used in a variety of ways to address pain, not only through the isophasal three-needle method. That approach was beneficial for stubborn problems, but in most cases, Manaka worked more flexibly. He would often begin with an ear point—at least 90% of the time—and then add other points depending on the patient's response.

For pain that does not change with range-of-motion testing, I have found Akabane's method useful. His approach focuses on identifying a focal point for pain, which you test with before-and-after movements. It can be applied very precisely. More generally, intradermals can be used as a single body point, a single ear point, or a combination of ear and body points. In some cases, adding a hand point to these combinations can also be effective.

I experimented extensively with the hand point model in the 1980s and early 1990s and found it interesting, but after moving to Europe, I stopped using it. In colder climates, such as here in the Netherlands, patients often wear gloves or keep their hands in their pockets for much of the year—anything placed on the hands is frequently lost as soon as they leave the treatment room. Because of this, I rarely use hand points now, preferring the flexibility of ear and body combinations, along with Akabane's focal-point method, to achieve reliable results.

CLOSING REFLECTIONS

As these vignettes show, contemporary practitioners apply Manaka's methods with creativity and care, always returning to the same foundation: safety, clarity, and responsiveness. Patients are guided to remove needles within safe timeframes, never press or rub them, and dispose of them responsibly. Dosage is adjusted thoughtfully—whether by choosing gentler tools, limiting retention, or accepting partial relief rather than risking overtreatment. And practical realities, from taping hand points to avoiding *ryu* in the ear canal, remind us that context matters as much as theory.

In short, the Golden Rules are not abstract instructions; they are the common thread running through each practitioner's story, ensuring that Step 4 treatment is effective, safe, and patient-centred.

IN PRACTICE: STEP 4—STORIES FROM THE CLINIC

We now return to Christine, David, and Margaret for their Step 4 treatments, the final part of their first session. In the next section, we'll show how their full treatments unfolded over the weeks and months.

As before, each instalment begins with a short recap of their earlier steps, then shows how symptomatic treatments were applied at this stage.

When applied, takeaway needles can provide powerful symptomatic relief, but the decision to use them depends on the patient's presentation, prognosis, and dosage tolerance.

CASE STUDY 1: SCIATIC PAIN

Christine, Female, 56

- **Chief complaint:** Right-sided sciatic pain, disturbed sleep
- **Notes:** History of migraines and old auto-accident injury; age-related abdominal hypotonia
- **Diagnosis:** Ren Dai (right-belt) (dominant right-sided Dai Mai reaction; Mixed Yin milder)

Step 1: Ren Dai (right-belt) with IPC (10 minutes)
Step 2: *Chishin* retained needling at bilateral GB 20 and GB 21; *chishin* with infrared (FIR) lamp on BL 23, BL 26, and lateral to BL 27 (mid-gluteal point)
Step 3: None
Step 4: *Chishin* at bilateral GB 20 and GB 21. Intradermal needle on *josen* (*shiqizhuixia*, M-BW-25); press tack (0.6 mm) bilaterally on BL 23

PRACTITIONER NOTE

Christine was treated locally with an intradermal on the spine and larger press tacks on both BL 23. Had another bladder point, such as BL 20, been selected, BL 23 and BL 20 would have been needled contralaterally to avoid placing two points on one meridian stream. This case shows how these needle types can be used flexibly for the branch treatment, without requiring Manaka's full isophasal trio.

CASE STUDY 2: NECK PAIN POST-WEIGHTLIFTING INJURY

David, Male, 39

- **Chief complaint:** Chronic right lateral neck pain with swelling between GB 9 and GB 10, radiating at times to the right shoulder and face
- **Notes:** Old weightlifting injury (8 years earlier); background pain rated 5/10 daily, rising to 8+/10 under stress
- **Diagnosis:** YWD

Step 1: YWD with IPC (10 minutes)
Step 2: BL 19, BL 22 with infrared (FIR) lamp
Step 3: N/A
Step 4: Shallow *chishin* needling into the swollen *ashi* point between GB 9 and GB 10 (right side). Pyonex press tack on the right ear *shenmen* (placement in the hairline was not possible). Taught him Korean hand microsystem massage for self-care at home

[Note: Moxa was not permitted in this clinic setting.]

PRACTITIONER NOTE

For clarity, the Step 2 heat treatment and the Step 4 *chishin* needling are listed separately, but in fact, they were applied at the same time. The press tacks were placed at the end of the session.

CASE STUDY 3: HIP DEGENERATION AND CHRONIC PAIN

Margaret, Female, 60

- **Chief complaint:** Chronic right lumbar and groin pain with hip joint degeneration; constant deep pain disturbing sleep and mobility
- **Notes:** History of lumbar fusion (L4–L5) with severe scarring; multiple cortisone injections with no relief; pain relieved by movement, pressure, and heat
- **Diagnosis:** YQR

Step 1: YQR with IPC (15 minutes)
Step 2: *Kyutoshin*—2 balls on GB 30, GB 31, GB 26
Step 3: *Sotai*—Prone Leg Flexion (PLF) and Waist Rotation (this Sotai for the waist will be covered in Vol. 2)
Step 4: *Kyutoshin*—GB 34 (right side only)

PRACTITIONER NOTE

As with David, the Step 2 heat treatment and the Step 4 *kyutoshin* at GB 34 were listed separately but were performed together during the session.

FINAL THOUGHTS

The cases in these instalments have been chosen because, for Step 4, takeaways were commonly used. However, in later chapters, we'll see how useful moxa can be in Step 4. As moxibustion and dosage are essential components of JAAM, we have focused on them in greater detail in the next part of the book, and the next batch of cases in Chapter 16 will illustrate these important concepts.

[Note: The full cases for these three patients can be found in Chapter 11.]

SUMMARY

- **Step 4:** Provides symptomatic relief after the root treatment of Steps 1–3.
- **Core method:** Isophasal treatment using ear, local, and hand points in resonance.
- **Principal tools:** Ryu (press spheres), empishin (press tacks), hinaishin (intradermals). Manaka's preference was intradermals. Advances in technology mean that minuscule Pyonex press tacks can now be used on the ear.
- **Dosage:** *Ryu* (mildest) → 0.3–0.9 mm *empishin* → *hinaishin* (strongest).
- Golden rules: Limit retention (3–7 days depending on climate), instruct patients not to press the needles, to remove them if uncomfortable, and dispose of them safely.
- **Auricular therapy:** The Chinese mapping uses an inverted foetus. You can map the spine on the antihelix. The ear was Manaka's priority system.
- **Korean hand therapy:** Involves mapping the whole body to the hand and applying intradermal and press spheres to address pain and systemic issues.
- **Clinical focus:** Check pain relief through ROM testing and palpation before insertion.
- **Contraindications:** Do not use with immunocompromised patients, take extra care with diabetic patients and avoid needling on their limbs.
- **Flexibility:** Contemporary practitioners adapt Step 4 with their own emphases, tools, and methods.

WHAT'S NEXT

We've been building the Four Step framework piece by piece. Chapter 11 marks a change of pace—bringing it all together in a series of clinical cases.

CHAPTER 11

CASE STUDIES PART 1: APPLYING THE FOUR STEPS

Now that you've explored the Four Steps in theory, it's time to see them in action through real clinical cases. Earlier, we used the metaphor of kitbags: each step offers a collection of tools, each with a specific clinical aim.

- Step 1 releases the yin anterior aspect of the body.
- Step 2 releases the yang posterior aspect; together, Steps 1 and 2 comprise the root treatment.
- Step 3 adjusts structural imbalances through Sotai counter-resistance movements.
- Step 4 focuses on symptom relief, including takeaways, additional needling, moxibustion, or other supportive measures.

Here are seven case studies. We begin with three familiar patients—Christine, David, and Margaret—whose first sessions were introduced in earlier chapters. We follow their progress over time, observing how the Four Steps were adapted from session to session. We then introduce four new patients to illustrate a broader range of clinical presentations and treatment approaches.

If reading seven consecutive case studies feels like a lot to take in, feel free to bookmark this chapter and come back to it later. As you continue to internalise the material from the other chapters, you will uncover more insights here.

We do, however, recommend that as a learning exercise, you work through each case with a pen and paper. For each one, you might pause and reflect:

- If the diagnosis is, for example, a YQR pattern, which points would you use and how would you connect the cords?
- Does the Step 2 treatment follow the textbook version? If not, how would you approach Step 2 yourself?
- What might Step 3 look like for this patient? Can you visualise it?
- How would you adapt Step 4 using the tools you've learned so far?

These case studies have been selected to reinforce the lessons of the previous chapters. There are another seven cases in Chapter 16, where the emphasis shifts to integrating ideas about dosage and moxibustion at Step 4.

CASE STUDY 1: SCIATIC PAIN

Christine, Female, 56

Occupation: Business consultant

PRESENTING CONDITION

Christine presented with right-sided sciatic pain, with occasional twinges in the left leg. The pain originated at the base of the right buttock and radiated down the stomach meridian above the knee. She experienced some weakness in the legs, especially on the right. The pain disturbed her sleep, waking her frequently and forcing her to change position frequently. Her neck and shoulders are often stiff.

RELEVANT HISTORY

- Duration: 2 months
- Advised to exercise, but no improvement
- No scans or diagnostic testing performed
- Avoids medication
- Previous long-term acupuncture treatment for migraines (over 9 years)
- Migraine treatment was effective; the patient ceased acupuncture 3 years ago after menopause
- Past migraine patterns mostly liver-related (CS, K3L, Mixed Yin)
- Auto accident at 32: head/face trauma, chronic neck and shoulder stiffness, occasional left arm numbness
- Managed previous back issues well with exercise

PALPATION

- Slight tension in the right subcostal region
- Right ASIS, SP 15, ST 25, and KID 16 are tight and jumpy
- Bilateral ST 26 stiff/sore; right ST 27 stiff
- Left ASIS tight
- REN above navel stiff; below navel flaccid (age-related pattern)

TREATMENT 1

Diagnosis: Ren Dai. Dominant right-sided Dai Mai reaction. Mixed Yin is also present but milder.

Step 1: Ren Dai (right-belt) with IPC (10 minutes)
Step 2: *Chishin* with infrared (FIR) lamp on BL 23, BL 26, and lateral to BL 27 (mid-gluteal point)
Step 3: N/A
Step 4: *Chishin* at bilateral GB 20 and GB 21. Intradermal needle on *josen* (*shiqizhuixia*, M-BW-25); press tack (0.6 mm) bilaterally on BL 23

TREATMENT 2 (3 WEEKS LATER)

Patient Response
Pain was significantly reduced. No radiating pain for two weeks. Some discomfort when standing too long.

Diagnosis: Mixed Yin pattern now dominant

Step 1: Mixed Yin with IPC (10 minutes)
Step 2: *Chishin* with infrared lamp (FIR) on BL 18, BL 23, and reactive points medial to GB 30
Step 3: N/A
Step 4: *Chishin* retained needling at bilateral GB 20 and GB 21. Intradermal needle on *josen* (*shiqizhuixia*, M-BW-25); press tack (0.6 mm) bilaterally on BL 23

TREATMENT 3 (2 WEEKS LATER)

Patient Response
Sciatic pain has fully resolved. After a stressful period, mild right leg pain returned down the stomach and bladder lines.

Diagnosis: Ren Dai pattern now apparent

Step 1: Ren Dai (right-belt) with IPC (10 minutes)
Step 2: *Chishin* with infrared (FIR) lamp on BL 18, BL 23, BL 26, and reactive points medial to GB 30
Step 3: N/A
Step 4: *Chishin* retained needling at bilateral GB 20 and GB 21. Intradermal needle on *josen* (*shiqizhuixia*, M-BW-25), press tack (0.9 mm) bilaterally on BL 26

TREATMENT 4 (3 WEEKS LATER)

Patient Response
Pain no longer wakes her. Some lingering stiffness and achiness in the lower back. Subcostal and Dai Mai reactions were greatly reduced.

Diagnosis: YWC

Step 1: YWC with IPC (right side,10 minutes)
Step 2: *Chishin* with infrared (FIR) lamp on BL 18 and BL 23
Step 3: N/A
Step 4: *Chishin* retained needling at bilateral GB 20 and GB 21. Intradermal needle on *josen* (*shiqizhuixia*, M-BW-25); press tack (0.6 mm) bilaterally on BL 23

TREATMENT 5 (3 WEEKS LATER)

Patient Response
Stable improvement. No daytime pain. One mild night episode of sciatic pain.

Diagnosis: YWC

Step 1: YWC with IPC (right side, 10 minutes)
Step 2: *Chishin* with infrared (FIR) lamp on BL 18 and BL 23
Step 3: N/A
Step 4: *Chishin* retained needling at bilateral GB 20 and GB 21. Intradermal needle on *josen* (*shiqizhuixia*, M-BW-25)

CONCLUSIONS AND REFLECTIONS

Bodily changes, such as ageing or childbearing, often trigger abdominal wall changes that manifest in different patterns. Manaka noted that changes in body musculature over the years tend to progress from hypertonia towards hypotonia (see *Chasing the Dragon's Tail*). With ageing, this is a gradual process that occurs over many years, whereas with childbearing, it can happen more rapidly over the course of one or more pregnancies. This abdominal softening reduces the visibility of previous patterns—for example, the reactions associated with the liver, such as right subcostal tension or tightness—while YQR-related patterns such as YQR, K3L, Mixed Yin, and Ren Dai become more apparent.

When the predominant pattern is treated successfully, a gradual return of abdominal wall tone can allow older or previously hidden liver patterns, such as CS or YWC, to re-emerge. These patterns, previously masked by hypotonia, become more apparent as tone improves. The likelihood of such hidden or older liver-related patterns can sometimes be anticipated not through palpation but through observation of the skin, including pigmentation, moles, vascular spiders, or petechiae.[145] In cases where a weakened abdominal wall presents with YQR-related patterns, improvement in tone and the subsequent surfacing of clearer liver patterns may be taken as a positive prognostic sign.

The K3L pattern is valuable as a broad-spectrum approach, particularly when the abdominal wall is soft. However, reliance on this shortcut alone is insufficient. As treatment progresses and abdominal tone improves, more specific and deeper patterns—such as CS or YWC—emerge, requiring precise and targeted treatment.

In this case, the patient responded well to treatment based on the Ren Dai pattern. This choice was appropriate given the right-sided Dai Mai reactions and concurrent right leg pain. Abdominal weakness below the navel was consistent with age and a long history of gynaecological issues. Initially, the pain was severe and disrupted sleep, but it stabilised quickly as the pattern shifted from Ren Dai to Mixed Yin.

---

145 Manaka, Y., Itaya, K., & Birch, S. (1995). *Chasing the Dragon's Tail: The Theory and Practice of Acupuncture in the Work of Yoshio Manaka*. Brookline: Paradigm Publications.pp. 129–131.

Christine had a wiry physique, unsuitable for *kyutoshin*. Treatment was carefully layered, combining IPC, *chishin*, FIR lamp, and minimal press tacks. *Josen* (*shiqizhuixia*, M-BW-25) proved to be a useful local point, and over time, even the nocturnal pain diminished.

Although for the sake of clarity, the *chishin* at bilateral GB 20 and GB 21 have been recorded at Step 4, they were inserted during Step 2. Some of the steps can be performed concurrently. This does not have to be a linear process.

CASE STUDY 2: NECK PAIN POST-WEIGHTLIFTING INJURY

David, Male, 39

Occupation: Corporate manager

PRESENTING CONDITION

David reported right lateral neck pain that began after a weightlifting injury 8 years earlier. There was a palpable swelling between GB 9 and GB 10, which occasionally radiated to the right shoulder with intermittent tingling into the face. He experienced a background pain level of 5/10 daily, which increased to over 8/10 under stress.

RELEVANT HISTORY

- High-stress managerial role
- Hypertension (controlled with medication)
- Hernia surgery 2 years ago
- Cholecystectomy 7 years ago

PALPATION

- Very tight along the Dai Mai bilaterally
- ASIS tender on palpation
- GB 34 on the right was also tender on palpation

TREATMENT 1

Diagnosis: YWD

Step 1: YWD with IPC (10 minutes)
Step 2: BL 19, BL 22 with infrared (FIR) lamp
Step 3: N/A
Step 4: Shallow *chishin* needling into the swollen *ashi* point between GB 9 and GB 10 (right side). Pyonex press tack on the right ear *shenmen* (placement at the *ashi* point in the hairline was not possible). Taught him Korean hand microsystem massage for self-care at home.

[Note: Moxa was not permitted in this clinic setting.]

TREATMENT 2 (FOLLOWING WEEK)

Patient Response
Despite a very stressful week, background pain reduced slightly to 4/10. No episodes of tingling radiating into the face or shoulder. Pain remained localised.

Treatment: Same as Week 1. Added breathing practice—low abdominal breathing for a minimum of 5 minutes daily.

TREATMENT 3 (FOLLOWING WEEK)

Patient Response
Stress from traffic before the appointment exacerbated the pain, but the background level remained steady at 4/10.

Treatment: Same as previous weeks.

TREATMENT 4 (FOLLOWING WEEK)

Patient Response
Slight decrease in pain behind the right ear (now 3.5/10). Reports improved ability to handle stress.

Treatment: Same as previous weeks.

TREATMENT 5 (FOLLOWING WEEK)

Patient Response
Reported significant improvement before a work trip. Background pain had decreased further before being aggravated by travel and meetings.

PALPATION

- Abdomen showed reduced tightness along the Dai Mai on the right
- Area below the umbilicus felt tight

Diagnosis: Ren Dai (right-belt)

Step 1: Ren Dai (right-belt) with IPC (REDLLL rule)
Step 2: BL 19, BL 22 with infrared (FIR) lamp
Step 3: N/A
Step 4: Shallow *chishin* needling surrounding a swollen *ashi* point between GB 9 and GB 10 (right side). Pyonex press tack on right ear *shenmen*; reviewed Korean hand microsystem—identified area that relieved pain when deeply massaged.

TREATMENT 6 (FOLLOWING WEEK)

Patient Response
Background pain reduced to <2/10 with occasional stress-related flares. Described himself as more "resilient" and "calm".

Step 1: Ren Dai (right-belt) with IPC
Step 2: BL 19, BL 22, and BL 23 with an infrared (FIR) lamp; added left BL 14
Step 3: N/A
Step 4: Shallow *chishin* needling at the *ashi* point between GB 9 and GB 10 (right side). Pyonex press tack on the right ear *shenmen*. The patient continued with Korean hand massage and low abdominal breathing for pain relief.

CONCLUSIONS AND REFLECTIONS

David presented with long-standing pain exacerbated by stress. A YWD pattern was observed on the abdomen, with strong tightness in the Dai Mai and associated tenderness in the right hip and GB 34.

Moxa was not permitted in this clinic, which limited available treatment strategies. However, a combination of IPC, local *ashi* needling, and auricular support using Pyonex press tacks yielded steady improvement.

While, for the sake of clarity for teaching, the Step 2 points with heat and the *chishin* in Step 4 are listed separately, they were applied together. Steps 2 and 4 were performed concurrently. The press tacks were administered at the end of the session.

Teaching David to self-manage via the Korean hand microsystem and abdominal breathing likely played a significant role in pain reduction.

By the sixth session, the background pain was significantly reduced, reactivity in the abdomen had eased, and the patient reported feeling more resilient overall. Additional use of local moxa may have further improved outcomes, had it been available.

CASE STUDY 3: HIP DEGENERATION AND CHRONIC PAIN

Margaret, Female, 60

Occupation: Retired

PRESENTING CONDITION

Margaret experienced back and groin pain associated with hip joint degeneration. The pain originated in the right lumbar region and referred into the right groin, with additional sacral discomfort. Her hip pain began 4 years earlier and had worsened over the past 2 months. The pain was constant, severe and deep, and limited her mobility. The pain was relieved by movement, pressure, and heat. She was particularly concerned about coping with an upcoming long-haul flight.

RELEVANT HISTORY

- Lumbar fusion at L4–L5 twenty-five years earlier, leaving severe scarring
- Hip degeneration confirmed by MRI 4 years earlier
- Previous cortisone injections for hip pain (with no lasting improvement)

PALPATION

- Very flaccid below the navel, slightly tight above
- Right ASIS was very sore

TREATMENT 1

Diagnosis: YQR

Step 1: YQR with IPC (5 minutes)
Step 2: *Kyutoshin*—2 balls on GB 30, GB 31, GB 26
Step 3: Sotai—Prone Leg Flexion (PLF) and Waist Rotation (this Sotai for the waist will be covered in Vol. 2)
Step 4: GB 34 (right side only)

TREATMENT 2 (FOLLOWING WEEK)

Patient Response
Pain relief was experienced on treatment day, but it did not last. Pain level unchanged. Dramatic improvement in range of motion.

Diagnosis: YWD (right)

Step 1: YWD with IPC on the right (10 minutes)
Step 2: *Kyutoshin*—2 balls on BL 25 (bilateral)
Step 3: Sotai—Prone Leg Flexion (PLF) and Waist Rotation (this Sotai for the waist will be covered in Vol. 2)
Step 4: *Kyutoshin*—GB 34 (right side only)

TREATMENT 3 (FOLLOWING WEEK)

Patient Response
Pain relief lasted 2 days. Range of motion greatly improved. Some groin pain recurrence.

Diagnosis: YWD

Step 1: YWD with IPC (15 minutes)
Step 2: *Kyutoshin*—2 balls on *josen* (*shiqizhuixia,* M-BW-25), BL 23, BL 25 (bilateral), GB 30 (right)
Step 3: N/A
Step 4: Press tacks on LIV 4, GB 40 (right), and *josen (shiqizhuixia*, M-BW-25)

TREATMENT 4 (FOLLOWING WEEK)

Patient Response
By the weekend: significant overall improvement; minimal pain; good range of motion. Patient reported "I feel much better in myself" after pain relief.

Diagnosis: YWD

Step 1: YWD with IPC on the right (15 minutes)
Step 2: *Kyutoshin*—2 balls on *josen* (*shiqizhuixia*, M-BW-25), BL 23, BL 25 (bilateral), GB 30 (right)
Step 3: N/A
Step 4: Press tacks on LIV 3, SP 5 (right), and *josen (shiqizhuixia*, M-BW-25)

TREATMENT 5 (FOLLOWING WEEK)

Patient Response
Improved gait. Pain 60% improved. Range of motion is nearly normal. No longer worried about flying.

Diagnosis: YWD

Step 1: YWD with IPC on the right (15 minutes)
Step 2: *Kyutoshin*—2 balls on *josen* (*shiqizhuixia*, M-BW-25), BL 23, BL 25 (bilateral), GB 30 (right)
Step 3: N/A
Step 4: Press tacks on LIV 4, ST 34 (right), and *josen* (*shiqizhuixia*, M-BW-25)

TREATMENT 6 (FOLLOWING WEEK)

Patient Response
Gait continued to improve. Pain was further reduced. Range of motion maintained. Occasional shooting groin pain.

Diagnosis: YWD

Step 1: YWD with IPC on the right (15 minutes)
Step 2: *Kyutoshin*—2 balls on *josen* (*shiqizhuixia*, M-BW-25), BL 23, BL 25 (bilateral), GB 30 (right)
Step 3: N/A
Step 4: Press tacks on LIV 3, and 2 reactive points in the groin area

TREATMENT 7 (FOLLOWING WEEK)

Patient Response
Back, hip, and groin pain have improved significantly. The stress of an upcoming flight triggered a headache.

Diagnosis: YWD

Step 1: YWD with IPC on the right (15 minutes)
Step 2: *Kyutoshin*—2 balls on *josen* (*shiqizhuixia*, M-BW-25), BL 23, BL 25 (bilateral), GB 30 (right)
Step 3: N/A
Step 4: Press tacks on GB 31 and GB 41 (right)

CONCLUSIONS AND REFLECTIONS

Initial diagnosis was YQR, based on early presentation, but was revised to YWD when the pain did not respond as expected. The pattern was treated unilaterally on the right side, corresponding to the location of the symptom.

Treatment frequency was increased due to time constraints, and Margaret received twice-weekly sessions in the final phase to prepare for her international travel.

Press tacks appeared to help maintain the treatment effect between visits, particularly for muscle pain. Distal and local reactive points were selected for both pain relief and to support the range of motion. Step 2 was often combined with Step 4, as needling these tight yang points achieved both the release of the yang aspect and relief of symptoms. Step 4 with press tacks included LIV 4, which helps release the groin and GB 40, which is the *yuan*-source point and treats the meridian directly.

The patient reported substantial improvement and was highly satisfied with the results. She left for an eight-week trip to the United States pain-free and planned to resume treatment upon return.

CASE STUDY 4. GLOBUS SENSATION AND DIGESTIVE ISSUES

Elizabeth, Female, 44

Occupation: Business owner

PRESENTING CONDITION

Elizabeth reported chronic digestive complaints along with plum stone throat (globus hystericus), describing a persistent sensation of a lump in the throat.

RELEVANT HISTORY

- Hiatal hernia
- Abdominal bloating
- Uterine fibroid
- Stomach ulcer
- Loose stools to diarrhoea
- Belching
- Flatulence
- Very obsessive and worries excessively

PALPATION

- Tight above the navel
- Very flaccid and cool below the navel
- Bilateral LU 1 and ST 12 reactive, KID 16
- Right ASIS sore

TREATMENT 1

Diagnosis: YQR

Step 1: YQR with IPC (5 minutes)
Step 2: Not given as we had run out of time
Step 3: N/A
Step 4: Ryu—stainless steel press ball at DU 11 for 4 days

TREATMENT 2 (FOLLOWING WEEK)

Patient Response
Plum stone throat had resolved until treatment day. Reported increased energy, calmness, and a strong sense of hope. Treatment coincided with premenstrual symptoms.

Diagnosis: YQR

Step 1: YQR with IPC (15 minutes)
Step 2: *Okyu*—3 cones on reactive points between T3 and T9 (Fukaya's psychosomatic treatment)
Step 3: N/A
Step 4: *Ryu*—stainless steel press ball at DU 11 for 4 days

TREATMENT 3 (FOLLOWING WEEK)

Patient Response
Plum stone throat resolved. During menstruation had sugar cravings, low energy, and early cold symptoms.

Diagnosis: YQR

Step 1: YQR with IPC (15 minutes)
Step 2: *Chishin* at BL 23 and BL 25 (bilateral) with infrared (FIR) lamp
Step 3: N/A
Step 4: *Hinaishin*—intradermal needles on the right ear *shenmen* and left ear Brain point (5 days)[146]

TREATMENT 4 (FOLLOWING WEEK)

Patient Response
Felt much better post-treatment. Developed cold-like symptoms 2 days later, with watery eyes and return of plum stone sensation. Digestion had improved.

---

146 Brain point lies within the cavum concha; see 'Beyond the Musculoskeletal Map' in Chapter 10.

PALPATION

- Right subcostal tension

Diagnosis: YWC

Step 1: YWC on the right with IPC and silver spike points (SSP) (10 minutes)

[Note: SSP are discussed in Chapter 17.]

Step 2: *Chishin* at BL 20, BL 18 (bilateral), and DU 12 with infrared (FIR) lamp. Additional *chishin*—DU 20, GB 20, GB 21
Step 3: N/A
Step 4: *Hinaishin*—intradermal needles on the right ear *shenmen* and left ear Brain point (5 days)

TREATMENT 5 (FOLLOWING WEEK)

Patient Response
Missed 1 treatment. Plum stone returned. Feeling premenstrual again.

Diagnosis: YWC

Step 1: YWC on the right with IPC and SSP (10 minutes)
Step 2: Japanese cupping: mild general whole-body treatment, abdomen (6 minutes), back (6 minutes)
Step 3: N/A
Step 4: Press tack on REN 12 for 2 days
Step 5: Home therapy—Chinese dietary advice: favour spleen-supporting foods and avoid liver-aggravating foods (see below)

CONCLUSIONS AND REFLECTIONS

Elizabeth's initial consultation was lengthy due to the complexity of her medical history. Based on the symptoms, a Yin Wei–Chong Mai pattern might have been expected, but the presentation was instead a clear Yin Qiao–Ren Mai. As treatment progressed, the Yin Wei–Chong pattern began to emerge.

The treatments proved beneficial, though their effects sometimes did not hold, likely due to her high anxiety levels. Improvements included better digestion, a strengthened immune system, and greater resilience, but the plum stone sensations tended to return when treatment intervals lengthened or coincided with emotional or hormonal fluctuations.

The course of treatment was interrupted by a trip to Canada, and symptoms related to the fibroid and menstrual cycle have not yet been addressed. Continuation is planned on her return.

This case also introduces a new concept—Step 5, or home therapy—which will be explored further in later books in the series.

CASE STUDY 5. THORACIC AND KNEE PAIN

Yudhi, Male, 61

Occupation: Property manager

PRESENTING CONDITION

Yudhi had chronic right-sided thoracic and scapular pain, constant at a level of 6/10, which had persisted for 17 years. He described it as wearing him down.

RELEVANT HISTORY

- C5–C6 fusion after herniated disc (17 years ago)
- Cervical degenerative disc disease
- Physically demanding job
- Work schedule requires a 2:30 a.m. wake-up

PALPATION

- YQD and YWD on the right side
- Right ASIS tenderness
- Right SI 10, ST 25, and ST 26 tender on palpation
- Right cervical vertebrae reactive

[Note: Moxa was not permitted in this clinic setting.]

TREATMENT 1

Diagnosis: YQD, YWD

Step 1: YQD, YWD with IPC, only on the right
Step 2: Infrared (FIR) lamp on back; *chishin* needling: bilateral BL 19, DU 20; right side: BL 43, BL 10, BL 40; left side: GB 43
Step 3: N/A
Step 4: Take-home auricular press tack on *shenmen*; taught Korean hand microsystem massage

TREATMENT 2 (FOLLOWING WEEK)

Patient Response
Pain reduced to 4/10. Sleeping through the night without waking in pain.

PALPATION

- Lustre improved on abdomen
- Dai Mai tightness, particularly at ST 25
- SI 10 is no longer tender
- Mild ASIS tenderness (right > left)

Diagnosis: YWD

Step 1: Bilateral YWD with IPC
Step 2: *Chishin* needling: bilateral BL 19, BL 22
Step 3: N/A
Step 4: Reviewed Korean hand microsystem; applied press tack to right mid-scapular *ashi* point with instructions to remove in 4 days

TREATMENT 3 (3 WEEKS LATER)

Patient Response
Thoracic pain reduced to 2/10. New complaint: acute medial right knee pain from squatting at work.

PALPATION

- Persistent tightness along the Dai Mai (especially ST 25)
- Midline tenderness, weaker below umbilicus
- Mild bilateral tenderness at LU 1–LU 2

C

Step 1: Ren Dai (right-belt) with IPC
Step 2: *Chishin* needling at bilateral BL 19 and BL 23 with infrared (FIR) lamp on back
Step 3: N/A
Step 4: Press tack to right medial knee *ashi* point; reviewed Korean hand microsystem for self-massage

TREATMENT 4 (FOLLOWING WEEK)

Patient Response
No thoracic/scapular pain. Right knee pain <1/10.

PALPATION

- Persistent Dai Mai tightness (especially ST 25)
- Tight above umbilicus, soft below
- Right-sided LU 1–LU 2 tenderness only

Diagnosis: YQD, YWD

Step 1: Ren Dai (right-belt) with IFC
Step 2: *Chishin* needling at BL 18, BL 19, BL 23, and BL 42 with infrared (FIR) lamp on back
Step 3: N/A
Step 4: Warm *enshin* stroked lightly down neck, back, and legs

CONCLUSIONS AND REFLECTIONS

Treatment 1 is interesting in that YQD, typically needled bilaterally, was needled only on the right. Together with YWD on the right, this kept the dosage of treatment down on the first treatment.

This case is also a good example of how MSA emphasises palpation over symptom differentiation. For example, from the perspective of other styles of acupuncture, such as Meridian Therapy or TCM, signs such as dark circles under the eyes, dark facial tone, and the emergence of knee pain suggest the involvement of the kidney meridian.

Even from the point of view of MSA, the cervical symptoms suggest a YQD pattern, as this is not only part of the Du Mai symptom picture, but also because the YQD secondary reactions include both sides of the cervical spine. In contrast with these clues from the symptom picture, the palpatory findings consistently indicated a YWD and YQR diagnosis, and this combination proved effective.

CASE STUDY 6. PELVIC PAIN AND ENDOMETRIOSIS

Grace, Female, 43

Occupation: Lawyer

PRESENTING CONDITION

Grace had suffered from chronic pelvic pain for 8 years. She experienced daily background pain, which she rated at over 4/10, and increased to 8/10 during ovulation.

RELEVANT HISTORY

- Fibroid (diagnosed 8 years ago)
- Endometriosis (diagnosed 3 years ago)
- Vulvodynia
- Dyspareunia
- Hydrosalpinx
- Overactive bladder (frequency and urgency)
- Gave birth 3 years ago

PALPATION

- Tightness on the midline above the navel
- Softness and pressure pain below the navel
- LU 1 and LU 2 tender (more pronounced on left)
- KID 16 tender on the left

TREATMENT 1

Diagnosis: YQR

Step 1: YQR with IPC (10 minutes)
Step 2: *Chishin* at BL 23, BL 25, BL 43, GB 12, DU 17 with infrared (FIR) lamp on back
Step 3: N/A
Step 4: Pyonex press tack on right ear *shenmen*; taught Korean hand microsystem massage

TREATMENT 2 (FOLLOWING WEEK)

Patient Response
Background pain reduced to 1.5/10. New complaint: right scapular pain.

PALPATION

- Right subcostals tight, and ST 25–27 reactive
- Softness and pressure pain below navel
- REN 17 tender

Diagnosis: YWC and YQR

Step 1: Mixed Yin with IPC
Step 2: *Chishin* at BL 18, BL 20 (bilateral) with infrared (FIR) lamp on back, right BL 43, SP 6, pressure pain point near left BL 25
Step 4: Pyonex press tack to right scapular *ashi* point

TREATMENT 3 (FOLLOWING WEEK)

Patient Response
Background pain slightly increased to 2.5/10 after a stressful week. Ovulatory pain is less than usual and shorter duration

PALPATION

- Tightness and tenderness in the right subcostal region
- Tenderness at CV 17
- Softness and pressure pain below the navel

Diagnosis: YQR and YWC

Step 1: Mixed Yin

Step 2: Bilateral BL 18 and BL 20 with infrared (FIR) lamp, plus right BL 43, bilateral BL 30, SP 6, and tender point near left BL 25

Step 3: N/A

Step 4: Reviewed Korean hand microsystem; prescribed home therapy with Pyonex press tack on right lower medial scapula *ashi* point and right ear *shenmen* point

TREATMENT 4 (FOLLOWING WEEK)

Patient Response

Pain reduced to 1.5/10.

PALPATION

- Tightness and tenderness at right subcostal region
- Tenderness at CV 17
- Softness and pressure pain below the navel

Diagnosis: YQR and YWC

Step 1: Mixed Yin

Step 2: Bilateral BL 18 and BL 20 with infrared (FIR) lamp, bilateral BL 31, and pressure pain point near left BL 25

Step 3: N/A

Step 4: Reviewed Korean hand microsystem; prescribed home therapy with Pyonex press tack on right lower medial scapula *ashi* point and right ear *shenmen* point

TREATMENT 5 (FOLLOWING WEEK)

Patient Response
Pain reduced to 1/10.

PALPATION

- Tenderness at left ST 25 and along the left Dai Mai
- Softness and pressure pain below the navel
- Tightness and tenderness at left LU 1, LU 2

Diagnosis: YQR and Dai Mai on the left

Step 1: Ren Dai (left-belt)
Step 2: Bilateral BL 19 and BL 23 with an infrared (FIR) lamp, bilateral BL 31
Step 3: N/A
Step 4: Reviewed Korean hand microsystem; prescribed home therapy with Pyonex press tack on right lower medial scapula *ashi* point and right ear *shenmen* point

TREATMENT 6 (FOLLOWING WEEK)

Patient Response
Pain maintained at 1/10.

PALPATION

- Tenderness at left ST 25 and along the left Dai Mai
- Softness and pressure pain below the navel
- Tightness and tenderness at left LU 1, LU 2

Diagnosis: YQR and Dai Mai on the left

Step 1: Ren Dai (left-belt)
Step 2: Bilateral BL 19 and BL 23 with infrared (FIR) lamp, bilateral BL 31
Step 3: N/A
Step 4: Reviewed Korean hand microsystem; prescribed home therapy with Pyonex press tack on right lower medial scapula *ashi* point and right ear *shenmen* point

CONCLUSIONS AND REFLECTIONS

At the end of this treatment period, Grace reported a significant reduction in chronic background pelvic pain and a reduction in both the duration and intensity of her ovulatory pain. She noted that her vulvodynia, a sharp, burning vulval pain, had disappeared by the third week. She also commented that she felt calmer overall and experienced a greater sense of well-being, despite the pressures of her very stressful job as a lawyer.

From a palpation perspective, tenderness below the navel when the patient is not menstruating is always a significant finding that calls for the inclusion of the YQR in the overall treatment. As we can see from the treatment arc, Grace was treated with YQR, Mixed Yin, and Ren Dai, all of which include YQR.

[Note: There's more about this presentation in Chapter 14.]

CASE STUDY 7. SCIATICA WITH NAIL PATELLA SYNDROME

Naoko, Female, 51

Occupation: Psychologist

PRESENTING CONDITION

Naoko had developed left-sided sciatica 3 months earlier after a fall. MRI confirmed a hernia at L5/S1, with pain radiating from the left sacroiliac joint down the GB meridian to the knee, foot, and big toe. The condition was progressively worsening. She relied on a stroller chair for walking support, had temporary relief from local injections, and managed day to day with paracetamol [acetaminophen] after discontinuing opiates. Twice-weekly physiotherapy gave only minimal improvement.

RELEVANT HISTORY

- Nail Patella Syndrome (a genetic disorder affecting nails and tendons)
- Multiple Achilles tendon surgeries (2 per side)
- Pre-eclampsia–induced kidney failure 13 years ago; bilateral kidney transplant in the lower abdomen
- On immunosuppressants and mild antihypertensives
- Ibuprofen is contraindicated due to kidney metabolism
- Menopausal (no menses for over 1 year; previously painful)
- Mother of 3 (2 via surrogate)
- Prior unsuccessful trial of Chinese acupuncture

From her medical history, it was clear she was likely to be sensitive.

PALPATION

- Right subcostal tightness
- Left ST 26–27 region tight and painful to pressure
- Left ASIS border stiff

[*Note: The scars from the kidney transplant surgery complicated the abdominal assessment.*]

TREATMENT 1

Diagnosis: CS

Step 1: CS with IPC (5 minutes)
Step 2: *Chishin* needling at GB 20 and GB 21, with infrared (FIR) lamp over BL 23, BL 25, and medial left GB 30
Step 3: N/A
Step 4: Intradermal at left ear, low back point; 0.6 mm Pyonex press tack at BL 23

TREATMENT 2 (FOLLOWING WEEK)

Patient Response
Pain improved; walking still difficult. Paracetamol [acetaminophen] use unchanged.

Step 1: CS with IPC (10 minutes)
Step 2: *Chishin* at BL 20, BL 23, and medial left GB 30 with infrared (FIR) lamp
Step 3: N/A
Step 4: Intradermal at left ear, low back point; 0.6 mm Pyonex press tack at BL 23

TREATMENT 3 (FOLLOWING WEEK)

Patient Response
Pain better but sleep worse; dizziness after physiotherapy.

PALPATION

- Pronounced tenderness at ASIS, ST 26 and KID 11

Diagnosis: YQD

Step 1: YQD with IPC (10 minutes)
Step 2: *Chishin* at GB 20, GB 21, BL 18, BL 23, and medial left GB 30 with infrared (FIR) lamp
Step 3: N/A
Step 4: Intradermal at left ear, low back point; 0.6 mm Pyonex press tack at BL 23

TREATMENT 4 (3 WEEKS LATER)

Patient Response
Pain improved; no longer used the stroller chair. Dizziness resolved after chiropractic.

PALPATION

Subcostal tightness and lower left quadrant jump reaction

Diagnosis: CS

Step 1: CS with IPC (10 minutes)
Step 2: *Chishin* at GB 20, GB 21, BL 20, BL 23, and medial left GB 30 with infrared (FIR) lamp
Step 3: N/A
Step 4: Intradermal at left ear, low back point; 0.6 mm Pyonex press tack at BL 23

TREATMENT 5 (11 WEEKS LATER)

Patient Response
Pain-free, walking normally; mild residual cough.

PALPATION

Subcostal tightness, midline tenderness and reactivity on right ST 25–ST 27

Diagnosis: Mixed Yin

Step 1: Mixed Yin with IPC (10 minutes)
Step 2: *Chishin* at GB 20, GB 21, BL 18, BL 23, and medial left GB 30 with infrared (FIR) lamp
Step 3: N/A
Step 4: 0.6 mm Pyonex press tack at GB 21; 0.3 mm Pyonex press tack at Stop Cough point near LU 5

CONCLUSIONS AND REFLECTIONS

Naoko responded well despite her complex medical history. A cautious approach with low-dose treatments was essential, given her sensitivity and history of kidney transplantation. Over the course of treatment, her sciatica resolved completely, mobility returned to normal, and she regained independence in daily activities.

This case illustrates how MSA can be effective even when applied with restraint: the root treatment (primarily CS) remained consistent, while branch treatments varied to address changing symptoms. The use of IPC, *chishin*, infrared support, and Pyonex press tacks provided safe and effective interventions. Her recovery reinforces the principle that steady repetition of root treatment, adapted to the patient's sensitivity, can produce durable outcomes.

CLOSING THOUGHTS

On reviewing these seven case studies, some clear themes emerge. Firstly, the Four Steps are not a rigid protocol but a flexible framework—more like four toolkits than a strict sequence. Each practitioner balanced structure with responsiveness, fulfilling the intent of each step while adapting to what the patient needed in the moment.

Secondly, the practitioner notes repeatedly highlight the value of feedback—every decision was guided by palpation changes, patient feedback, and clinical observation, ensuring the approach was not mechanical but alive to the patient's needs. We can also imagine that the patients experienced these palpatory changes first-hand, and this would have been a helpful added benefit of the palpation. As those abdominal reactions softened for the practitioner, the patients, too, were able to experience physical changes taking place during the session.

Thirdly, we see how supportive measures, whether with takeaways or simple advice, can extend the effects of treatment into daily life and help patients consolidate their gains.

These themes underscore the spirit of Manaka's system: freedom within the structure of the Four Steps with a focus on economy, adaptability, and sensitivity to the needs of the patient. The Four Steps provide the framework, but it's the practitioner's presence, listening, and creativity that make them effective.

With this foundation established, we now turn to Part 2 of the book, which begins with a detailed exploration of moxibustion—both theory and practice. We will look more closely at how Japanese traditions of *okyu* and *kyutoshin* can be woven into the Manaka system as powerful additions to Step 4. And there are still more case studies to come—some presented in a standalone chapter like this one, others woven into subsequent chapters.

WHAT'S NEXT

Part 2 starts with the last of our Context chapters—a broad overview of the theory of moxibustion, comparing different kinds of moxa and exploring how moxibustion might work.

PART 2

MOXIBUSTION

CHAPTER 12

CONTEXT: INTRODUCING JAPANESE MOXIBUSTION

If a condition does not respond to needling, it should be treated with moxa.

—*Ling Shu*, Chapter 73[147]

Moxibustion should be used for conditions that do not respond to medicine or acupuncture.

—*Yi Xue Ru Men*[148]

Dr Manaka leaned heavily on moxibustion in his system. We have already seen how he used *kyutoshin* at Step 2 and *okyu* at Step 3, and both could also be applied at Step 4. In Step 4 practice, Manaka relied more on *hinaishin* for symptomatic relief, whereas his close associate Kazuko Itaya applied *okyu* more widely. In later volumes in this series, we will also see how Manaka developed specialised *okyu* treatments that could be used at Step 1 in place of ion pumping.

---

147 *Ling Shu*. Quoted in Auteroche, B. et al. (1992). *Acupuncture and Moxibustion: A Guide to Clinical Practice*. Edinburgh: Churchill Livingstone. p. 75.

148 Li, S. Yixue rumen [The Rudiments of Medicine]. Ming Dynasty. Quoted in Auteroche, B. et al. (1992). *Acupuncture and Moxibustion: A Guide to Clinical Practice*. Edinburgh: Churchill Livingstone. p. 75.

Chapters 12 and 13 will review moxibustion in general terms and explore how Japanese practice diverges from traditional Chinese approaches in terms of conceptualising dosage and the perception of moxibustion as a 'heating' therapy. We will focus on *okyu* small-cone moxibustion and broaden our understanding of *kyutoshin*, giving us more options and tools to apply during the Four Steps, especially at Step 4.

One of the striking features of Japanese practice is the way it treats dosage—how much stimulation is delivered—as a central component of treatment. We have described Manaka's approach as "maximum effect with minimum intervention" and Japanese refinements of *okyu* small-cone moxibustion reflect this philosophy. Dosage is not an afterthought: it shapes the manufacturing of moxa, the way cones are rolled, and the choice of technique. As we go through this chapter, we will keep dosage in mind—it explains why Japanese moxibustion looks and feels different from its Chinese counterparts.

MOXA BASICS

Moxibustion is a Traditional Chinese Medicine (TCM) therapy that involves burning dried mugwort (moxa) on specific points on the body. It plays an important role in the traditional medical systems of China, as well as those of Tibet, Japan, Korea, Vietnam, and Mongolia. It is one of the oldest forms of therapy, originating from China and predating acupuncture. The earliest acupuncture texts—the *Huang Di Nei Jing, Suwen,* and *Ling Shu*—contain information about it.

Moxibustion was in use as a therapeutic tool before acupuncture was formalised in the *Huang Di Nei Jing*. It is discussed there alongside needling, and in later centuries, both modalities continued to be practised in parallel. Several centuries later, during periods when acupuncture became less prominent, moxibustion gained greater traction, with specialist literature emerging in the seventh century and dedicated moxa-only treatises appearing by the late twelfth century.

The Chinese word for moxibustion is *jiǔ* (灸), which means 'to burn or cauterise'. The herb most often burned in historical and contemporary practice is mugwort (Artemisia vulgaris), but after the Jin and Tang eras, the scope of moxibustion was broadened with the introduction of medicinal substances used in conjunction with mugwort.[149]

Moxibustion can be applied to broad regions and meridian points, stimulating the circulation and promoting a smoother flow of qi and blood. In TCM, it is indicated for conditions associated with cold, yang deficiency, or dampness. It is considered especially effective for chronic and deficient presentations, as well as in geriatric care.

Historically, there have been more than fifty methods of applying moxibustion.[150] Moxa can be rolled and applied in a cigar form, shaped into cones, or placed onto the end of a needle. It can be burned in containers such as moxa boxes or Ontake and applied to intermediaries such as salt, ginger, garlic, onion, or chives. Moxibustion does not use mugwort exclusively; heat can also be applied by burning mulberry wood, peach wood, or rush pith. Moxibustion 'without heat' can be applied by using vesicatory medication.

This huge variety of techniques means that it is difficult to discuss the effects of moxa in general terms, unless we are specific about the particular moxa technique. Thus, when we say that moxa is "good for immunity", we need to specify what kind of moxa technique we are referring to. Modern Chinese texts tend to describe moxa as heating, whereas Japanese texts tend not to. Which moxa techniques are heating, and which are warming or merely stimulating?

ACUPUNCTURE AND MOXIBUSTION

> *Moxibustion and acupuncture needle treatment are totally different kinds of stimulation. When we use a needle, the needle is metal, and we insert it into your skin, with the contact of the metal to your skin, but moxibustion is heat, and heat basically burns your skin, and that's a totally different*

149 Auteroche, B., et al. (1992). *Acupuncture and Moxibustion: A Guide to Clinical Practice*. Edinburgh: Churchill Livingstone.

150 Ibid. p. 75.

> *stimulation. If you combine two different kinds of stimulation like that, if you have two different tools and if you connect two tools, two very good methods, you can make more efficiency. So, needle stimulation and moxa/ heat stimulation don't conflict with each other; they help.*
>
> —Junji Mizutani[151]

In China, moxibustion has had three main roles:

1. To treat intractable diseases
2. For longevity
3. To prevent disease

According to the *Great Compendium of Acupuncture and Moxibustion*, officials often travelled with two or three unhealed moxa scars on their bodies as protection against malaria, epidemics, pestilences, and ulcerating sores. It says, "*If you wish to be safe, never allow the* zusanli *points to become dry*."[152]

In this context, the classics refer to direct moxa, a cone placed on the skin and burned all the way down. In Chinese traditions, these cones may be quite large, and the burns and subsequent blisters they produce can be substantial.

In the 1950s, with the formalisation of TCM, a hierarchy was established in which herbal theory sat at the top, while acupuncture and moxibustion were considered subordinate. As a result, moxibustion in China has been interpreted largely through a herbal lens.

---

151 Kivity, O. (2018). 'Japanese Acupuncture: What's So Unique?' *European Journal of Oriental Medicine*, 9(2). p. 21.

152 Needham, J. & Lu, G.-D. (1980). *Celestial Lancets: A History and Rationale of Acupuncture and Moxa.* Cambridge: Cambridge University Press. p. 181.

In herbal medicine, warm diseases are treated with cooling herbs, never with warm ones. By analogy, moxibustion—because it involves burning a herb—was categorised as a warming therapy, to be used like a warming herb for patients with cold conditions. From this perspective, warm diseases should not be treated with moxibustion, as this would be adding yang to yang, heat to heat.

This view makes sense if we are talking about large cones that scar the skin or a moxa box. Moxa boxes produce such intense heat that they must be moved frequently to avoid burns, leaving the skin sweaty and red. However, as we have seen, the term *moxibustion* covers a wide range of methods. In JAAM, some are not regarded as warming at all, but as stimulating.

Chinese texts describe the actions of moxibustion in much the same terms as herbs. *Acupuncture: A Comprehensive Text* lists its functions as:

- Opens the twelve primary meridians
- Courses through the three yin
- Regulates qi and blood
- Expels cold and dampness
- Warms the uterus[153]

Acupuncture and Moxibustion: A Guide to Clinical Practice says it:

- Warms and moves qi and blood
- Strengthens kidney yang
- Expels wind and disperses cold
- Invigorates the blood and dissolves toxins[154]

By contrast, in Japan, the theory and practice of acupuncture and moxibustion developed independently of herbal theory. More importantly, moxibustion came to

153 Shanghai College of Traditional Medicine (1985). *Acupuncture: A Comprehensive Text.* Seattle: Eastland Press. p. 438.

154 Auteroche, B., et al. (1992). *Acupuncture and Moxibustion: A Guide to Clinical Practice.* Edinburgh: Churchill Livingstone. p. 76.

be practised as a therapy in its own right. This is one of those areas of specialisation in JAAM that we mentioned in Chapter 3, and it yielded novel and original approaches.

Pioneers such as Takeshi Sawada and Isaburo Fukaya often treated patients using moxa alone, applying it in situations where herbal theory would have proscribed it. Dr Shimetaro Hara, practising in the pre-antibiotic era, used moxa to treat tuberculosis. Sawada did likewise. Fukaya applied it for fevers.

It was used for red, swollen, arthritic joints, although in such cases it is applied proximally, or surrounding the site of inflammation, rather than directly on it. The legacy of these masters is that the scope of moxibustion in JAAM is much broader than in TCM. It is also less theoretical and more empirical than acupuncture, even Japanese acupuncture. Moxa was also widely used as a home treatment. This did little for its reputation. Because parents were often unskilled in its application, generations of Japanese children grew up experiencing it as painful. Dr Hara helped to reframe this folk therapy. He was the first medical doctor we know of to train formally in moxibustion, and he conducted ground-breaking research into its humoral effects (see below). His work helped elevate moxibustion's status from a folk remedy to a respected medical practice. Dr Hara also advocated daily moxa for longevity, and in 1991, he died at the age of 108, the oldest man in Japan.

Moxibustion in Japan can thus be summarised as follows:

- A specialised treatment, often applied without acupuncture
- A home treatment by lay people
- Used for a wide range of conditions, both internal and external, including hot conditions
- Less theoretical, more empirical

APPLICATION

These differences between Chinese and Japanese perceptions of moxa appear not only in the theoretical aspects of moxibustion but also in practical terms: its application and manufacture.

> *When I lived in Malaysia, a colleague showed me his small-cone moxa technique, which he'd learned in China. He rolled small tapering cones about 7 mm tall. They were wide at the base and narrow at the top, and he used much force to compress the moxa as he rolled. While I admired the speed, proficiency, and uniformity with which he rolled these cones, they were the antithesis of what Japanese teachers had taught me. The wide base meant that more heat would be delivered to the skin. The high degree of compression meant that the cone would burn longer and more slowly, again delivering more heat. He usually used a greener, coarser moxa to make his cones and marvelled at the quality of my Japanese gold moxa. Unrefined moxa burns at a higher temperature than refined gold moxa. Thus, on all counts, his moxa cones were going to deliver more heat for longer than mine.*
>
> —Oran Kivity

Stephen Birch explained these differences in an interview on YouTube:

> *When I first learned acupuncture, moxa was either this crude, green powdery stuff that you put into a metal thing and you massage somebody with this metal thing and it was really, really hot or it was sticks of smelly moxa that you would hold near the point and it would get really, really hot, or you cut pieces off these sticks and you stick it on the handle of the needle, and it got really, really hot.*
>
> *My first teacher, Tin Yau So, had been working in China before at a time when there was basically no functional health care system in China, so he had to use the tools available to treat whatever was happening, whoever came for treatment.... He would take relatively large, hard, compressed balls of moxa—the smallest being like an adzuki bean or a mung bean and then the largest being like a kidney bean—and he would place it on the skin and burn it down to the skin and basically leave a clear scar. So when I first learned about moxa it was any of those things and it was really, really hot and sometimes really, really uncomfortable ...*

> *The Japanese are very good at taking somebody's idea and kind of playing with it to make it better and more functional, so instead of making a round ball of moxa, you make your moxa shape like a grain of rice, so that the contact point on the skin is much smaller... and you don't roll it hard, you roll it softly, so it burns more quickly; it's moulded softly to shape, so when it burns down—yes there's a pinch of heat, but it's not the same kind of burning sensation or really, really hot sensations.*
>
> —Stephen Birch[155]

This description highlights how Japanese refinements to moxibustion techniques shift the experience from something harsh and painful to something more subtle and tolerable.

MOXA TECHNIQUES ON A SPECTRUM

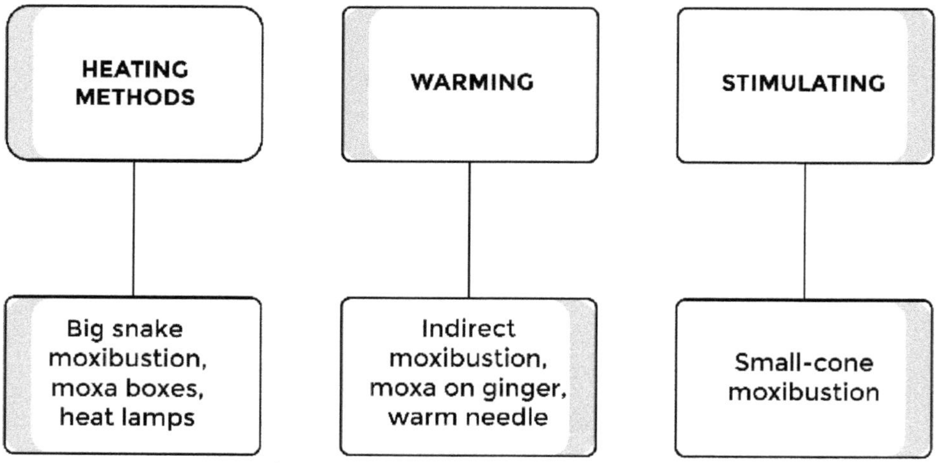

Figure 12-1: A spectrum of moxibustion techniques.

Moxa techniques can be divided into two broad categories: direct and indirect.

155 Kivity, O. (2018). 'Japanese Acupuncture: What's So Unique?' *European Journal of Oriental Medicine*, 9(2). p. 22.

Direct moxa is applied directly to the skin. Cones may be rolled into a wide range of shapes and sizes, from the large balls described by Stephen Birch to pyramid-shaped cones about 1 cm high, or narrow cones ranging in size from a sesame seed or grain of rice up to 7 mm in height. Direct moxa can be scarring (including blistering or suppurative techniques) or non-scarring.

Indirect moxa is burnt away from the skin, or through an intermediary. Moxa-on-the-needle methods, such as *kyutoshin* in JAAM or *wenzhen* in TCM, are indirect, as are moxa on salt in the navel, moxa on ginger, and moxa boxes and Ontake. Using a moxa stick is also indirect, since the skin is warmed from a distance. Even with press moxa methods using a stick such as *oshi kyu* (Chinese *shi'an jiu*), a sheet of cloth is placed between the moxa and the skin.

The most extreme indirect moxibustion technique is a Chinese method known as Long Snake Moxibustion (*Cheng She Jiu*). A thick mound of crushed garlic is laid along the entire length of the spine. Various powdered herbs are placed on top of the mound, and then moxa is placed on top of these. The cones are lit and replaced for several rounds, producing profound heat and blistering. This is a very uncomfortable treatment. The blisters are then pierced, drained and bandaged. This treatment is thought to raise immunity, as it is on the sea of yang, the Du Mai.[156]

We can now see the difficulty of talking about 'the effects of moxibustion'. Clearly, a technique like *Cheng She Jiu* will have markedly different effects than using a moxa stick, Ontake, or half-rice-grain-sized moxibustion. What we see in the diversity above is a spectrum of moxibustion techniques. At one end are heating methods, such as moxa boxes and *Cheng She Jiu*. In the middle are warming techniques such as *kyutoshin* or moxa on ginger, and at the other end are stimulating techniques, such as small-cone moxibustion or Ontake.

---

156 Kivity, O. (1992). *Lecture on Clinical Moxibustion*. Shandong University of Traditional Chinese Medicine Teaching Hospital, Jinan, China. Personal notes.

COMPARING *KYUTOSHIN* AND *WENZHEN*

We saw in Chapter 8 that the Chinese and Japanese versions of warm needle are practised differently and feel quite different. In Chinese acupuncture, copper-wound needles conduct heat strongly, and a segment of a moxa stick is used, burning hotter and longer than loosely rolled semi-pure moxa. Radiated and conducted heat are therefore greater and more prolonged in *wenzhen* than in *kyutoshin*.

Even with the same technique, there is a spectrum from heating to warming, depending on the grade of moxa, the density and size of the moxa cone, and the needle design.

GRADES OF MOXA

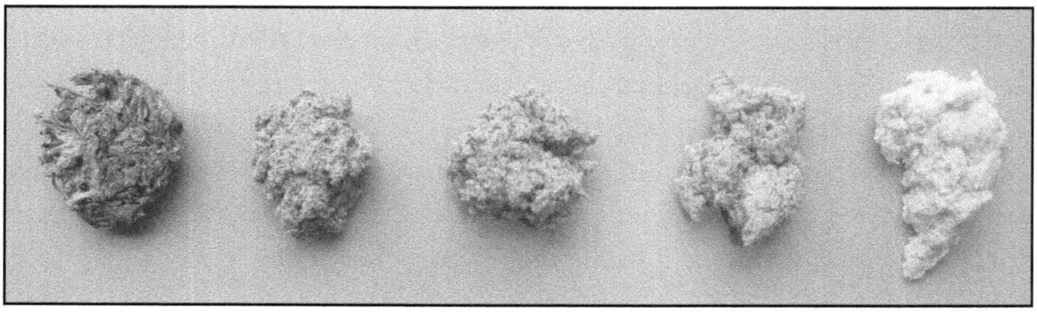

Figure 12-2: Samples of Japanese Moxa. Left to right: processed mugwort (1st stage); processed mugwort (2nd stage); coarse moxa for indirect moxibustion; semi-pure moxa for indirect and direct moxibustion; refined moxa for direct moxibustion.[157]

Both Paul Movsessian and Oran Kivity have visited Yamasho, a traditional moxa manufacturer in Japan, established in 1895. Yamasho produces three general grades of moxa: coarse, semi-pure, and refined.[158]

---

[157] Image sourced from Wikimedia Commons. Released under the Creative Commons CC0 1.0 Universal Public Domain Dedication.

[158] To see Oran Kivity's site visit to the Yamasho moxa factory, view: *Japanese Acupuncture Today*. (2022). Episode 7: 'Making Moxa—Inside Yamasho' [Video]. Available at: https://youtu.be/D44d9AS_Ltk?si=V9e3_BHL2BJhLdUf

COARSE

Coarse moxa is dark green. It contains small fragments of twig and leaf, mixed with trichomes—the fine, downy hairs on the underside of the leaves. Because it burns at a relatively high temperature, it is mainly used in indirect methods, such as moxa on garlic or in a moxa box. This is the grade Yamasho uses in its platform moxa cones and is similar to the material used in Chinese moxa sticks.

SEMI-PURE (MEDIUM GRADE)

Semi-pure moxa is a lighter green, with fewer impurities and a higher proportion of trichomes. It's refined enough for rolling balls of moxa for *kyutoshin* or large-cone moxa (*chinetsukyu*). It can be compressed securely into bamboo tubes, making it ideal for the percussive strokes of Ontake. Yamasho's best-known medium grade is Wakakusa.

PURE MOXA (FINEST GRADE)

Pure moxa, sometimes called gold moxa, is yellow and so refined that no leafy material remains, only trichomes. It burns at a relatively low temperature, especially if the cones are rolled loosely.

The different burning temperatures of each grade of moxa are summarised in Table 12.1.[159]

[159] Young, M. (2023). *The Moon over Matsushima: Insights into Moxa and Mugwort.* 2nd ed. London: Sayoshi Books. p. 221.

Table 12.1: Burning temperatures of different grades of moxa.

TYPE OF MOXA	BURNING TEMPERATURE
Chinese coarse moxa	450°C
Wakakusa semi-pure	430°C
Yomei Gold Mountain moxa	400°C

This high degree of refinement underpins a key difference between TCM and JAAM. While Chinese moxa is often greener and less refined, limiting its use to primarily indirect techniques, Japanese gold moxa is a specialised tool. Its purity allows for direct application on the skin, fundamentally expanding its therapeutic scope beyond the TCM canon and enabling the treatment of a far wider array of conditions. Together with the specialisations of moxa-only practitioners, such as Isaburo Fukaya, we can utilise moxa to treat a wide range of symptoms and conditions.

SMALL-CONE MOXA THEORY

> *I believe that already more than a century ago, in Japan, you see the beginning of physiological studies of the biological effects of moxa that show distinct differences between moxa and needling. When you burn down with moxa to the skin, it triggers production of red and white blood cells in a way that needles don't. When you burn moxa down to the skin and cause small tissue damage, it triggers these immunological changes, which happen on a larger scale and more diversely than you tend to see with simple needling alone, and if you understand how to use these... it gives you a very broad-ranging set of tools.*
>
> —Stephen Birch[160]

160 Kivity, O. (2018). 'Japanese Acupuncture: What's So Unique?' *European Journal of Oriental Medicine*, 9(2). p. 21.

In JAAM, a distinction is often made between two levels: the qi level and the blood level. Acute problems are said to be at the qi level, and chronic problems are said to be at the blood level. Direct small-cone moxibustion is more effective for blood-level conditions and generally beneficial for organic problems and difficult, complicated, and stubborn diseases. It can soften indurations in muscle tissue, relieve contracture, and improve mobility. It warms, moves, and stimulates. It maximises capillary action and revitalises tissue. It can be applied to soften tight spots that were not released by needling. For this reason, you can see why the *Ling Shu* quotation at the start of the chapter states that if a cold condition does not respond to needling, it should be treated with moxa. Moxa treats chronic, stagnated conditions at the blood level.

Sadly, moxibustion has not been researched as much as acupuncture. The first modern scientific publication on moxibustion was written by the Japanese physician Shimetaro Hara, who conducted intensive research about the haematological effects of moxibustion in 1927. *Chasing the Dragon's Tail* cites many more recent pieces of research. Some research has been published in the *North American Journal of Oriental Medicine* (*NAJOM*). Merlin Young, the author of a definitive book on moxibustion, *The Moon over Matsushima*, and co-founder of the Moxafrica moxibustion charity, has stated that moxibustion has little appeal to modern researchers, appearing more barbaric and less plausible than needling. It is hard to get funding to research the effects of deliberately burning patients' skin! However, Moxafrica has successfully completed research into *okyu* and drug-resistant TB.[161]

This kind of direct small-cone moxibustion appears to be beneficial across a range of areas. It has been said to assist the body to:

- Return to homeostasis, with increased resistance to disease and improvement in sleep, appetite, and general well-being
- Regulate the autonomic nervous system
- Regulate the bowels
- Improve blood circulation and mobility

161 Young, M. (2023). *The Moon over Matsushima: Insights into Moxa and Mugwort*. 2nd ed. London: Sayoshi Books. pp. 331–360.

- Soften hardened tissue, relieve hard knots due to overuse and repetitive movement that causes degeneration and hardening in the tissues, reduce inflammation, and relieve pain
- Increase longevity

DOSAGE

As we saw at the beginning of the chapter, a central principle of Japanese moxibustion is the careful control of dosage—achieving maximum effect with minimal stimulation. Japanese *okyu* exemplifies this. The rolling method is very light, so the moxa wool is not compressed, resulting in less heat. The base of the moxa cone is narrow, which reduces its surface area and delivers less heat. Furthermore, in the manufacturing process, moxa is refined to an extremely high degree. It takes 100 kg of mugwort to make 4 kg of gold moxa.[162] The moxa wool is super-refined, allowing it to burn at a lower temperature. Thus, minimal stimulation is emphasised at all stages, starting even at the manufacturing process, and continuing to the rolling technique and even the shape of the cone. There's a wonderful unity of purpose from theory to manufacturing and to application. Considering the dosage helps us understand the physiological mechanisms discussed next.

MECHANISM

Historically, direct moxibustion was performed using large cones that were burned all the way to the skin, leaving scars. In the twentieth century, under the influence of practitioners such as Takeshi Sawada and Isaburo Fukaya, much smaller cones were used, including rice-grain-sized and half-rice-grain-sized. Thus, moxa was always used to damage the skin, but with modern refinements, the cones were much less damaging. Thus, the practice can be understood as a sophisticated biological conversation between a controlled injury and the body's innate healing systems. The mechanism is not singular but multi-layered, engaging the immune, nervous, and sensory systems simultaneously.

---

[162] *Japanese Acupuncture Today*. (2022). Episode 7: 'Making Moxa—Inside Yamasho' [Video]. Available at: https://youtu.be/D44d9AS_Ltk?si=V9e3_BHL2BJhLdUf

MICROBURNS AND DENATURED PROTEINS

At its most fundamental level, moxibustion works by creating a precise, controlled microburn. Simply put, the body doesn't like getting burned and reacts. *Okyu* creates a microburn, triggering a local inflammatory response. But crucially, this local trauma then provokes a powerful, systemic anti-inflammatory response.

This process has a good analogy in your kitchen. Consider what happens when you boil an egg. The heat damages or denatures the protein in the egg, causing it to solidify. Similarly, the heat from moxa damages proteins in the skin. One theory, based on Dr Hara's work, is that this creates denatured or *heat-shock proteins*. These denatured proteins seep into the bloodstream in minute amounts. Although harmless, the body identifies them as foreign (histotoxins or antigens), stimulating the production of red and especially white blood cells and increasing phagocytosis (the immune system's clean-up process).

TRIGGERING THE IMMUNE SYSTEM

This triggered immune response is measurable and potent. Examination of skin tissue after moxibustion stimulation reveals an increased migration of helper T-cells and natural killer cells from surrounding blood vessels, both of which are essential for activating a broad biological immune response.[163] The result is a cascade of systemic changes: an increase in red blood cells and haemoglobin, a higher sedimentation rate, and rises in blood glucose and calcium.

Critically, moxibustion not only stimulates the immune system but also regulates it. This regulatory effect is powerfully demonstrated in historical and modern treatments for tuberculosis. Both Dr Shimetaro Hara and Takeshi Sawada routinely treated TB with blistering moxibustion, and this work has been replicated by the British charity Moxafrica, founded by British practitioners Merlin Young and Jenny Craig. They found that microburns trigger immunological changes, which, for patients with drug-resistant

163 Kazuo, T. (2002). 'Examination on the Immunological Effects of Moxibustion Treatment', *NAJOM*, 9(25). pp. 13–16.

TB, can render standard drugs effective again. The drug-resistant TB starts to respond to the medication. Simply put, daily moxibustion triggers an immune response sufficient to make the TB drugs effective once again, much like placing a plank under a car wheel that is spinning in the mud, providing the traction the immune system needs to fight back.

PAIN MODULATION AND RELAXATION

Parallel to the immune response is a profound effect on the nervous system. The initial burn causes pain, which itself triggers the body's own analgesic response. The body has many reflexes that respond to pain stimuli, which can help reduce the experience of pain. Furthermore, certain methods, such as the small-cone Japanese style, appear to specifically activate the parasympathetic nervous system—the 'rest and digest' state. This leads patients to relax, their blood pressure to reduce, and their appetite to increase.

NEW RESEARCH INTO TRP CHANNELS

Recent research, presented by Merlin Young, has begun to shed light on how moxibustion might interact with the body's sensory systems.[164] One promising line of inquiry concerns transient receptor potential (TRP) channels. These protein structures sit on the surface of nerve and skin cells, acting like molecular gatekeepers. When triggered by heat, pressure, or specific chemicals, they open to let calcium ions enter the cell, setting off a cascade of physiological responses, including pulling your hand away from a hot object. These are the same channels that make chilli peppers feel hot (TRPV1) and menthol feel cool (TRPM8).

Some TRPs are directly involved in pain signalling, and when they become overactive, they can get 'stuck in the on position'. Like a telephone receiver left off the hook, the line is constantly busy, and no other signals can get through—almost a definition of chronic pain. Three specific TRP channels are linked to chronic disease, and it seems that they may have a special relationship with moxibustion:

---

164 Young, M. (2023). *The Moon over Matsushima: Insights into Moxa and Mugwort*. 2nd ed. London: Sayoshi Books.

TRPV1: Activated by heat (around 43°C–52°C) and by capsaicin, the fiery component of chilli. When desensitised, it can reduce pain signals. Small-cone moxa appears to work partly through this pathway.

TRPA1: Normally causes strong pain responses. It can, however, be inhibited by borneol and cineole.

TRPM8: Triggered by menthol and borneol. It creates cooling sensations and counterbalances TRPV1, helping to reduce pain when TRPV1 is firing.

The most remarkable part of the TRP–mugwort story is that while one of these TRPs is triggered by heat, such as that given by an *okyu* microburn, the other two are triggered *only* by a tiny shortlist of chemicals. Bizarrely, of the 200 or so chemicals in mugwort, the two most abundant are borneol and cineole. The most prominent components of mugwort inhibit TRPA1 and activate TRPM8. At the same time, the heat of burning moxa desensitises TRPV1.

In other words, moxa doesn't just warm the skin; it may be engaging with the body's chemistry in highly specific ways, modulating pain and sensation through multiple distinct channels simultaneously. This also suggests that the constituents of mugwort are an essential factor in promoting the immune and neurological response, which might explain its extraordinary longevity as the herb of choice for moxibustion.

A SYNERGISTIC SYSTEM

The growing body of research suggests that different moxa techniques may act through different physiological mechanisms. Just as there's a spectrum of moxa techniques, ranging from heating to warming and to stimulating, there's also a range of effects in the body. On the one hand, the challenge for the future is to determine which methods influence which receptors and systems, and how best to apply that knowledge in practice. On the other hand, we already have a vast canon of effective *okyu* techniques that were proven effective before the development of contemporary theories on their mechanism.

Ultimately, moxibustion is a holistic intervention; it creates a controlled injury to regulate immunity, modulates pain through precise chemical and thermal pathways, and prompts a state of nervous system relaxation, all working in concert to stimulate the body's powerful self-healing capabilities.

DIRECT MOXA IN MSA

Manaka considered direct moxibustion so useful that he taught methods for its use in his Four Step protocol. Table 12.2 illustrates how these techniques align with each of his Four Steps.

Table 12.2: Direct moxa during the Four Steps.

STEP 1	As an alternative treatment that can be used in place of an ion-pumping treatment, direct moxibustion can be applied as a whole-body, non-pattern-based root treatment.	We will examine this in Vol. 2.
	Moxa on DU 20 can be applied when the abdomen is very reactive, ticklish, or hard to palpate.	This is a good workaround when your patient jumps every time you palpate the belly.
	Okyu can be applied concurrently with Step 1 to supplement the body's energy; for example, treating ST 36 and REN 12 while the cords are in place. Alternatively, you can use symptomatic moxa points, such as those for diarrhoea or food poisoning, treating Step 4 during Step 1.	Treatment does not have to be linear. Doing moxa during Step 1 can save time considerably.
STEP 2	*Okyu* can be used as an alternative to *kyutoshin*. *Okyu* can be applied with meridian stretching techniques (Vol. 2).	
STEP 3	*Okyu* can be applied with Sotai.	
STEP 4	*Okyu* and *kyutoshin* (especially *okyu*) can be applied for symptom relief (see below).	

SUMMARY

- Dosage as a central plank: Japanese practice is built on the principle of maximum effect with minimal stimulation, from refining moxa wool to rolling and applying the cones.
- Different traditions: While TCM frames moxa as a heating therapy bound to herbal theory, Japanese practitioners developed it as an empirical treatment, often used independently and for hot conditions.
- Refinement: Japanese innovations transformed crude, painful methods into tolerable ones, greatly expanding their therapeutic range.
- A spectrum of methods: Techniques range from heating (moxa boxes, Long Snake Moxibustion) and warming (*kyutoshin*, moxa on ginger moxa) to stimulating (small-cone *okyu*, *Ontake*).
- Action on the blood level: *Okyu* is especially valuable for chronic blood-level conditions, softening indurations, regulating function, and moving stasis.
- Mechanism: Microburns from *okyu* mobilise and regulate the immune system, trigger natural pain-relief mechanisms, and activate the parasympathetic nervous system.
- TRPs: Moxa may be engaging the body's chemistry in precise ways, such as through its chemical constituents borneol and cineole, not just through its warmth.

WHAT'S NEXT

The next chapter takes us out of the theory and into the fire, where we'll explore the practical skills of *okyu* and *kyutoshin*.

CHAPTER 13

PRACTICAL MOXIBUSTION

With all we've written about the theory of moxibustion, it could be tempting to think of it as something very abstract. In reality, moxibustion is a series of very embodied processes, from palpating for points to rolling, placing, and lighting cones, all accompanied by the glow of the incense stick and the distinctive scent of the smoke.

Many practitioners avoid direct moxa, intimidated by its technical demands. To explain the process, the first part of this chapter is a practical guide to mastering *okyu*—from rolling the perfect cone to extinguishing it at the precise moment. We will demystify the procedures and show how, once again, skilled palpation is the key to unlocking its powerful clinical effects. You will learn the intricacies of rolling, placing, and burning moxa and find dynamic 'alive' points that transform a textbook point location into an effective one.

The second part of the chapter returns to *kyutoshin*. While we have so far explored it as a Step 2 treatment, we will now learn how to adapt and use it effectively within Step 4.

DIRECT MOXIBUSTION: *OKYU*

This technique involves the use of super-pure or gold moxa, from which all the particles and leaf fibres have been removed, leaving only the trichomes, the tiny hairs on the underside of the leaf. We saw how this reduces the intensity and consistency of the moxa burn. The high-quality wool also makes it easier to roll tiny cones, which are burnt directly on the skin. These vary in size:[165, 166, 167]

Table 13.1: Moxa cone descriptions.

NAME	DESCRIPTION / DIMENSIONS
Thread moxa	Very fine, like a thread
Sesame size	Minuscule pieces
Half rice grain	Small pieces
Rice grain size	Can vary in size: • **HEIGHT:** 2–3 mm • **SMALL:** Base 1 mm • **MEDIUM:** Base 1.5–2 mm • **LARGE:** Base 2.5 mm

If you consider a standard moxa cone, about the size of your thumbnail, it is shaped like a triangle. As it burns down, progressing from the apex to the broad base, the heat diffuses sideways, warming the surface of the skin.

Rice-grain moxa is a different shape. Rather than triangular, it is cylindrical, or tapered, like a toothpick. It can be rolled with two different configurations at the base.

1. Flat base
2. Tapered or pointed base

---

165 Mizutani, J. (1998). *Practical Moxibustion Therapy*. Vancouver, BC: NAJOM.

166 Shinma, H. (2015). *The Treasure Book of Points: Fukaya Kyu*. Tokyo: Shinma.

167 Kivity, O. (2025) *Lecture on Fukaya Kyu*, by Felip Caudet, Jakarta, Indonesia. Personal notes.

The base shape affects the penetration of heat. A pointed base directs heat deeper into the body. A flat base spreads the effect more superficially. The wider the base, the more heat the patient feels. Thus, when rolling cones, it makes sense to have a narrow base or a slightly pointed one.

ACTIONS

- It is said to help treat problems more at the blood level (as compared to needling, which is often said to act more at the qi level).[168]
- It is recommended for all chronic, complex or complicated conditions.
- It has been found to increase blood cell counts, especially white blood cells, thus strengthening immunity.

POINT LOCATION

BACK TO PALPATION: FINDING THE ALIVE POINT FOR MOXIBUSTION

In Japan, the concept of living and functioning points is often attributed to Takeshi Sawada (1877–1938), one of the most renowned moxa practitioners of the twentieth century. Points are more than anatomical landmarks; they are manifestations of a functional problem in the body. Normally dormant, they become active as problems develop. In JAAM, point location based solely on anatomical knowledge is considered to be less effective than point location based on skilled palpation. This concept, the dynamic reflection of developing problems, is often translated as the *presently alive*, *currently alive*, or simply, the *alive point*.

The Japanese Meridian Therapy authority Shudo Denmai writes, "When qi stagnates... the point becomes depressed or protrudes. Qi, which is invisible, is thus transformed into a 'quality' that can be palpated and distinguished."[169]

---

[168] Fukushima, K. (1991). *Meridian Therapy*. Tokyo: Toyo Hari Medical Association.

[169] Shudo, D. (2003). *Finding Effective Acupuncture Points.* Translated by S. Brown. Seattle, WA: Eastland Press. p. 5.

These qualities were defined by Isaburo Fukaya, another influential moxa practitioner, who said that points are only effective for moxibustion when they display two palpable reactions: pressure pain and induration. Indurations are chronic, hard, knotted areas, usually formed over a long time.

The alive point may not correspond exactly to the anatomically described locations given in the textbooks, and those descriptions themselves vary between Chinese, Japanese, and Western sources.

Felip Caudet, a Spanish specialist in Fukaya moxibustion, likens the process of finding a point to visiting a friend. You may have the number and name of their area, but it is only a rough indication of where they live. In practice, you must locate the actual house in that area and read the nameplate on the door.[170]

In acute conditions, an entire area may feel tender. Sawada suggested treating the 'real tender point' at or near the site of the original injury, often with multiple cones applied over a short time. Chronic findings, such as indurations, call for fewer cones, repeated over a longer period.

Points are not static, rooted in local anatomical structures; they move. Some shift only within a small radius of the textbook location, others over a larger area. Each time the patient returns for their next visit, the particular alive point may have moved a little or even disappeared as it is resolved.

The alive point can only be located by skilful palpation. As Shudo says, it takes "effort and ingenuity" to find it. And if the point isn't alive, don't use it! He reminds us that acupuncture points came first, and textbooks came later. It's better to learn points from the body than from books.[171]

This emphasis on palpation and looking for changes brings us back to our earlier discussion in Chapter 3 on abnormal tissue findings.

---

170 Kivity, O. (2025) *Lecture on Fukaya Kyu*, by Felip Caudet, Jakarta, Indonesia. Personal notes.

171 Shudo, D. (2003). *Finding Effective Acupuncture Points.* Translated by S. Brown. Seattle, WA: Eastland Press. p. 7.

> *What* [the sages] *called 'joints' are where the spirit moves and passes in and out. They are not just skin, flesh, tendons, and bones.*
>
> —Ling Shu, Chapter 1[172]

An acupuncture point is not mere skin and flesh nor tendons and bones, but it is where qi meanders in and exits out. The most important idea in this passage is that points are understood as products of qi movement along the meridians, rather than as structures defined by the physical body. Despite the discussion of palpation, induration, and pressure pain, the key to point location is to consider it not as a simple mechanical task but as something more—engaging with the patient's vitality and energy flow.

PERFECTING YOUR MOXA

Rolling moxa to the proper shape, size, and consistency is a skill attained only with hours of careful practice. In Japan, students in acupuncture school spend many hours learning and perfecting their moxa rolling, placing, and burning techniques, so they can pass their difficult practical exams. In the West, this level of repetitive diligence is less common, though still very important, as we need to attain a general level of skill to use moxa effectively and repeatedly without unnecessarily burning our patients. When applying *okyu,* the following points should be observed:

- Generally, the patient should feel the moxa as slightly hot but not uncomfortable. When applied correctly, the heat of the moxa is generally like a brief pinprick. Sometimes it even elicits the same stimulation sensation as a needle.
- If the cone is rolled too large or compressed too tightly, it burns hotter and longer, which can be uncomfortable for the patient. Keeping cones consistent in size and density allows you to produce a steady, predictable dose of heat each time.
- This consistency gives you much greater control over the total dosage delivered.

172 Unschuld, P. U. (2016). *Huang Di Nei Jing Ling Shu: The Ancient Classic on Needle Therapy.* Berkeley: University of California Press. p. 45.

- Perfecting the delivery technique requires frequent practice in moxa rolling. You might set tasks for yourself, using a practice board. A practice board can be a piece of paper with crosses on it, where you place your moxa, or a wooden ice cream stick, where you can place and burn your cones. Try to achieve a goal such as rolling and placing twenty moxa cones in a row that are all the same size and consistency.

With these principles in mind, we can now look at practical rolling methods.

ROLLING MOXA

The moxa cone or punk sizes listed above are tiny, ranging from thread-sized to rice-grain-sized (usually the largest size used). The piece of moxa should be shaped either in a thin rod shape or like a grain of rice. It is essential to ensure that when the piece of moxa is placed on the skin, it stands upright with minimal contact. The base should be narrow. A wide base is counterproductive because the bigger footprint feels hotter as the cone burns down.

It's perhaps better to think of 'shaping' the moxa cones, rather than 'rolling' them, although this is indeed the action. When rolling the cones out between the thumb and index finger, do it as if leaving a 1 mm space between them, and avoid adding any pressure with the fingers. The heat of the burning cones can vary significantly, depending on how they are rolled.

When shaping moxa cones, roll the moxa as gently as possible. Softly rolled cones have more airspace, burn faster, and feel cooler. Tightly rolled cones, on the other hand, burn longer and feel hotter. Remember: Your rolling technique directly shapes the patient's experience.

PROCEDURE

Rolling and applying moxa cones requires a certain degree of manual dexterity. There are many ways to do this. Below are three options. Which one you favour is entirely up to you. Many practitioners in Japan are competitive about their moxa rolling skills and shun moxa rolling tools, such as cork boards, as an easy way out. Still, you are not rolling cones to win a competition, but to treat your patients, so choose the method that suits you best.

ROLLING

Option 1) Place a small piece of moxa in the palm of your non-dominant hand. Use the outer edge of your dominant hand to roll a thin, long sausage shape or thread, using very light pressure.

Place the sausage on the side of your index finger and use your thumb to roll it forward, extruding it a little at a time. With the other hand, gently pull pieces off so you avoid compressing them and making them dense. The base of each cone should be as narrow as possible. A narrow base delivers less heat to the skin, reducing the risk of an unwanted burn.

The moxa is soft and delicate, so avoid crushing it by gently holding it and pulling it off to separate a piece. The part of the cone that is separated from the moxa thread will have loose fibres and be shaggy after being pulled apart. Place the cone gently on the skin so that the ends of these fibres rest on the skin. Doing this creates a small space between the skin and the cone, making the heat sensation even softer.

Option 2) Break off a small lump of moxa and place it between your thumb and index finger. Imagine rolling a toothpick lightly between your fingers and using the same motion to roll the lump. It will eventually become a thin sausage, which you can extrude between your fingers. The key to getting started with this technique is starting with a very small lump of moxa, like a green lentil or small dry bean.

Option 3) An alternative technique, recommended by Canada-based moxa exponent Junji Mizutani, is to use rolling boards made of cork or balsa wood. These produce even threads of moxa. If you get sticky hands, this is a useful addition to your toolkit. Once you have a long thread rolled, place it between your thumb and index finger and extrude it, as above. To some degree, using a cork rolling board is a simple hack for producing uniform moxa cones, taking much of the labour out of applying *okyu*. However, even when using boards, the above points about cone shape and density should still be observed.

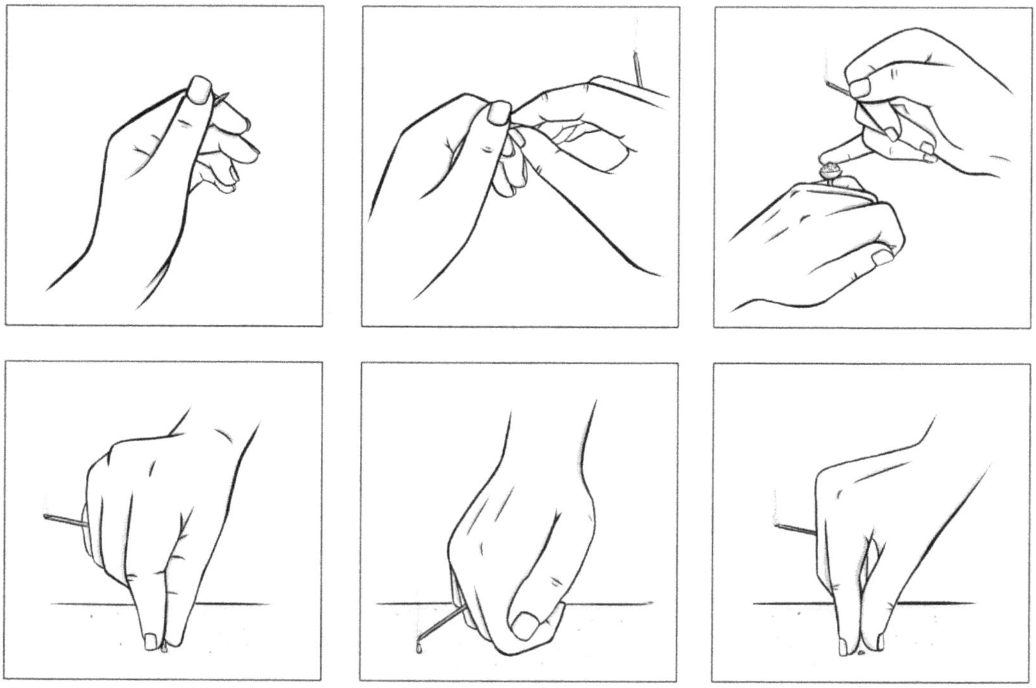

Figure 13-1: Rolling, placing, lighting and cowling.

PLACEMENT

Each finger has a role. Use the little finger of your dominant hand to moisten the point with water, so the moxa adheres to the skin. It is best to dedicate one finger to this role, so the others stay dry. Many Toyohari practitioners wear a moxa ring on one finger, a simple ring that holds moistened cotton wool. You can use this to wet your little finger.

Use the index finger and thumb on your dominant hand to set the cones in place and to extinguish the cone at the right time (see below). Most Japanese practitioners keep the incense stick between the third and fourth fingers of their dominant hand, allowing them to place, light, and extinguish each cone with the same hand. The other hand is used to provide a steady supply of rolled moxa wool.

Try to place the cones lightly, so the base remains narrow.

LIGHTING

To light the moxa, use an incense stick. The hottest part of the incense stick is not the tip, but the junction between the unlit part and the glowing ember. Roll the lighted incense stick over the top of the cone: rolling it helps prevent the moxa from sticking to it. If you don't roll the incense stick, it might adhere to the cone and lift it away from the skin. It's also important to keep the end of the incense stick free of ash: the more ash there is, the greater the chance the cone will stick to the incense stick.

EXTINGUISHING

There are different styles for extinguishing the moxa, which can be summarised by the percentage of the cone that you allow to burn before extinguishing it. The rationale is simple: the 70–80% style produces a strong pinch of heat without damaging the skin, while the 100% style is allowed to burn down to provoke an immune response through micro tissue damage (remember the idea of denatured proteins in the last chapter, like the protein of an egg that changes with boiling).

In the 70–80% style, the cone is pinched out before it reaches the skin. This approach is often chosen to relax tight muscles or reduce pressure pain reactions. Techniques such as placing each cone on the ash of the previous one can help moderate the heat reaching the skin.

In the 100% style, the cone is allowed to burn all the way down, deliberately causing a tiny burn. This added burning action stimulates the immune system and microcirculation. Here, the aim is not to reduce the heat reaching the skin, but rather to minimise discomfort—for example, pressing around the smouldering cone with a bamboo tube, as taught in Fukaya style.

Each style, therefore, has a clear rationale and its own management techniques, with the choice depending on the patient's condition and therapeutic goals. Table 13.2 summarises each style.

Table 13.2: Summary of cone extinguishing methods.

STYLE	METHOD	MAIN EFFECT	TYPICAL USE	MANAGEMENT TECHNIQUE
70–80% style	The cone is extinguished before reaching the skin.	Pinch of heat without tissue damage	Relaxing tight muscles, reducing pressure pain reactions	Reduce heat reaching the skin (e.g. place on ash, pinch off early).
100% style	The cone burns down completely to the skin.	Pinch of heat plus burning action from micro tissue damage	Stimulating the immune system, enhancing microcirculation	Do not reduce heat; instead, reduce sensation (e.g. press around the cone with a bamboo tube).

As explained above, the choice between the 70–80% style and the 100% style depends on the therapeutic goal and the patient's condition. Within the 70–80% style, you can further moderate the dosage by extinguishing the cone earlier or later, which is especially important for more sensitive patients. For example, you can burn to 40%.

Here are three ways to extinguish the cone. With all three, the moxa should feel hot but not burning, sometimes like a pinprick or even like a needle.

[Note: These terms are not translations from Japanese manuals but are simple-to-remember English labels for the actions, taken from *The Moon over Matsushima*.[173]]

1. *COWLING*

Gently pinch the index finger and thumb of your dominant hand together and then lower them to the burning cone, like a canopy or candle snuffer. Roll the thumb and index finger over the burning cone. The canopy restricts the flow of air without touching the cone. This technique is called *cowling*, as your fingers form a hood or cowl over the cone. It also leaves a residue of ash on the skin that acts as insulation and a base for the next cone.

---

173 Young, M. (2023). *The Moon over Matsushima: Insights into Moxa and Mugwort*. 2nd ed. London: Sayoshi Books.

2. *SNATCHING*

Watch the cone burn carefully, and when it has burned down sufficiently, usually to 80%, use your thumb and index finger to snatch it away. This technique means that no cushion of ash is retained for the next cone, so you need to moisten the skin again with the little finger of your dominant hand.

3. *STAMPING*

This is a slightly more vigorous technique. As the cone reaches 80%, stamp down on it with the fourth finger of your dominant hand. This usually results in a greater perception of heat compared to the other removal techniques.

ROLE OF EACH FINGER DURING APPLICATION

Each finger has a distinct role as you shape and place the cones. Table 13.3 summarises their roles during moxa application.

Table 13.3: Role of each finger.

NON-DOMINANT HAND	DOMINANT HAND
Your thumb and index finger work together to shape and extrude the moxa, creating an ongoing supply of moxa thread, while your dominant hand is busy lighting the moxa.	Index finger and thumb pinch off small pieces of the thread and place the cones gently on the point.
The little finger wears the moxa ring, which includes a shallow dish to contain wet cotton wool.	The little finger makes contact with the moxa ring and moistens the point before the first cone is placed.
	The incense stick is held between the third and fourth fingers. The whole hand rotates slightly to roll the incense stick over the top of the cone, preventing adhesion.
	Cowling: Use the thumb and index finger.
	Snatching: Use the thumb and index finger.
	Stamping: Use the fourth finger.

The first cone is the most important one to get right, because this is the one that feels hottest to the patient. Subsequent cones do not feel as hot, first because patients become accustomed to the sensation, and second because the ash from the first cone acts as insulation. For the first cone, use a small, lightly rolled cone between the size of a sesame seed and half a rice grain.

SHIUNKO

Some practitioners do not moisten the skin with water; instead, they prefer to use a herbal paste of Chinese origin, made from sesame oil and various herbs, which is used for healing skin wounds, such as burns. In Japan, this is called *shiunko* ointment. This usage may have started in the West and has recently been adopted by some practitioners in Japan. Once you've decided which points to use, apply a little *shiunko* on each. The herbal component of the ointment protects the skin and helps prevent moxa scarring. It also acts as an adhesive, allowing the moxa cone to stand easily on the skin.

Some practitioners use a matchstick or needle guide tube to dab on small amounts. Others fill a small syringe with it and squeeze out small dots on the skin. It is best to apply as little *shiunko* as possible. If the paste is applied too liberally, the heat can build up in the oil, causing the temperature to rise, which might injure the skin.

Paul Movsessian notes that as *shiunko* creates a barrier between the burning moxa cone and the skin, the application of *okyu* with *shiunko* should be considered an indirect moxa technique.

DOSAGE

In JAAM, moxa is usually applied in odd-numbered sequences, such as 3, 5, or 7 times. This number does not relate to the actual number of cones, but rather to the number of cones the patient perceives. It may take five cones for the patient to feel heat three times. For points that are insensitive to heat, multiple moxa applications may be necessary before the patient experiences any sensation. Insensitivity to heat at a point is a confirmatory sign that moxa is appropriate. The greater the insensitivity, the more severe the problem. In these situations, it's tempting to increase the size of the moxa cones to get a reaction. In fact, that is counterproductive. The patient's reactivity to the sensation of heat generated by your standard cone size is a helpful gauge for assessing effectiveness and prognosis.

The general principle is that if heat is felt, apply cones until it is no longer felt. Some practitioners say that the sensation of heat turns into a sensation of coolness when the point has been sufficiently treated.[174] If heat is not felt, keep applying cones until it is. This is a helpful approach for local treatments.

---

174 Baek, S. (1990). *Classical Moxibustion Skills in Contemporary Clinical Practice*. Boulder, CO: Blue Poppy Press.

Another approach described by Mizutani involves applying as many cones as necessary to cause the skin around the point to turn red.

Palpation is also useful as a feedback mechanism. It can be helpful to repalpate after treatment: diminishing tenderness or induration is a reliable sign that the point has been treated sufficiently.[175]

PRECAUTIONS AND CONTRAINDICATIONS

Direct moxa, such as *okyu*, can trigger biological reactions to the heat stimulation, as well as small-scale tissue damage from the burning moxa. In most patients, this can be very helpful. But in patients who are in poor physical condition, such as those who are terminally ill or in a state of exhaustion, triggering those biological reactions can use energy reserves they do not have and can cause them to feel worse. Thus, it is better to avoid doing 100% style *okyu* on, for example, terminally ill patients in the last stages of life, to avert this risk.

Dr Hara suggested that if *okyu* is selected with the aim of strengthening the patient, it is better to use much milder forms, such as the 70–80% style, applied carefully and comfortably. This helps gradually build up the patient's reserves over time, using a minimal number of points. This gentler, milder stimulation approach can also be helpful for terminally ill patients if applied judiciously.

Merlin Young, when practising moxa on drug-resistant TB patients during the first Moxafrica project, reported that for one patient who was terminally ill, he did two cones only, from a protocol of ten points. The patient improved remarkably, was walking within two days, and discharged himself a short time afterwards. "Just two cones as a total treatment for a dying man—and definitely no blistering involved. We had to accept that Dr Hara may have been right."[176]

---

175 Mizutani, J. (1998). *Practical Moxibustion Therapy*. Vancouver, BC: NAJOM.

176 Young, M. (2023). *The Moon over Matsushima: Insights into Moxa and Mugwort*. 2nd ed. London: Sayoshi Books. p. 249.

The 100% style of *okyu* should not be used on patients taking immunosuppressant drugs or who have problems healing. For example, it should not be applied to the extremities of diabetic patients or others with peripheral neuropathy. Patients with this condition can't report if the moxa is hot, and if you do burn the skin accidentally, the circulation at the extremities may be so poor that they are unable to recover. Milder (70–80%) styles do not cause burns per se, but you must have good technique to apply them to the affected areas. If you're not yet skilled with your technique, it is better to avoid these affected areas. It can, however, be helpful to apply *okyu* proximal to the affected areas to help stimulate increased circulation to them.

Finally, there are several other practical considerations and contraindications for small-cone moxibustion:

THE FACE

You may notice at the end of a long day of moxibustion that your fingers look yellow, like those of a hardened smoker. Moreover, your patient's skin may have tiny yellow stains where the cones were. Sometimes, if your moxa rolling or timing was not up to standard, patients return with small blisters. For these reasons, it's not advisable to perform small-cone moxibustion on the face. It may discolour the skin or, even worse, damage it. There are other moxa methods that are far better for treating the face, such as Ontake.

BLOOD VESSELS

Avoid direct moxibustion over large blood vessels, especially if they are swollen or distended.

FASTING

If you work with the Muslim community, this is a regular occurrence, at the very least annually during Ramadan. Fasting is not, however, exclusive to people of faith. Workaholics and recreational drug users may also not eat for long periods. Many people practise intermittent fasting.

The key thing to remember is that fasting makes people's energy much more volatile, so you must be alert to this when treating. Thus, if you are aware that someone is in a fasted state, you should skip moxa or reduce the dose considerably by using the milder forms.

AFTER HOT BATHS OR SAUNAS

The *Zhen Jiu Da Cheng* cites hot baths as a contraindication.[177] Hot baths and modern saunas open the pores and disperse defensive qi, while direct moxibustion draws yang qi to the surface and consolidates defensive qi. If the pores are already open, applying moxa can allow wind or cold to enter more easily, or cause the heat to penetrate too deeply, leading to dryness, irritation, or blistering.

In modern times, Dr Hara noted that moxa stimulates a mild immune response, and exposure to moisture or excessive heat soon afterwards may interfere with this process.

INEBRIATION

The classics list intoxication as a contraindication to moxa. They are referring to alcohol, but of course, this contraindication includes intoxication from any source, be it recreational drugs or shamanic potions. Once again, the reason is that when intoxicated, people's energy is volatile and can react much faster than you anticipate.

CHILDREN

This book does not describe the treatment of children. Paediatric moxibustion is a highly specialised area and should only be undertaken by practitioners with the appropriate training. Without that education, it is not safe to apply *okyu* to children.

177 Yang, J. (1601/1963 reprint). *Zhen Jiu Da Cheng (Great Compendium of Acupuncture and Moxibustion).* Beijing: Renmin Weisheng Chubanshe

DURING *KYUTOSHIN*

During Step 2, as the moxa is burning merrily on the needles, you may be tempted to release a few tight points on the upper back with *okyu*. There's no energetic reason why you shouldn't, but there are sound practical arguments for not doing so. One of the rules of doing *kyutoshin* is that you avoid startling the patient or moving the needles. Palpating for tender, tight points on the upper back, or accidentally burning a cone to the skin so that the patient jumps, are risks that can easily be avoided.

Instead, you can set up the *kyutoshin* on the lower back, ready to go, but don't light the balls. Then palpate the upper back and release reactive points with *okyu*. When this process is complete, simply light the balls on the *kyutoshin*. This rapid transition from one moxa approach to another can feel extremely relaxing.

USES, INDICATIONS AND POINTS OF INTEREST

Okyu can be used at each of the Four Steps. This section is focused on its use as a branch treatment at Step 4. Below is a list of approaches and points that have been found to be particularly effective for specific conditions. For more extensive information on conditions that can be treated with *okyu*, refer to *Chasing the Dragon's Tail, Japanese Acupuncture: A Clinical Guide* and *The Moon over Matsushima*.[178, 179, 180]

178 Manaka, Y., Itaya, K., & Birch, S. (1995). *Chasing the Dragon's Tail: The Theory and Practice of Acupuncture in the Work of Yoshio Manaka*. Brookline: Paradigm Publications.

179 Young, M. (2014) The Moon over Matsushima - 'the Single': Clinical Moxibustion Treatments. Kindle edition. Available at: https://www.amazon.co.uk/dp/B00N98FXE8

180 Birch, S., & Ida, J. (1998). *Japanese Acupuncture: A Clinical Guide*. Brookline: Paradigm Publications.

INFLAMMATION AND FEVER

Inflamed areas, such as swollen knees or patches of skin inflammation, respond very well to moxa. You can apply one thread-sized moxa about every 1 cm around the area. With time, the surface area of the inflammation will decrease. Each session, you can move the moxa cones inwards, in a contracting perimeter. The moxa facilitates absorption and reduces inflammation.

For acute myofascial pain, concentrate on the most tender points and burn as many cones as needed until the warmth is felt deeply. With chronic muscle fatigue, light stimulation on multiple points can be beneficial. This releases the tight muscles associated with sympathetic over-stimulation; in other words, when the patient is stressed.

TENDINITIS, CONTUSIONS, SPRAINS AND BOILS

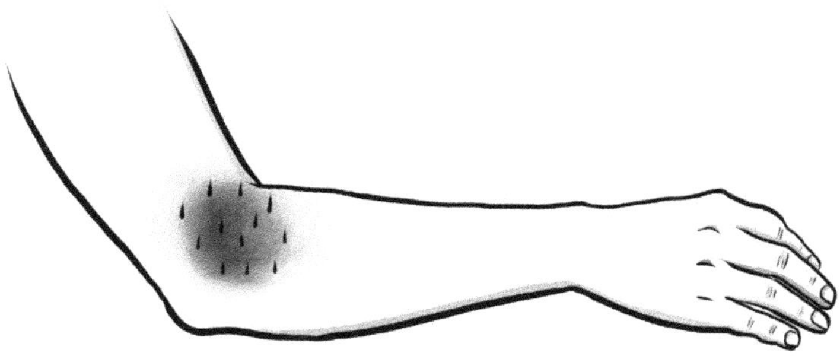

Figure 13-2: Placement of small moxa cones for tendinitis, contusions and sprains, combining both edge and centre applications.

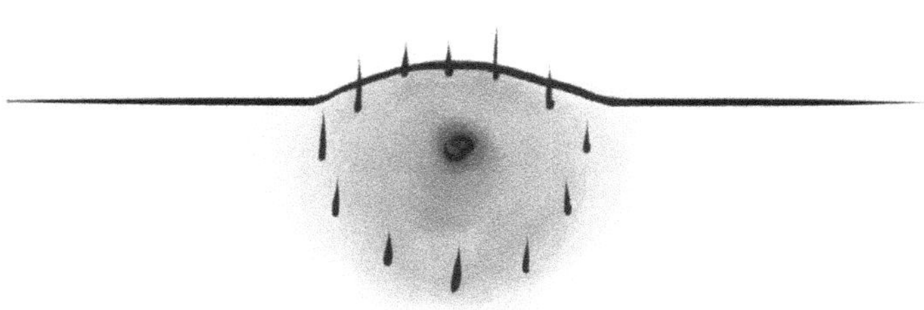

Figure 13-3: Placement of cones for boils (surround moxa).

Check for and mark the area with the strongest tenderness reactions on palpation. Apply *okyu* once to tender points around the edges of this marked area, then apply multiple single small cones within the area itself. Use a total of 20–25 points, combining both edge and centre applications.

Roll very fine thread-sized pieces and let them burn all the way to the skin. The sharp heat disperses inflammation and swelling.

For boils, surround the area of inflammation. Do not apply to the centre of the inflammation.

FUKAYA'S PYSCHOSOMATIC TREATMENT

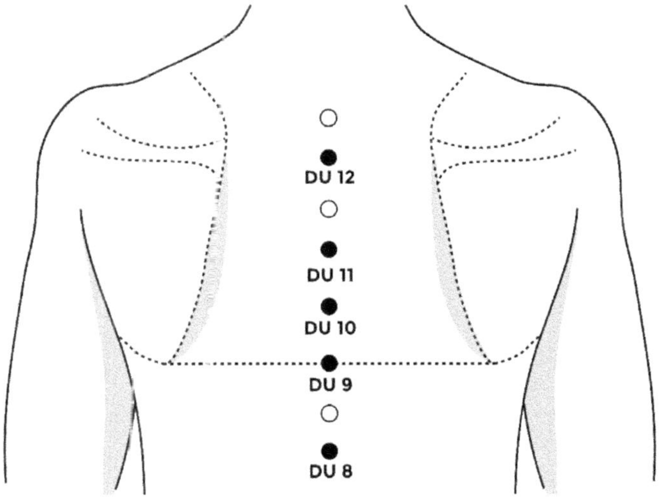

Figure 13-4: Fukaya's psychosomatic treatment points.

These reactions can appear in many situations where the patient is experiencing emotional difficulties—not only anxiety, but also depression, stress, grief, and anger. They can occur in other physical states, such as high blood pressure or menopausal hot flushes, for which they are helpful. The treatment is thought to regulate the body's response to emotional and physiological stress through the spine and nervous system.

URANAITEI (裏内庭)

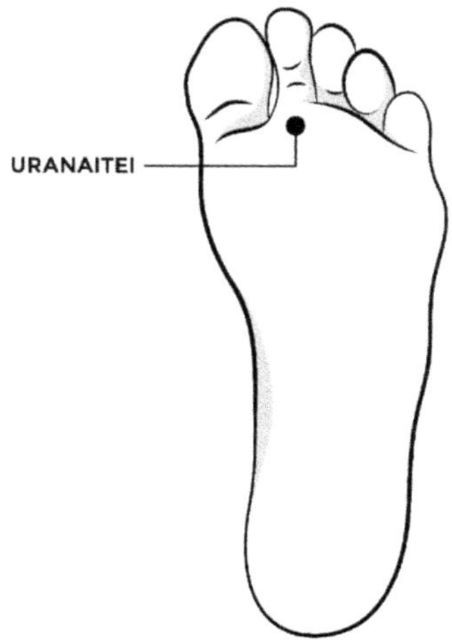

Figure 13-5: Uranaitei—"Beneath ST 44", where the tip of the pad of the second toe would touch the sole if bent.

Neiting (内庭), known in Western notation as ST 44, is called *Naitei* (内庭) in Japanese. The Japanese name for this extra point on the plantar surface of the foot is *Uranaitei* (裏内庭), which means 'beneath *Naitei*'. To locate it, bend the second toe towards the sole until the tip of the pad touches. This is where you palpate for the point. If the toe is not flexible, simply extrapolate an arc to where the pad would touch.

Another way to find it is to make an inverted equilateral triangle with the plantar crease at the base of the second toe. If the crease is the base of the triangle, the point is at the apex.

This point is commonly used for food poisoning, overeating, and food allergies.

SHITSUMIN (失眠)

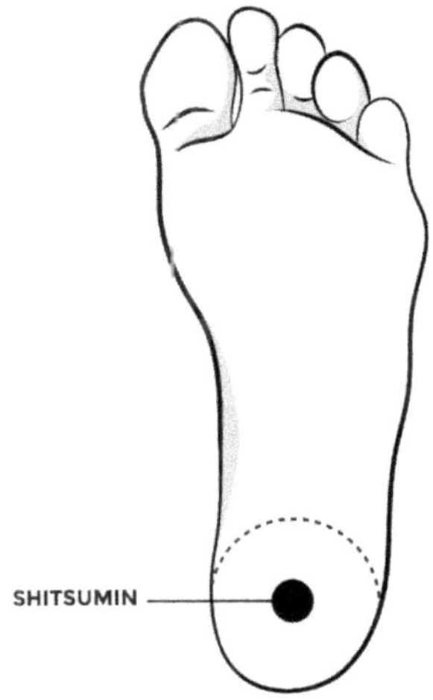

Figure 13-6: *Shitsumin*—insomnia point.

Shitsu means 'to lose', and *min* means 'sleep', so the name literally translates as 'loss of sleep', usually rendered as 'insomnia point'.

Shitsumin is located on the plantar surface of the foot, at the centre of the heel. As its name implies, it is commonly used for insomnia, with other indications noted by various sources, including oedema of the lower leg and high blood pressure.[181]

TRANSFER MOXA: *KAN NUKI NO KYU*

This technique involves treating a pair of points on opposite sides of a limb; for example, PC 6 with TB 5 at the wrist.[182] Usually, one yin point is paired with one yang. Both cones are burnt at the same time, so that the pinch of heat is perceived at both points simultaneously. Transfer moxa is used to reduce inflammation in the joints (e.g. for knee inflammation, SP 10 with ST 34, or SP 9 with GB 34) or to warm cold extremities.

181 Becker, M. (n.d.). Japanese Direct Moxa: Extra Foot Points. Unpublished manuscript. Available at: https://www.scribd.com/document/869096355/Moshe-Becker-Moxa-Points-Foot

182 This technique is also known as *tsuranuki no kyu*.

In practice, it is easiest to roll one cone slightly longer than the other and place both on the skin. Light the longer cone first, then time the ignition of the shorter cone so they burn down to the skin simultaneously. In this way, the patient feels a pinch of heat on both sides of the limb as you extinguish them. In this context, stamping is arguably the easiest method to extinguish the cones.

If coordinating the timing proves difficult, the same effect can be achieved by alternating quickly between the two points, applying one cone at a time in rapid succession.

Table 13.4 lists yin–yang pairs for different parts of the body.

Table 13.4: Transfer moxa combinations.

RHEUMATOID ARTHRITIS	Treat proximally to the inflammation. Treat the yin and yang sides in the adjacent areas.
LEG	
Knee	SP 10 + ST 34
	SP 9 + GB 34
Ankle	KID 6 + BL 62
	SP 6 + GB 39
ARM	
Shoulder	PC 2 + SI 9
Elbow	LU 4 + LI 12 LU 6 + LI 10
Wrist	PC 6 + TB 5
Fingers	LI 4 + SI 3 or SI 4 (an exception to the yin–yang rule)

Additionally, the following back-*shu* points can be used for treating rheumatoid arthritis (RA).

- RA affecting the upper body: BL 15
- RA affecting the lower body: BL 27

The idea of BL 15 and BL 27 as the key points in RA is worth considering. Why should the heart and small intestine, both associated with imperial fire, be involved in an autoimmune disease such as RA? Various authors have speculated on this, though no single explanation has gained universal acceptance. Nevertheless, treating the heart–small intestine axis appears to be a key component of approaches to rheumatoid arthritis; therefore, BL 15, the back-*shu* of the heart, and BL 27, the back-*shu* of the small intestine, are useful points to consider.

MOXA PROTOCOLS

The remainder of this chapter is designed as a clinical reference guide. You will find two distinct listings of information to support your practice:

1. ***Okyu* Treatments:** The first section catalogues a wide range of conditions and the points commonly treated with *okyu*. While extensive, this list is not exhaustive. We encourage you to use the principles of palpation detailed earlier—finding 'alive' points distinguishable by pressure pain and induration—to explore beyond these suggestions and develop your own clinical insights.
2. ***Kyutoshin* Treatments:** The second section provides information on clinical uses of *kyutoshin*. Remember, just as with *okyu*, palpation remains the key to locating points. Use the cross-fibre method described in Chapter 8 to locate the most reactive and effective points to needle.

These listings can serve as a good starting point for your Step 4 treatments, and we hope they will be a valuable resource for you to return to time and again.

Table 13.5: ***Okyu*** **indications.**

CONDITION	**TREATMENT**	**AUTHORS' INSIGHTS**
CIRCULATORY		
CVA	Start treatment 1 month after the stroke. For motor problems, check the *jing*-well points for insensitivity. Treat the most insensitive points. Fukaya recommends alternative *jing*-well points at the tip of each digit.	
Yeast infection under the nail	Find a point on the midline of the nail, at the junction of the central and distal thirds. Burn moxa until the patient feels the heat. If heat is felt quickly, the prognosis is better. Have the patient apply 2–3 times per day. This is also useful for blackened nails following bruising (see case below).	
Oedema of the lower limb	*Shitsumin* (*Shimian*—centre of the heel). [See previous section for the location of this point.]	

DERMATOLOGICAL		
Hives	LI 15	
Stye	Sawada's LI 2, on the radial side of the proximal interphalangeal joint on the affected side. Treat the same side as the stye.	
Skin conditions	Check pressure pain on LI 4, LI 10, LI 11, and LI 15. Select the most tender point. Apply cones until pressure pain reduces.	
DIGESTIVE		
Food poisoning or acute gastroenteritis	*Uranaitei* [see previous section for the location of this point]. Use *okyu* on the insensitive side until the patient feels the heat. This may need many applications. Once the heat is felt, continue until the patient feels it 5–10 times. The patient should feel an immediate result.	

Chronic gastritis (including heartburn)	BL 17, 18, 20 (Six Flowers). Instead of discrete knots, this often presents as very hard, tight bands running parallel to the spine, extending from at least BL 17 down to BL 20. Locate the reactive points along these bands and treat them 5–7 times. For hyperacidity, use BL 14 or BL 15 instead of BL 17; for ulcers, use BL 21 or BL 22 instead of BL 20.	The 6 flowers in the title of this technique refer to the 6 blisters formed by the application of moxa. However, in contemporary practice, blistering moxibustion is not necessary. Moderate your treatment according to the patient's strength.

DIGESTIVE		
Diarrhoea Acute Chronic	 Acute The *navel clock* Imagine a clock around the navel that includes KID 16 and REN 7 and 9. Palpate around the clock and treat any tender points you find. Chronic Palpate in a larger circle around the navel that includes ST 25 and REN 12 and 5, and treat tender points. Additionally, if reactive, add SP 6 and BL 25 and 27.	
Constipation	Sawada's HT 7, located at the wrist between the small intestine and heart meridian.	
Abdominal pain, stomach pain, and diarrhoea	ST 34	The most straightforward technique for diarrhoea is ST 34. However, Fukaya's navel clock, described above, is also highly effective.

GYNAECOLOGICAL AND OBSTETRIC		
Breech position	BL 67 and SP 6—treat the less sensitive side daily.	
Pregnancy care	To treat mother and foetus in preparation for labour, apply daily moxa at SP 6 from the beginning of the 5th month. 5th month—5 on each side 6th month—7 on each side 7th month—9 on each side 8th month—11 on each side 9th month—13 on each side When labour begins, apply 30–50 cones on SP 6. If the contractions are false, they will stop; otherwise, they will strengthen and stabilise. Continue where possible during labour.	No one can afford the time and money to come for daily treatment for 4 months, so this means taking a little time to train the parents in placing and lighting moxa. This is where cork rolling boards are helpful, as they significantly reduce the learning curve for moxa. This is a very effective treatment and involves partners who may otherwise feel detached from the pregnancy. It also helps expectant mothers with sleep, anxiety, and urinary symptoms, so it is well worth the time to teach it to couples.

Menopause	Palpate and treat the most reactive out of Fukaya's psychosomatic points. [See description in previous section.] Add SP 6 and SP 10 if tender. Daily treatment if possible.	
MUSCULO-SKELETAL		
Stiff shoulders	Presenting with digestive problems: GB 21, BL 43, and BL 17. Neck and shoulder with no underlying pathology: SI 11, BL 43, SI 14, SI 15, BL 10, GB 21, and GB 20. 50-year-old shoulder, with stiffness and pain, presenting unilaterally. Difficulty abducting—treat intrascapular region, TB 12, SI 9, SI 10, SI 11. Difficulty extending backwards—LU 4, LU 1, *jianqian* (Ex-UE 13), LI 14.	

Osteoarthritis	Do not apply *okyu* directly over inflamed joints. Instead, treat using one of the following approaches: Manaka-style: Apply single cones to tender points arranged in a rough circle around the affected joint (e.g. knee). Fukaya–Sawada style: Use transfer moxibustion as described above.	
Sore and stiff neck	BL 10	
Arm pain	BL 43	
Tight occiput	BL 32	

NEUROLOGICAL		
Intercostal—neuralgia	Back Check the upper and mid-back for pressure pain, especially slightly lateral to the intervertebral spaces at the level of the nerve roots. Front Palpate and treat reactive points in the intercostal space of the affected nerve branch. Sides Mid-axillary line, especially the left side around the 8th and 9th rib and around LIV 13.	
RESPIRATORY		
Asthma	Look for a reactive point lateral and superior to BL 17.	

High fever, colds, and flu	DU 14 As a preventive measure, apply 7 cones daily. At onset, apply 20 cones. To lower the temperature, apply 20–30 cones. If already established, apply 20–30 cones.	
Rhinitis	DU 14	
Sinus infection, nasal congestion, rhinitis	Tender point around DU 23	Place the wrist crease at the tip of the nose and palpate for a tender point on the Du Mai where the middle finger comes to rest.
Sore throat	LU 5 Palpate 1 *cun* proximal to the textbook location.	
PSYCHOLOGICAL		
Insomnia 1	*Shitsumin* (*Shimian*—centre of the heel) [See previous section for the location of this point.] Treat the insensitive side until the patient starts to feel heat.	To distinguish which side is insensitive, burn 1 cone of identical size on both sides and ask the patient which side feels hotter; that side is more sensitive. Choose the insensitive side for the remaining procedure.

Insomnia 2	Find a tight, knotted area around BL 17.	
Anxious and neurotic patients	Fukaya's psychosomatic treatment (sometimes called Fukaya's anxiety points or neurogenic points) [See previous section for a description of this area.] Check the intervertebral spaces between T3 and T9 on the Du Mai for reactive points: If one space is distinctly reactive, apply at least 9 *okyu* until the reaction lessens. If several spaces are reactive (e.g. T5, T6, T7) with no single one standing out, apply at least three cones on each.	Sometimes a point can be stubborn and resist release. In such cases, ask the patient to arch their back and inhale, holding the breath while the moxa is lit. As the moxa is extinguished (usually by stamping), have the patient exhale and lower back down onto the table. Combining moxa with movement and breathing can help release stuck points. [Note: This is a variation of a Sotai movement that will be studied in Vol. 2.]

OKYU AND BLOOD STASIS

> *A patient came with back pain. During his first session, while the ion-pumping cords were on, I noticed that his right big toenail was completely black. He mentioned that he'd dropped a door on it when doing some home renovation. I applied several small moxa cones, burning them down completely, but after seven, he had not felt any sensation of heat, so I stopped.*

He returned six months later, full of praise for the moxa treatment, with a pink and healthy toenail. I was surprised, because a toenail will typically take about six months to grow back anyway. "No, you don't understand", he said. "I dropped the door on it ten years ago!"

This single episode taught me right away about the remarkable, blood-moving properties of okyu. Following physical trauma, this man had had blood stasis in one toe for ten years. It responded immediately to just seven small moxa cones.

—Oran Kivity

KYUTOSHIN REVISITED

While *okyu* is powerful, the needle-moxa technique introduced in Step 2 can also be adapted and expanded for use as a focused treatment in Step 4.

As ever, finding reactive points is the key to effective treatment. For *kyutoshin*, this often requires cross-fibre palpation, as described in Chapter 8.

GENERAL INDICATIONS

- Tight areas, pressure pain points, and painful conditions
- Stiff joints or muscles, contusions or injuries
- Diarrhoea, bloating, oedema, and similar symptoms, especially when accompanied by signs of diminished circulation such as palpable coldness in the abdomen or feet
- Numbness, tingling and/or paralysis anywhere in the body
- Indurations

Kyutoshin can be applied to help treat induration-like reactions in tight bands of muscle. When doing this, take care to needle slightly to the side of the hard knot, inserting instead into the surrounding muscle tissue. Advance the needle until you feel something hard, and then withdraw just a little. Apply 2–3 rounds of moxa and recheck the induration.

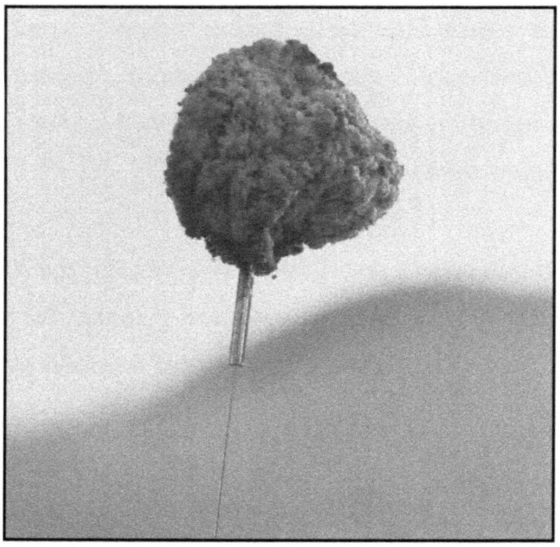

Figure 13-7: *Kyutoshin* at Step 4.

For example, for diarrhoea, palpate the areas around REN 10, REN 12, REN 14, ST 25, ST 26, ST 27, and REN 4, REN 6 for the most tender points. Needle at least one point on each side of the umbilicus and apply 2–3 rounds of moxa. Adding ST 36 to this treatment is also effective.

CONTRAINDICATIONS

For the needle to support the weight of the moxa ball, it typically needs to be inserted to a depth of approximately 1 cm. While this is suitable for the lower back, it is not appropriate for the upper back, where the lungs lie close beneath the surface. For this reason, *kyutoshin* on the upper torso requires special attention and precautions. Always be cautious with needle depth and review the point indications if you wish to insert the needle perpendicularly.

- Do not apply *kyutoshin* over the torso without paying attention to the appropriate needle depth.
- Use shorter needles with smaller balls of moxa to reduce the risk.
- Never apply *kyutoshin* to very thin patients.
- Points on the torso, such as GB 21 and LU 1, may require special adaptation due to the constraints of safe needle depths and angles of insertion; either include these precautions or omit such points from treatment.

CLOTHES PEG MOXA

A workaround for *kyutoshin* on the upper torso is to use *clothes peg moxa*. Insert a short 30 mm needle perpendicularly with a shallow insertion depth. Attach a small clothes peg to the needle at the insertion point; the peg lies horizontally on the skin at 90° to the needle, acting as an anchor to keep it upright. You can then place the moxa ball securely without fear of the needle toppling over. Taping the needle with micropore tape can also provide similar support.

FIFTY-YEAR-OLD SHOULDER: *GOJUKATA*

Gojukata is a Japanese term for 'frozen shoulder'. The name literally means 'fifty-year-old shoulder' because it is a common ailment that affects people in this age group. This term includes frozen shoulder and adhesive capsulitis:

1. Check the shoulder range of motion (ROM) with the patient to locate tender points. Needle the most sensitive points, usually one or more of LI 15, TB 14, or points between these two. Apply up to three rounds of moxa, repeating the ROM test after each round to judge its effectiveness.
2. A more anatomical approach uses muscle groups:
   In the prone position, for latissimus dorsi, palpate and treat reactive points around BL 22 and BL 13. For the rhomboids and levator scapulae, palpate and treat reactive points around BL 43 and SI 14. For infraspinatus, treat reactive points around TB 15, LI 16, and SI 11.
   In the lateral recumbent position, palpate and treat reactive points on the deltoid at LI 15, LI 14, TB 13, infraspinatus at TB 14, and supraspinatus at LI 16.
3. In the supine position, treat LU 1.

HEADACHE OR HEAVY FEELING IN THE HEAD

Kobe Akabane recommended this procedure for a sensation of heaviness in the head. It can also be helpful for headache, vertigo, and neck mobility issues related to flexion/extension and/or rotation. Needle BL 10 and GB 20 on the affected side. Apply 2–3 rounds of moxibustion and repeat until the patient notices improvement.

HYPERTENSION

Although moxibustion is contraindicated for hypertension in the TCM canon, in JAAM, there is no such restriction; both *okyu* and *kyutoshin* are considered beneficial. Apply 2–3 rounds of *kyutoshin* on the following points: BL 10, GB 20, GB 21, preferably at least two times a week. You can close the treatment with seven *okyu* at ST 36.

[Note: For points over the lungs, such as GB 21, see the contraindications section and workaround above.]

WEAKNESS IN THE LOWER BURNER

When there are problems with the lower burner, especially those involving the kidney meridian, BL 32, BL 33, or BL 34 may be treated instead of, or in addition to, BL 23 and BL 52. In chronic disorders, BL 51, or the point just lateral to it, *pigen*, is often tight and sore. If you find this response, treating these reactive points can be helpful.

[Note: *Pigen* (Ex-B4) is located on the back, 3.5 *cun* lateral to the lower border of the spinous process of the L1.]

SIMPLE *KYUTOSHIN* TREATMENTS

Table 13.6 outlines key points and strategies for using *kyutoshin*. These points are chosen for their broad therapeutic effects, which include reducing pain and tension, as well as promoting the circulation of qi and blood. They offer reliable options for local treatment at Step 4. Not every point needs to be used; let palpation guide your choices, and keep in mind that, especially with *kyutoshin*, less is often more.

Table 13.6: *Kyutoshin* points and protocols.

Anorexia	Palpate and treat pressure pain points (PPP) on the sides of the navel and the right subcostal region. On the back, treat BL 20 and DU 9, if reactive.
Asthma	Treat the *Huatuo-jiaji* points level with DU 14, BL 13, and BL 17, and treat SI 11 with Ontake or a tiger warmer.[183]
Backache and herniated disc	Check *josen* (*shiqizhuixia*, M-BW-25) below L5, BL 25, BL 29, or GB 30.
Carpal tunnel	PPP on the large intestine meridian
Cold, flu, and *taiyang* symptoms	DU 14 and BL 12
Haemorrhoids	PPP at the perianal area, or SP 7 LU 7 (often paired with SP 7)
Gastroptosis and stomach atony	With the patient supine, palpate a wide navel clock with a radius of 12–15 cm and treat pressure pain points. With the patient prone, treat reactive points on the lumbar area. Close with ST 36.
Inducing labour	SP 6

183 A tiger warmer is a small handheld moxibustion device: a metal tube with a spring-loaded inner sleeve that holds a smouldering moxa stick. Heat is applied through the tip, and the intensity is adjusted by moving the burning moxa closer to or further from the skin.

Knee pain	Look for pressure pain reactions around the knee at LIV 8, SP 9, GB 34, *neixiyan* (EX-LE4), and *waixiyan* (EX-LE5). Check the thigh at rectus femoris (ST 32 and ST 34, vastus medialis (SP 10), a point two fingers above SP 10, and vastus lateralis (GB 33).
Menstrual cramps	SP 8
Sciatica	Look for PPP from below L2 to L5, or just slightly lateral. Treat PPP around the PSIS. Treat GB 30 and the most reactive point in the buttock on the same side as the pain.
Sciatica during pregnancy	GB 31, GB 38, and GB 39
Whiplash	PPP from BL 17–BL 11

FINAL THOUGHTS

In this section, we've seen how moxibustion can be used as a branch or supplemental treatment, alongside any of the Four Steps. Moxa is very useful! In a YouTube interview, German Toyohari practitioner Sascha Groebe advises, "If you don't smell smoke from a clinic, run a mile!" His words capture the heart of moxibustion: it's not an optional extra, it's essential.[184]

[184] *Japanese Acupuncture Today*. (2015). Episode 2: Moxibustion [Video]. Interview with Sascha Gröbe and Merlin Young. Available at: https://www.youtube.com/live/uvFZFJrOoDE

Small-cone moxibustion is harder to learn than *kyutoshin*. It takes patience and practice, but it's worth every hour you invest. Once you get the feel for finding the alive point, rolling, placing, and lighting the cone, you'll see just how powerful this simple little practice can be. Learn it well, use it often, and both you and your patients will reap the rewards.

SUMMARY

- **Moxibustion is a practical art**: Its effectiveness depends on embodied skills, including palpation, cone rolling, shaping, placement, and lighting.
- **Cone size and shape matter**: A wide base delivers more heat to the skin's surface, while a pointed base allows heat to penetrate more deeply.
- **Delivery technique shapes outcome**: Loosely rolled cones burn cooler and quicker; tightly rolled cones burn hotter and longer.
- **Management of burning styles is essential**: Extinguish at 70–80% for stimulation without skin damage, or allow a 100% burn for immune activation.
- **Alive points are the key**: Look for pressure pain and induration, which mark the points most responsive to treatment.
- **Points can move**: Alive points shift or disappear as conditions resolve, so palpation must always guide treatment.
- **Precautions matter**: Avoid direct moxa on inappropriate sites, such as the face and blood vessels. Insert with care over the lungs. Be cautious with patients who are fasting or intoxicated.
- **Small-cone moxibustion takes dedication**: It is harder to learn than *kyutoshin*, but mastery rewards you with confidence, versatility, and powerful results.

WHAT'S NEXT

Part 3 is about fine-tuning—refining your diagnosis and tailoring treatment to each patient. We'll cover the secondary reactions, symptom differentiation for difficult abdominal patterns, and the all-important question of dosage: the Goldilocks Zone of treatment.

PART THREE

FINE-TUNING

CHAPTER 14

FINE-TUNING YOUR DIAGNOSIS

INTRODUCTION

Up to this point, we've explored techniques that can be applied at various stages of the Four Steps. These final three chapters are about fine-tuning: sharpening your use of pattern recognition, dosage, and workflow. In this chapter, we revisit Step 1—pattern recognition—and learn how to refine it further when the picture is unclear.

Diagnosing the *hara* is sometimes straightforward. A single round of palpation might reveal a classic Cross Syndrome (CS), and your treatment choice is obvious. At other times, several patterns may present at once, each with equal reactions. Which one do you pick?

To answer that, we'll consider two final sets of differentiation tools and some other fine-tuning strategies:

1. Secondary reactions (points and areas beyond the primary reflexes)
2. Symptomatology (the traditional Eight Extras symptom pictures)
3. Other fine-tuning strategies, such as counterflow qi and discomfort below the navel

SECONDARY REACTIONS

HISTORICAL CONTEXT

We had a brief encounter with the secondary reactions in Chapter 5, but until now, we've mostly discussed differentiation using the primary points and areas. Here, we return to the secondary reactions in more detail. Let's begin with a little historical context.

When Manaka developed his system, he identified four primary patterns: YQR, YQD, YWC, and YWD. He then added CS, the combination pattern of YWC and YWD. Thus, his system began with a limited range of options at Step 1—only five patterns in total. Because this was a small diagnostic set, nearly every patient presented with one or more of them, often in combinations such as CS with YQR, YWC with YQR, YQR with YWD, or, as we will see in Vol. 3, YQR with YQD (Qiao Connection).

Manaka prioritised the primary reflex areas and points, but when findings were ambiguous, he used *secondary reactions*—additional points on the neck, trunk, arms, and legs—as tools for further differentiation. These are not designed for routine palpation, but as tiebreakers when more than one pattern presents.

EVOLUTION TO COMBINATION PATTERNS

Since Manaka's passing, his system has continued to evolve. Stephen Birch and Brenda Loew introduced combination patterns—Mixed Yin, K3L, and Ren Dai—because overlapping patterns were so common. Sometimes, it felt more economical simply to treat the combination.

> *I got tired of choosing between YQR and Cross Syndrome because many people had both. I wondered if there was a way to make things easier.*
>
> —Stephen Birch[185]

[185] Kivity, O. (2024). Notes from authors' meeting.

Combination patterns are convenient, but on busy clinic days, when there isn't time for extended palpation, they can become the default choice. A fair way to describe this is the *all-in-one approach*: a practical way of covering overlapping patterns in a single treatment.

Manaka described diagnosis as finding "the most significant paradox in the body".[186] Stephen Birch later refined this principle to finding the "most significant bias". The all-in-one approach provides us with valuable treatment tools to clear multiple reactions at once; however, sometimes focusing on a single pattern, the most significant bias, would serve the patient better. The secondary reactions provide a way to refine the decision between treating multiple patterns or one.

DECISION PRINCIPLES

When you detect multiple patterns nested together, first check the strength of reactions on the primary areas, then the primary points. This may help you distinguish which pattern is more important to treat.

If they feel the same, move on to the secondary reactions. If one pattern shows particularly strong secondaries, this suggests it is the body's dominant bias and should be treated as a single pattern.

On the other hand, if the secondary reactions are weak or evenly distributed across several patterns, this points towards using a combination pattern. In these cases, the all-in-one approach—treating overlapping patterns together—may be the more appropriate choice.

Secondary reactions, in this sense, act as a compass. They help us decide whether to sharpen the focus onto one clear pattern or to broaden the treatment with a combination when no single pattern stands out.

---

186 Matsumoto, K., & Birch, S. (1988). *Hara Diagnosis: Reflections on the Sea*. Brookline: Paradigm Publications. p. 365.

This shift reflects the evolution of the system. Manaka originally used secondaries to distinguish among his four primary patterns, which he treated one at a time. With the development of combination patterns such as Mixed Yin, K3L, and Ren Dai, their role has expanded: today, they also guide us in deciding between treating a single pattern and using an all-in-one approach.

For example, if you are considering K3L, you can check the secondaries for YWC, YWD, and YQR. If the secondaries for YQR are strongly reactive and the others only mildly so, it suggests that YQR is the more significant bias and should be treated separately. Conversely, if no one pattern shows clearly stronger secondary reactions, K3L would be the better choice.

The primary areas and points are located on the torso. By contrast, the secondary reactions are more widespread, appearing in four regions: the neck and shoulder, trunk, arms, and legs. Manaka's original list of points, first published in English in *Chasing the Dragon's Tail*, is presented in Table 14.1, ordered by region.[187]

Table 14.1: Secondary reactions.

PATTERN	NECK/SHOULDER	TRUNK	ARM	LEG
YQR	ST 12, ST 9	ASIS (anterior superior iliac spine), KID 11	LU 3, LU 4	KID 8
YWC	ST 11, REN 22	GB 24	—	SP 6, KID 9
YWD		KID 16, SP 15, BL 23 (posterior belt line)	—	—
YQD	Cervical spine, sides of vertebrae	SI 9–10 area, PSIS (posterior superior iliac spine)	—	—

187 Manaka, Y., Itaya, K., & Birch, S. (1995). *Chasing the Dragon's Tail: The Theory and Practice of Acupuncture in the Work of Yoshio Manaka*. Brookline: Paradigm Publications. p. 139.

As we compared notes for this chapter, it became clear that each of us approaches the secondary reactions in a different way. Much of this comes down to palpation style and how we each gather diagnostic information. With that in mind, let's examine the secondary reactions for each pattern and consider how each author considers them.[188]

YIN QIAO REN (YQR)

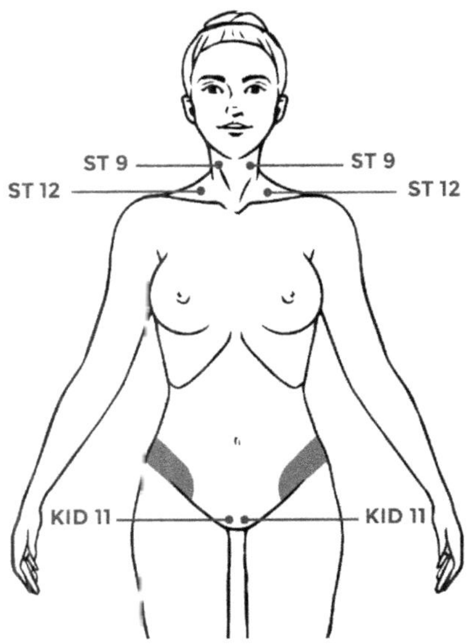

Figure 14-1: YQR secondary reactions on the neck and trunk.

[188] Kivity, O. (2024). Notes from authors' meeting.

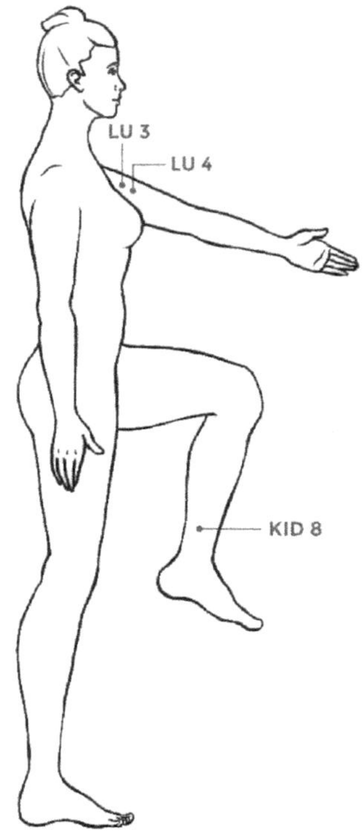

Figure 14-2: YQR secondary reactions on the upper and lower limb.

Tenderness or jump reactions at the ASIS can be misleading. As a primary reaction, it leads us to YQD or YWD, but sometimes it's secondary to YQR. Checking other secondaries, such as ST 12 or LU 3, can clarify the picture.

[Note: In Japan, the lung meridian on the upper arm is understood to flow along the *medial* border of the biceps brachii rather than the lateral border. Accordingly, LU 3 and LU 4 are palpated on the medial aspect of the arm, not the lateral.]

PRACTICAL TIPS

> *At ST 12, the healthy finding is a soft hollow. With chronic imbalance, it fills out, creating a bump that's tender. This is a clear YQR indicator.*
>
> —Stephen Birch

A normal, healthy finding at ST 12 is a soft depression in the supraclavicular fossa. In cases of chronic imbalance, the tissue starts to feel abnormal, filling out and creating a slight bump instead of a depression. This raised and uneven texture is often tender on palpation and is an indicator of chronicity. This kind of reaction suggests YQR.

—Stephen Birch

ST 9 either feels healthy and soft or stiff and hard. If it's stiff and hard, it's often tender as well.

—Paul Movsessian

I don't find the reactions on the neck easy to read, but I like LU 3 and LU 4, which I go to routinely. For me, they're pretty reliable indicators that can help support or discount the possibility of YQR.

—Oran Kivity

YIN WEI CHONG (YWC)

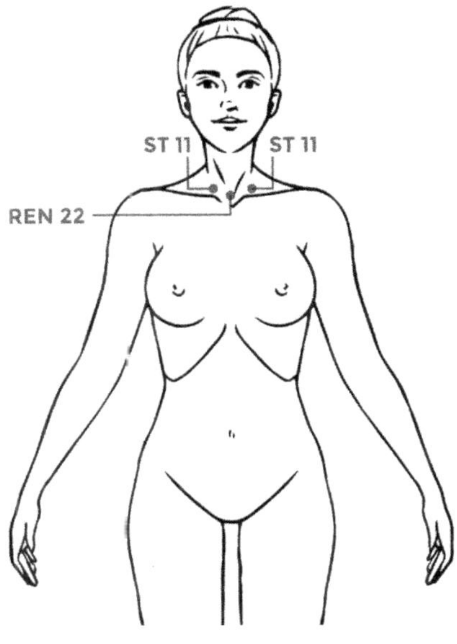

Figure 14-3: YWC secondary reactions on the neck and trunk.

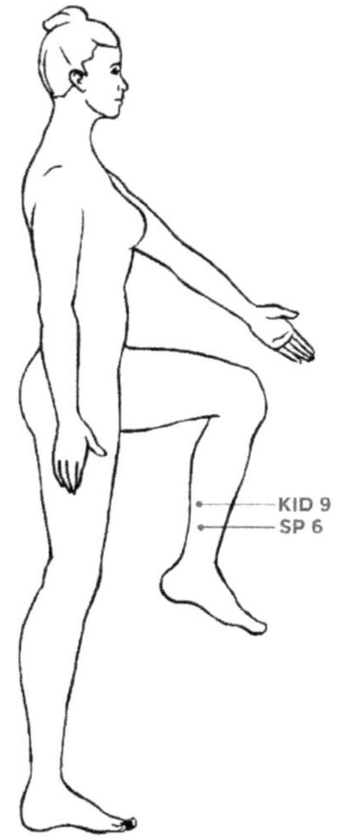

Figure 14-4: YWC secondary reactions on the leg.

With tightness under the subcostals, the YWC is one of the least ambiguous findings on the *hara* and extra differentiation with the secondary points is seldom required. Although Manaka listed LIV 14 and GB 24 as secondary reactions, in practice, they add little: LIV 14 lies at the centre of the subcostal region itself and is therefore not assessed separately, and GB 24, although listed, is rarely palpated or clinically necessary. For this reason, the authors tend to rely on the primary subcostal area as the clearest diagnostic indicator. After observing Manaka in clinic, Stephen Birch also checks ST 11 and REN 22.[189, 190]

189 In JAAM, LIV 14 is on the subcostal margin directly below the nipple and thus is part of the 'subcostal' reaction indicative of YWC, extending from roughly ST 19 to LIV 13).

190 Manaka originally listed GB 24 as a reflex point for YWD. However, as Stephen Birch found that this very rarely shows, this was dropped from the list of primary points. Given its relationship to YWD, it doesn't seem so useful as a secondary reaction to YWC.

PRACTICAL TIPS

REN 22 is a clear indicator for this pattern, and can feel markedly sore or reactive, becoming less so when the cords are placed.

—Stephen Birch

If I'm trying to decide between a YQR pattern and a YWC pattern, while I'm on the neck, it's a simple matter to palpate ST 12 [for YQR] *and then move medially to ST 11 and REN 22* [for YWC]. *When I'm on the legs, I can compare KID 8* [for YQR] *and KID 9* [for YWC]. *So, it's pretty easy to compare these points, just moving from one to the other in each region.*

—Paul Movsessian

SP 6 is reactive on so many patients that I find it hard to use as a tiebreaker in this context.

—Oran Kivity

YANG WEI DAI (YWD)

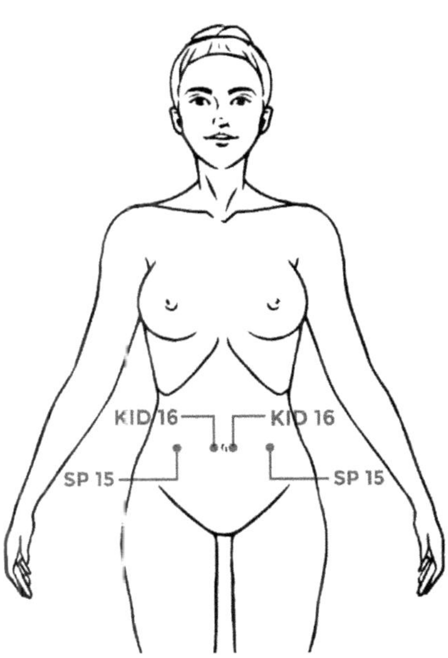

Figure 14-5: YWD secondary reactions on the anterior trunk.

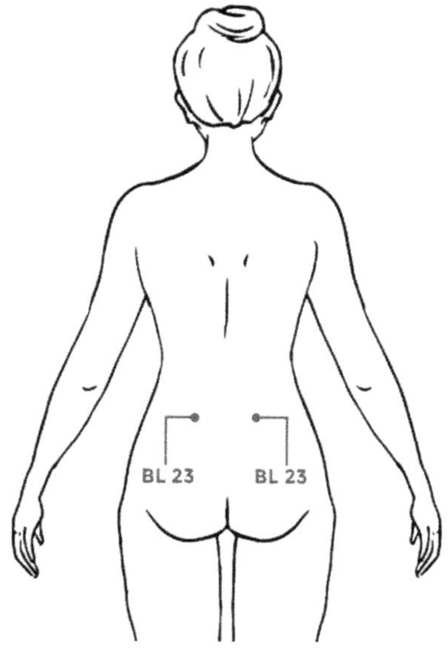

Figure 14-6: YWD secondary reactions on the posterior trunk.

Interestingly, the YWD pattern secondaries are found only on the trunk. Given the horizontal nature of the Dai Mai, this makes perfect sense: we palpate for reactions along a line from KID 16 to SP 15 and across to BL 23. In practice, however, the points Manaka listed as 'secondary'—SP 15 and KID 16—sit squarely within the primary belt region and are better understood as part of the main diagnostic area rather than true secondary reactions. The only secondary finding outside the belt is BL 23.

The Dai Mai naturally spans from ASIS to ASIS at the level of the navel, which means ST 25, SP 15, KID 16, and the ASIS already fall within the primary area. Once these are identified, little further palpation is required, other than deciding the side of treatment.

PRACTICAL TIPS

> *Sometimes, when the anterior reactions, such as the ASIS, are not strong, I like to check BL 23 to determine left or right.*
>
> —Oran Kivity

Reactions at BL 23 can only be considered together with reactions on the front line. If they're a singular finding, they're not necessarily indicative of YWD.

—Brenda Loew

If I find the ASIS alone is reactive, I lean towards YQD. If I find the ASIS plus the belt line is reactive, it points towards YWD.

—Marian Fixler

YANG QIAO DU (YQD)

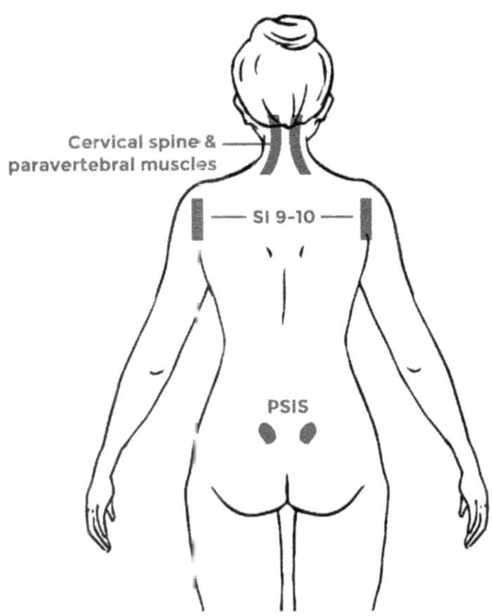

Figure 14-7: YQD secondary reactions on the posterior trunk.

The ASIS comes up in three of the basic patterns. It's a secondary reflex for YQR and a primary reflex for YWD and YQD. When you can't interpret the ASIS reaction, the secondary points of YQD are the easiest way to break the deadlock. When the patient is supine, slip your hands under the neck and palpate the sides of the cervical vertebrae. They are frequently reactive in this pattern and not reactive in a YWD or YQR pattern. You can also slide your hands under the shoulder and palpate the SI 9–SI 10 area. These areas are reliable indicators of a YQD pattern.

PRACTICAL TIPS

In my experience, the area from SI 9 to SI 10 is always reactive when a YQD pattern requires treatment. Pressure pain along the cervical vertebrae is a significant indicator to select this pattern.

—Stephen Birch

Both Paul Movsessian and Brenda Loew check the PSIS before and after ion pumping, sliding their hands under the back when the patient is in a supine position.

CROSS SYNDROME (CS)

What do we do for CS? While it may seem logical to use secondary reactions for YWC and YWD, Manaka did not do this, and Stephen Birch observes that it is not necessary. The pattern of upper right quadrant reactions with lower left quadrant reactions on the abdomen is enough.

In summary, the process of differentiation moves step by step. The primary areas alone can help you decide, as in CS, and the primary points can help confirm a diagnosis. When things are less clear, the secondary points act as our tiebreakers. Finally, we turn to symptoms—the last tool in our kit—for weighing and refining our choice.

SYMPTOMS

When more than one of the four patterns is present in a patient, we first check the secondary patterns and then review the symptoms. These two procedures are crucial. Together, they provide reliable evidence to support the corresponding pattern.

—Stephen Birch

We already know that to decide a pattern, the primary area and both corresponding primary points must be reactive. Sometimes that's enough. In more complex situations, we have learned to check the secondary reactions to see which of the candidate patterns do and which do not have secondary reactions. We pick the one that does.

After palpating the secondary reactions, if the picture remains confusing, and more than one pattern is still feasible, then we turn to Manaka's fourth differentiation strategy. The symptoms help us decide. Stephen Birch describes this Four Step protocol, from primary areas and points to secondary reactions and symptoms, as a foolproof system. This section explores how to use symptoms as a final differentiating tool.

CONTEXT

Manaka's use of the Eight Extraordinary Vessels to treat at the root level was a modern innovation. Traditionally, broad symptom pictures were allocated to each of the Eight Extras. These comprised long lists of symptoms associated with just four pairs of points. The Extras were presented and used as ways to treat at the branch level, even just one symptom within the broad range of indications; for example, for asthma, treating the Ren Mai.

> *If we think about this treatment style, it is really broad; it's like trying to catch a single rabbit in a field with a massive net.... The Extraordinary Vessel is the massive net, the symptom the rabbit.*[191]

For Manaka, the effects of the Extras on the octahedral structure were more important than their effects on symptoms. Table 14.2 summarises the symptoms, discussed in *Chasing the Dragon's Tail*, that he considered most important for differentiating patterns.[192]

---

191 Matsumoto, K., & Birch, S. (1986). *Extraordinary Vessels*. Brookline, MA: Paradigm Publications. p. 72, quoting Gao Wu, *Zhen Jiu Ju Ying* (1529).

192 Manaka, Y., Itaya, K., & Birch, S. (1995). *Chasing the Dragon's Tail: The Theory and Practice of Acupuncture in the Work of Yoshio Manaka*. Brookline: Paradigm Publications. pp. 145–146.

Table 14.2: Eight Extraordinary Vessels symptomatology.

REN MAI	Head: toothache; ear, nose, and throat problems Chest: asthma, bronchitis, lung problems Lower abdomen: gynaecological problems; haemorrhoids Mental: neurosis
YIN QIAO MAI	Lower abdomen: gynaecological problems; urination problems; intestinal problems Legs: cold feet
CHONG MAI	Chest: heart problems Upper abdomen: stomach problems; liver and gall bladder problems Lower abdomen: gynaecological problems; problems of the anus Legs: cold feet Mental: neurosis
YIN WEI MAI	Chest: heart problems, palpitations Upper abdomen: stomach problems Mental: nervousness, psychological problems, insomnia
DAI MAI	Lower abdomen: gynaecological problems; menstrual problems; problems in the lower abdomen generally Lower back: feelings of cold or aching in the lower back
YANG WEI MAI	Head: dizziness, headache, trigeminal neuralgia, ear and eye problems Neck: whiplash General: sweating problems, fatigue
DU MAI	Spine and brain: epilepsy, problems in the spine and neck General: fatigue, superficial invasion of cold or external qi; early stages of catching a cold (*Shang Han Lung Taiyang* stage of disease) Mental: neurosis, insomnia
YANG QIAO MAI	Spine and brain: whiplash, epilepsy, speech disorders, trigeminal neuralgia Torso: shoulder pain, lumbar pain General: unusual sweating

CROSS SYNDROME	Head and neck: head, eyes, ears, nose, and throat problems, especially on the left Upper abdomen: liver problems, digestive problems (especially intestinal) Lower abdomen: gynaecological problems Musculoskeletal: shoulder problems, low back problems, sciatica (especially of the left leg)

CLINICAL APPLICATIONS

How can we integrate these indications into our pattern selection? Manaka suggested that in some situations, the symptoms could be used to choose a pattern. This can be useful in two situations:

1. When palpating the abdomen is difficult or awkward
2. When differentiation by palpation is problematic, because two patterns present equally

For example, in the final months of pregnancy, it is very hard to palpate the abdomen. The same is true of professional bodybuilders with rock-hard six-packs and patients with extensive scarring on the abdomen. Some patients, for cultural reasons, may not permit abdominal palpation without the presence of a chaperone. In these cases, it makes sense to have another set of indicators to help you decide the pattern.

Thus, if you're treating two women in late pregnancy, you can use their symptoms to guide you. If one patient has posterior sciatica, you might select the YQD pattern. If the other has shortness of breath, you might consider the YQR pattern. It is worth mentioning that even in pregnant women, when the primary areas are difficult to palpate, the Manaka-*mu* points can still be useful.

Finally, we should consider that symptom matching is useful not only for patients who are hard to palpate but also for everyday patients who present with more than one pattern. For example, if a patient presents with both a YWD pattern and a YQD pattern, you can consider their symptoms and the meridian pathways involved. For example, if they have sciatica on the gall bladder meridian, you could treat YWD, and if it is on the bladder meridian, you could choose YQD. If they have a temporal headache, you could choose YWD. If they have poor flexion and extension of the neck, you could choose YQD.

Let's consider a patient whose *hara* presents with both subcostal tightness and midline reactions. We can't decide between a YWC and a YQR pattern. However, she experiences digestive problems, including bloating and undigested food in her stool. This points us in the direction of YWC. Conversely, if she has wheezing or shortness of breath, we would lean towards YQR.

Thus, basic theory can influence our choice. Typically, it is not the primary selection tool but simply a weighting factor that helps filter the palpatory information. It comes into its own more when palpation is not an easy option; for example, with women in the last months of pregnancy or teenagers who flinch at the slightest touch (see below).

ADVANCED APPLICATIONS

Some experienced practitioners use this symptom list to refine their application of the Extraordinary Vessels by adjusting polarity within the master-couple pairs—for example, emphasising one vessel and its symptom picture more strongly by reversing the clip placement. These refinements require a deep familiarity with the Eight Extras and their symptomatology and sit beyond the scope of this book. We'll come back to these more advanced ideas in the future.

OTHER FINE-TUNING STRATEGIES

FINE-TUNING ACCORDING TO DIRECTION

Manaka also emphasised another principle for pattern selection, which is the prevalence of counterflow symptoms such as red face, cold feet, headache, and tight shoulders (*katakori*).

Counterflow qi refers to the condition where the patient's qi tends to rise with little provocation and is a condition that can overlay and complicate other general patterns. It can predispose towards conditions such as cardiovascular disease (high blood pressure, stroke, myocardial infarction, etc.) and conditions such as chronic headaches. It is often related to emotional problems, both as a cause and an effect. It commonly presents with:

- Cold feet
- Tight shoulders, reddened complexion or headache
- Emotional instability
- Tightness and warmth above the navel; coldness and softness below the navel

In these cases, it makes more sense to select patterns with a downward flow, where the black clip is on the arm and the red clip is on the leg, and to choose the Wei Mai patterns over the Qiao patterns.[193]

YQR REACTIONS ABOVE OR BELOW THE NAVEL

The most common manifestation of YQR is stiffness, hardness, discomfort, or pressure pain above the navel (mostly between REN 10 and REN 12) with softness below the navel. Sometimes this presents as a general hardening in the upper abdomen with softening in the lower.

In elderly patients, another pattern can appear: a soft lower abdomen with a stiffened, rounded upper back, shoulders slumped forward, and the neck projecting ahead. Most often, however, the reaction to the loss of abdominal tone is not up–down but front–back. When the lower abdomen loses tonus, a frequent secondary reaction is tightening of the lower back muscles, perhaps due to compensatory changes in posture and movement.

---

193 Matsumoto, K., & Birch, S. (1988). *Hara Diagnosis: Reflections on the Sea*. Brookline: Paradigm Publications. pp. 373–374.

Sometimes, in addition to these typical midline reactions above the navel, YQR presents with pressure pain *below* the navel. Less commonly, but significantly, YQR presents as pressure pain below the navel without any upper abdominal signs.

If pressure pain below the navel is found during menstruation, it is normal and not especially significant. But if the same finding appears in a male patient or a non-menstruating female, it becomes highly significant and prioritises the use of YQR.

In such cases, YQR should be included in the final pattern selection—either on its own or as part of a combination pattern such as Mixed Yin, K3L, or Ren Dai. Birch emphasises that this presentation represents a more severe form of YQR pattern that is better addressed directly with a matching pattern.

DESENSITISING JUMPY PATIENTS

Sometimes, patients are very ticklish or sensitive to palpation. This is especially true of teenagers and wiry or thin patients with less body fat. In these cases, Manaka suggested burning a single rice-grain-sized cone on DU 20, which very often calms the patient and helps the abdomen relax, enabling the normal palpation sequence.

Direct moxa on the head is simpler than it sounds. Part the hair around the point and place a small drop of *shiunko* ointment there. Roll a slightly longer thin cone of moxa and place it on the point.

Another method uses electrostatic adsorbers, one of Manaka's alternative polarity devices. We'll introduce them in Chapter 17. If you have one, place the black (negative) probe on DU 20 and have the patient hold the red (positive) probe. This simple trick can sometimes reduce abdominal ticklishness or jumpiness.

CASE STUDY 8: STROKE RECOVERY

Ziva, Female, 63

Occupation: Retired journalist

PRESENTING CONDITION

Ziva had suffered an ischaemic stroke 4 years earlier, which left her with loss of mobility in her right arm and leg. Her whole right side went numb, she lost sensation in her face, and she was unable to speak clearly. At the time of presentation, she could walk with a stick, but she could not control her right foot and ankle and had to place them carefully with each step. Her right arm had recovered somewhat more than her leg, though it still felt heavy and was difficult to lift.

RELEVANT HISTORY

- After the stroke, for the first 6 months, she had TCM acupuncture 5 times a week. Following this, she had it 3 times a week for almost the whole 4 years. She still has TCM acupuncture once a week and physiotherapy 3 times a week.
- Her back gets sore because of the way she walks.
- Her bowels are good. She occasionally misses a day.
- Sleep is good unless she overeats.
- She's slim, but she says her appetite is 'too good,' and she has very good self-control.

PALPATION

- There is midline tightness below the sternum to about REN 12.
- Both ASIS are very jumpy.
- LU 1 and LU 2 areas are tight; KID 16 is also tight. ST 26 and KID 11 are both tight.
- ST 12 feels quite hard and lumpy, no reactions at ST 9, LU 3, LU 4.
- SI 9 to SI 10 feel painful, the whole back of the neck is painful, and the PSIS is reactive.

TREATMENT 1

Diagnosis: YQD

Step 1: IPC: YQD with IPC and silver spike points (SSP) for 5 minutes

[Note: SSP are discussed in Chapter 17.]

Step 2: Ontake along the bladder meridian on each side of the spine and the back of the legs
Step 3: N/A
Step 4: *Okyu* on 4 tight tender points in the intrascapular region (3 cones on each) and 1 cone on each of the *jing*-well points of the 5 toes on the right (on the tip of the toes, rather than at the corners of the nail)

TREATMENT 2 (FOLLOWING WEEK)

Patient Response
Ziva was delighted. She had not mentioned that she'd had a stiff neck for 4 years, but this had disappeared in the week, and she was able to turn her head with ease. Her arm felt stronger, and she felt an improvement in her foot mobility.

PALPATION

- Midline tightness below the sternum to about REN 12 was present but less pronounced.
- Both ASIS are very jumpy.
- LU 1 and LU 2 areas are tight; KID 16 is also tight. ST 26 and KID 11 are both tight.
- ST 12 feels quite hard and lumpy, no reactions at ST 9, LU 3, LU 4.
- SI 9 to SI 10 feel painful, the whole back of the neck is painful, and the PSIS is reactive.

Diagnosis: YQD

Step 1: YQD for 5 minutes with IPC and SSP
Step 2: Ontake along the bladder meridian on both sides of the spine, focusing on BL 27, BL 28, and the backs of the legs
Step 3: N/A
Step 4: *Okyu* on 4 tight tender points in the intrascapular region (3 cones on each) and 1 cone on each of the *jing*-well points of the right hand and foot; 3 cones of ST 36 bilaterally

TREATMENT 3 (FOLLOWING WEEK)

Patient Response
Really happy celebrating her new neck mobility. Sleeping better than before. Feels her waistline has shrunk, perhaps because she is no longer so gassy. Her shoulder is looser, but her elbow still feels tight. She has lower back soreness on the left. Her leg feels stronger and her movement a little smoother.

PALPATION

- Midline tightness below the sternum to about REN 12 is more pronounced. It feels like a typical YQR pattern.
- Both ASIS are very jumpy.
- LU 1 and LU 2 areas are tight; KID 16 is also tight. ST 26 and KID 11 are both tight.
- ST 12 feels quite hard and lumpy, no reactions at ST 9, LU 3, LU 4.
- SI 9 to SI 10 feels painful; the whole back of the neck is painful, and the PSIS is reactive.

Diagnosis: YQD

Step 1: YQD for 5 minutes with IPC and SSP
Step 2: Ontake along the bladder meridian on both sides of the spine, focusing on BL 27, BL 28, and the backs of the legs
Step 3: N/A
Step 4: *Okyu* on 4 tight tender points in the intrascapular region (3 cones on each) and 1 cone on each of the *jing*-well points of the right hand and foot; 3 cones of ST 36 bilaterally

TREATMENT 4 (FOLLOWING WEEK)

Patient Response

She went back home after treatment and napped for a couple of hours. Her ankle feels looser, and her toes have more movement. When she takes a step and places her foot, some pain that she had not previously reported has eased considerably. The back of her neck feels tight today, and although her shoulder is much looser, she feels tightness in her arm.

PALPATION

- Midline tightness below the sternum to about REN 12 is pronounced. It feels like a typical YQR pattern.
- Both ASIS are very jumpy.
- LU 1 and LU 2 areas are tight; KID 16 is also tight. ST 26 and KID 11 are both tight.
- ST 12 feels quite hard and lumpy, no reactions at ST 9, LU 3, LU 4.
- SI 9 to SI 10 feels painful; the whole back of the neck is painful, and the PSIS is reactive.

Diagnosis: YQD

Step 1: YQD for 5 minutes with IPC and SSP
Step 2: Ontake along the bladder meridian on both sides of the spine, focusing on BL 27, BL 28, and the back of the legs. Ontake along the large intestine and stomach meridians. Ontake around the back of the neck.
Step 3: N/A
Step 4: *Okyu* on 4 tight tender points in the intrascapular region (3 cones on each) and 1 cone on each of the *jing*-well points of the right hand and foot; 3 cones of ST 36 bilaterally

CONCLUSIONS AND REFLECTIONS

Ziva presented with two patterns that showed equal evidence in the primary points and areas. The ASIS was a confusing indicator because it appears in the YWD pattern and as a secondary reaction in YQR. By weighing the secondary reactions, it was possible to break the tie: the YQD pattern emerged as the most pronounced. In the second week, YQR was less pronounced, but in weeks three and four, the two primary patterns had to be distinguished, once again, using the secondary reactions.

We can also consider Ziva's treatment options in terms of symptoms. Of the two patterns, YQD, with its connection to the spine and brain, seems more relevant to stroke recovery than YQR. Had her secondary reactions been more or less equal, then her presentation and symptoms would have led to the selection of YQD.

Because Ziva appeared frail, SSP were selected. These are non-insertive silver terminals that are taped to the skin and then connected with IPC and are considered less strong than needling. As treatment progressed, it became clear she tolerated moxa well, so the dosage was gradually increased. She reported napping after treatment but without any ongoing exhaustion, indicating the dose was appropriate.

The moxa treatments followed Fukaya's advice to check the intrascapular area for upper limb problems and to release tight points. On the side of her stroke, many exquisitely painful points were found. Treatment focuses on two or three in each session.

It is hard not to compare the results from just four non-invasive MSA treatments with the years of acupuncture she had previously received. After this short series, she broke through a long-standing plateau of pain, stiffness, and restricted range of movement.

At the time of writing, she has completed four sessions and is very keen to continue.

SUMMARY

- **Historical application:** Originally, Manaka's system focused on five primary patterns, treating them individually. The secondary reactions were important tiebreakers to distinguish between this narrow set of options.
- **Evolution of combination patterns:** Over time, Stephen Birch and Brenda Loew developed combination patterns, such as Mixed Yin, Ren Dai, and K3L, to address the frequent co-presentation of patterns, simplifying decision-making on busy days but sometimes leading to a fast-track, all-in-one approach for everything.
- **Palpation preferences:** The authors have different preferences for secondary points in clinical practice, but points such as ST 12, ST 11, REN 22, and the posterior neck are useful for differentiation, as are the reactions at the back of the axilla, specifically SI 9 to SI 10.
- **Fine-tuning and decision-making:** The secondary reactions remain essential for decision-making and fine-tuning your treatment. They prevent reliance on combination patterns as a fast-track default approach and guide you to address the "most significant bias" in the body.

- **The Eight Extras symptom pictures**: These provide a final layer of filtering, deployed when two patterns present equally through palpation, or when palpation is difficult and yields unclear findings.
- **Midline pressure pain below the navel:** If the patient is not menstruating, midline pressure pain below the navel is significant and should always be treated by selecting a pattern that includes YQR.

WHAT'S NEXT

In a nineteenth-century tale, a little girl called Goldilocks finds three bowls of porridge: one is too cold, one is too hot, and one is just right. In the next chapter, we'll explore dosage in the same spirit—don't treat too much, don't treat too little, but find a dose that's just right.

CHAPTER 15

DOSAGE AND THE GOLDILOCKS ZONE

Continuous effort should be made to perform therapy using the minimum number of acupuncture points possible.... Although the amount of stimulation may be increased when the need arises, care must be taken not to exceed the individual's limit, beyond which unnecessary side effects arise.

—Yoshio Manaka[194]

MAXIMUM BENEFIT WITH MINIMAL INTERVENTION

In *Moxa in Motion*, Oran Kivity introduced the idea of the Goldilocks Zone through the familiar tale of Goldilocks and the Three Bears. It describes a range that is neither too much nor too little, but just right for a particular function.[195]

---

194 Ibid. p. 116.

195 Kivity, O. (2020). *Moxa in Motion with the Ontake Method: Rhythmic Moxibustion Methods from Japan for Mind-Body Healing*. London: Sayoshi Books.

The idea that there is a limit to treatment "beyond which unnecessary side effects arise" is crucial to understanding dosage in acupuncture. In Western medicine, drug dosage is related to several criteria, with age and body weight being the most important. For example, a doctor may prescribe a child a quarter of an aspirin pill, and an adult two whole pills. An elderly or frail patient may need only one.

We can derive two important concepts from this. Firstly, each patient has a unique Goldilocks Zone for dosage of treatment: not too much, not too little, but just right. Secondly, patients can be divided into two categories: sensitive and robust.

If these two categories sound familiar, it is because TEAM often discusses weak and strong, deficient and excess types. In Japanese, these are referred to as *kyo* (deficient) and *jitsu* (excess). These are pathological states. However, beyond the meaning of 'excess', *jitsu* has another meaning relating to health: 'robustness' or 'strength'. Someone who is *jitsu* can be said to be in 'rude good health', strong and full of life. In clinical practice, this means that robust patients can tolerate acupuncture much better than sensitive patients. Thus, we need to do two things:

1. Identify patients as either robust or sensitive and treat them accordingly.
2. Recognise the signs, both good and bad, that show we have given sufficient treatment.

ADVANTAGES OF A GRADUALIST CLINICAL APPROACH

A few years ago, an elderly patient of mine borrowed her neighbour's car while hers was being repaired. Her own car was an antiquated and sedate automatic, a real-life example of the 'one careful lady owner' that you read about in the classified ads for second-hand cars. Her neighbour's car, also automatic, was far more powerful and highly tuned. Within thirty seconds of starting the engine, she had accelerated through her garden gate, just managing to brake outside her living room patio doors. She ended up with a few bruises, a sprained wrist and some injured pride.

—Oran Kivity

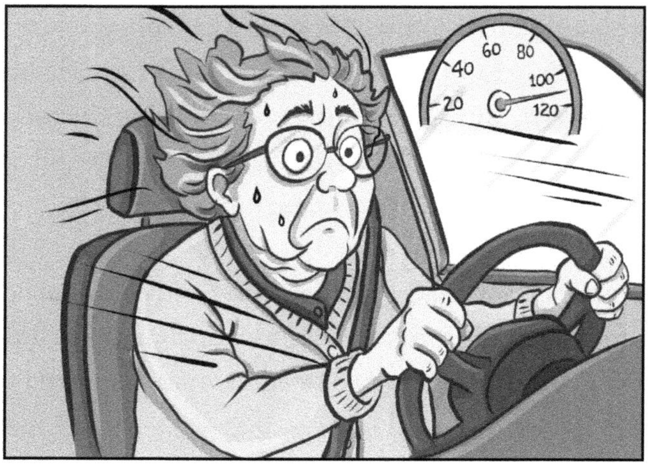

Figure 15-1: Fast cars can overshoot the destination.

Slow cars and fast cars offer the same outcome: they both get you to where you want to go. Similarly, both low-stimulation and strong-stimulation methods aim to improve your patients' energy. One crucial difference is that slow cars and low-stimulation methods give you much more control over the journey. Without that control, you may overshoot badly, especially when treating sensitive patients.

'Overtreatment' can have many adverse consequences, including fatigue, nausea, lightheadedness, or aggravated symptoms. The late Akihiro Takai, former president of the Toyohari Association of Japan, stated that he believed 90% of adverse reactions in his clinic over his forty years of practice were due to overtreatment.[196]

DR MANAKA'S GRAPH OF STIMULUS AND REACTION

Dr Manaka first explained this concept in *Chasing the Dragon's Tail*. Figure 15-2 shows his model for contrasting strong and mild methods of treatment.[197] There are three horizontal bands representing insufficient, adequate, and excessive dosages of

196 Kivity, O. (2000). *Lecture on Dosage* by Akihiro Takai. Toyohari Summer School, Tokyo. Personal notes.

197 Manaka, Y., Itaya, K., & Birch, S. (1995). *Chasing the Dragon's Tail: The Theory and Practice of Acupuncture in the Work of Yoshio Manaka*. Brookline: Paradigm Publications. p. 119.

treatment. An insufficient dose will not cause a curative effect. Too much will cause adverse reactions. Our ideal treatment dosage should fall in the Goldilocks Zone: not too much, not too little—but just right.

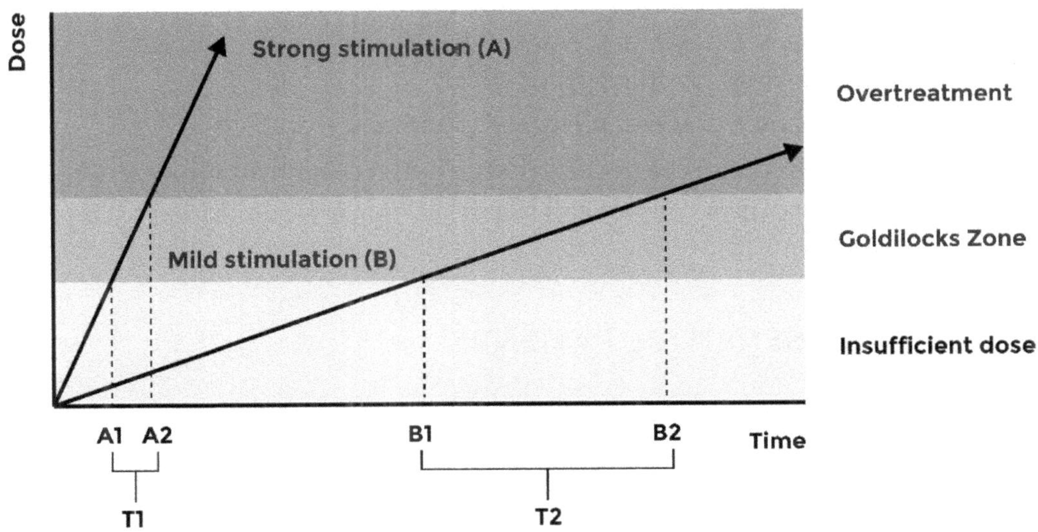

Figure 15-2: The Gold locks Zone for an average patient.

Treatment A, which uses strong physical stimulation, can quickly arrive at the correct dosage, but, like the neighbour's powerful car, can easily overshoot, causing adverse reactions. If we measure from the time the dosage reaches the Goldilocks Zone (A1) to the time it exceeds it (A2), we can see that the time is quite short (T1).

Treatment B, utilising low-intensity stimuli, employs a series of carefully monitored, low-dose interventions to achieve an effective level of stimulation. In this instance, if we measure from the same two points, B1 and B2, we can see there is much more time to monitor the effects of the treatment (T2) and stop at the right time. There is less chance of overtreating the patient.

We have already seen that Manaka saw the meridian system as a low-energy system that responds best to low-energy interventions (like whispering in a library, not yelling at a football match). Now we see a more pragmatic, clinical reason to apply treatment in incremental steps. Manaka researched and developed devices and techniques that apply small or minute stimuli to the meridian system. Each step is monitored for its effect, with feedback mechanisms specific to the method used.

This approach is taken for all patients, but particular care should be taken for sensitive patients, which includes the elderly, the very young, and anyone who might react strongly to standard treatment.

The benefits of this gradualist, gentle approach to treatment include:

- Greater control over therapeutic effects
- Increased time to assess and regulate treatment
- A reduction in adverse reactions from incorrect treatment and overtreatment
- Increased patient comfort and relaxation from low-stimulation techniques

IDENTIFYING SENSITIVE PATIENTS

Some patients are more sensitive than others. Who are they, and how can we recognise them? To plan dosage and treatment, it's important to identify such patients from the outset. Often their appearance gives the first clue—they may look weak, thin, or fatigued.

Age is another key identifying factor. We must assume that the very young and the very old are more sensitive. Of course, we will encounter robust elderly patients from time to time, but as a general rule, it is safe to assume that the older they are, the more sensitive they will be. If it seems obvious that a ninety-nine-year-old with back pain should be treated more gently than a thirty-year-old, it is worth noting that by the same principle, a sixty-year-old should be treated more gently than a fifty-year-old. Likewise, a weak or tired-looking fifty-year-old should be treated more gently than a healthy-looking patient of the same age.

Infants and children are also extremely sensitive to treatment and require very different treatment methods and dosages from adults.

Age is therefore at the top of the list as an indicator for sensitivity, although many other signs might warn you that certain patients are more sensitive than others:

- They have been ill for a long time.
- They have a history of a complex disease like cancer and its treatment.
- They have a history of psychological or emotional issues, which may include long-standing events from their past or more recent ones. If they start crying during the pre-treatment chat, it is a clear indication to do a light treatment.
- They are literally sensitive: They 'feel' things. They can 'sense' things. They receive 'guidance'. Some spiritually inclined individuals are highly sensitive and require minimal intervention.
- They do a great deal of work on themselves and their own qi. This includes so-called therapy junkies and other people engaged in yoga, Tai Chi, meditation, personal growth work, and counselling.
- They are artistic, creative, or reflective.
- They talk a lot, and it's hard to get them to relax.

Koryo Nakada, another former president of the Toyohari Association, reported that volubility is a very obvious indicator of sensitivity. In a lecture on dosage, he said unequivocally, "If a patient talks a lot, use fewer needles!"[198]

Why would this be? We all know patients who talk a lot—some are just naturally voluble. Others are nervous about treatment, and in those cases, it is wise to take note and "use fewer needles".

There's a second group of patients, however, who talk at length but offer little relevant information. They may mishear our questions, wander off into unrelated detail, or become emotionally re-stimulated by the conversation.

This kind of volubility is a pathology in itself. In simple terms, it points to an energy imbalance. It is a volatile state and must be treated with particular caution. At its extreme, it can verge on psychosis. Here, reducing dosage is the first step to successful treatment.

---

198 Kivity, O. (2010). *Lecture on Dosage* by Koryo Nakada. Toyohari Summer School, Tokyo. Personal notes.

The example of volubility helps us understand the range of conditions that lead to sensitivity. At first glance, the list may appear odd. Why should we group together people with past trauma and those who invest in their health through Tai Chi or yoga? One seems traumatised, the other healthy.

But when we look more closely, the connection becomes clear. Many people with trauma are drawn to self-cultivation practices. However, whether people do meditation, have a chronic disease, or talk a lot, what they have in common is an energy system that is unusually sensitive to nudges—either because it is finely tuned or somewhat out of balance.

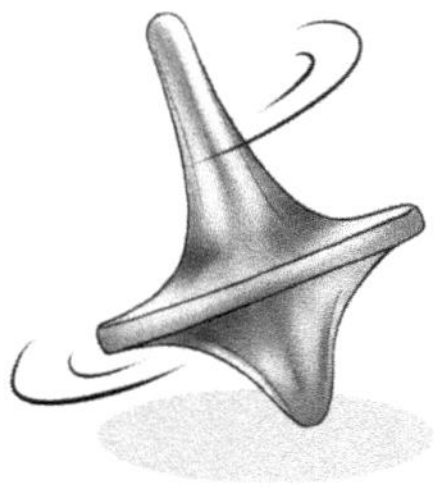

Figure 15-3: This spinning top is sensitive to nudges.

Imagine a child's spinning top. When it begins to lean or wobble, only the gentlest nudge is needed to bring it back into balance. Push too hard and it topples, leaving the patient worse off. Overtreatment is the same: by applying too much force, we overshoot the optimal zone and push the patient into counter-reaction.

THE GOLDILOCKS ZONE FOR SENSITIVE PATIENTS

Using Manaka's model of treatment, Stephen Birch modified Manaka's original graph to represent the characteristics of sensitive patients.[199] We can see in Figure 15-4 that they present quite differently. The Goldilocks Zone undergoes two crucial changes. First, it is lower on the y-axis (vertical) than that of a normal, robust patient. Less

[199] Birch, S. (2011). *Shonishin: Japanese Pediatric Acupuncture*. Stuttgart: Thieme Medical Publishers. pp. 19–23.

treatment is needed to achieve an adequate dose. Second, it is narrower on the y-axis than a robust patient's zone. This means that, just like the elderly patient in the powerful car, it is now even easier to give too much stimulation and to overshoot in a shorter time (T1).

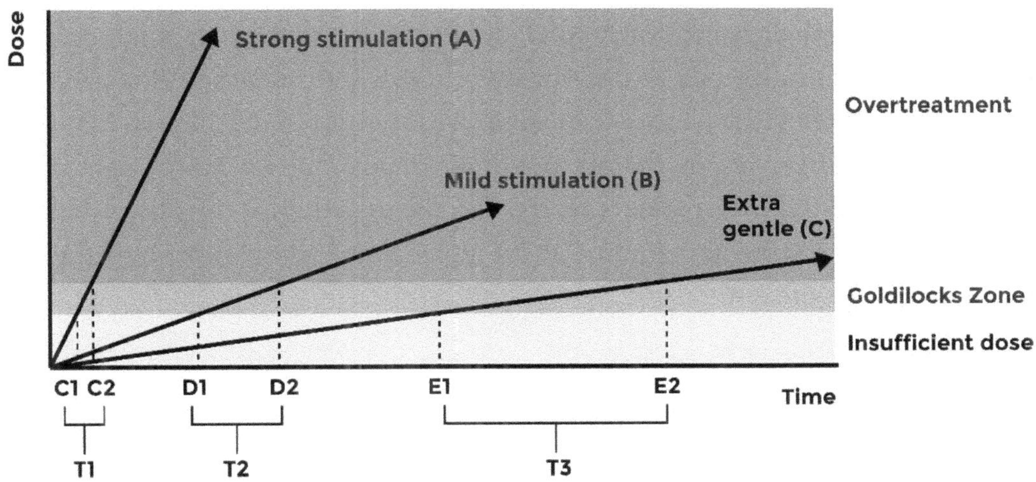

Figure 15-4: The Goldilocks Zone for a sensitive patient.

Even with normal, mild stimulation (B), T2 is shorter. Thus, with this kind of sensitive or hyper-sensitive patient, it makes sense to use an even gentler gradient of treatment, meaning that you should apply extra gentle methods of stimulation (C).

THE JITSOMETER THOUGHT EXPERIMENT

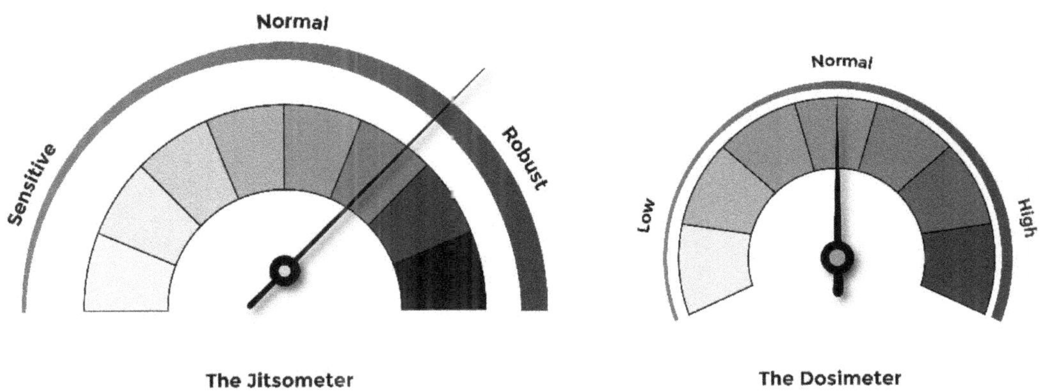

Figure 15-5: The jitsometer and dosimeter are mental constructs to estimate strength and dosage.

As we have seen, while *jitsu* primarily signifies 'excess' in the context of imbalance (pathology), contrasting with the fragility or weakness implied by *kyo*, its broader meaning of 'substance', 'strength,' or 'solidity' means it can also be thought of as a term for robustness or vitality. A *jitsu* individual, therefore, could be seen as strong, full of life, and able to tolerate treatments like acupuncture more robustly than one who is *kyo*.

The *jitsometer* is a thought experiment that you can perform before you start treatment. If the word *jitsu* can be used to describe the strength and robustness of a patient's energy system, then the jitsometer is a mental construct, a dial that can estimate that strength. If the dial is zero on the left, five in the middle, and ten on the right, then the farther to the right the needle is on the dial, the more robust the patient is. The farther to the left the needle is on the dial, the more sensitive the patient is and the less treatment you should give.

Practising the Manaka system in class often involves students working together in small groups of 3–5 around a practice table. One student lies on the table, serving as the model for examination and practice. This collaborative setup enables the group to collectively assess the model's condition, often reaching a consensus on the approximate jitsometer level. Oran Kivity remarks that in group practice, there is usually widespread agreement by the treating group about the model patient's jitsometer score. This suggests that this is an intuitive, common-sense process. Once you have grasped the concept of dosage and the Goldilocks Zone, it becomes relatively easy to place people on a continuum.

GRADUALISM: START LOW AND BUILD UP SLOWLY

Despite our best efforts and accumulated experience, there will inevitably be cases where the initial evaluation is incorrect, as in Kivity's case below. For most patients, however, determining the appropriate dose is relatively straightforward, especially when following Manaka's model.

A critical part of this model is *gradualism*, which involves starting with a conservative dose and increasing it only as needed. This approach enables practitioners to fine-tune dosage, avoid overtreatment, and tailor treatment to each individual. In practice, this means:

- Lower initial dose: Always begin with a reduced dose at the first visit, regardless of the patient's perceived sensitivity.
- Response monitoring: If the patient shows improvement, maintain the same dose at the next visit, rather than increasing it.
- Plateau management: If progress stalls in later sessions, consider carefully increasing the dose to stimulate further change.

Gradualism prioritises starting conservatively. Start low and build up slowly: by addressing the complexity of dose judgment in this way, you will be able to develop and maintain accurate and individualised treatment plans.

THE DOSIMETER THOUGHT EXPERIMENT

The next thought experiment tool is the *dosimeter*, another mental needle gauge in a direct relationship to the jitsometer. In science, a dosimeter is a device used to measure exposure to radiation. In this context, we will use it to refer to an internalised intuitive dial that indicates the amount of stimulation with acupuncture and moxibustion you should provide to your patient. If someone scores high on the jitsometer, you can set your dosimeter to one point below that and feel free to treat root and branch with any method within the Four Steps. If someone scores low on the jitsometer, you must adjust the dosimeter downwards by one point, reducing treatment time, focusing more on the root, and using less stimulation. For example, a score of 5 on the jitsometer will enable a treatment strength of 4 on the dosimeter. We will revisit all the techniques used in the Four Steps shortly and see how we can moderate their dosage.

As a rule of thumb, most patients will fall somewhere around 4–6 on your dial and can be treated with a dosage of 3–5. Those who score below two on the jitsometer, however, can be considered hypersensitive and should be treated with great care.

These two thought experiments offer simple ways to picture sensitivity and guide dosage in learning, practice, and teaching.

TODAY I'M FRAGILE: UNUSUAL SENSITIVITY

The jitsometer lets us classify most patients, in our mind's eye, into three groups:

1. Robust (7–10)
2. Normal (4–6)
3. Sensitive (1–3)

- If you judge someone to be 7–10, start with a dose of 5–6 and gradually increase until you reach the level that gives the best effect.
- If you judge the patient to be in the 4–6 range (normal), start with a dose of 3 at the first treatment, then build up as needed.
- If you judge the person to be a 1–3, start with a dose of 1 during the first treatment, then carefully and slowly increase the dose as needed to the required level. This may mean that your Step 1 is completed in seconds and Step 2 in just a few short minutes.

It is important to remember that these energy states are constantly in flux. If a patient comes to see you who is usually a robust 7 on the jitsometer, but tells you tearfully that his wife just left him, it absolutely makes sense to downgrade his rating immediately.

The same thinking applies to a normal patient who is jetlagged—your mental jitsometer and dosimeter should dial down. This gives us a new category: *unusually sensitive patients*, individuals who are usually robust or normal but now present as sensitive. We now have four categories of patients:

1. Usually robust
2. Usually normal
3. Usually sensitive
4. Unusually sensitive

This fourth category means that patients who are usually at one point on the sensitivity spectrum may, on a given day, be less robust and more sensitive than usual. A patient's sensitivity can increase for many reasons, including:

- Recovery from illness (cold, flu, etc.)
- Conflict at work or home
- Poor sleep
- Jet lag
- Stress, overwork, bereavement, or other emotional trauma
- Accident

This principle also applies to sensitive patients. On some days, they may become even more sensitive, and this unusual situation will test your skill to the utmost to find a meaningful dose of treatment without overtreating.

Thus, you should never take your patients' sensitivity for granted. Always consult your jitsometer before treatment and adjust your dosimeter accordingly.

FEEDBACK MECHANISMS AND WARNING SIGNS

There are several feedback mechanisms to assess the effectiveness of treatment:

- Relief of pressure pain on treatment points and the hara
- Improved mobility of affected joints
- Relief of symptoms
- Patient feedback
- Pulse changes (improvements in quality when monitored regularly)
- Improved skin lustre (skin feels smoother)

These same feedback mechanisms can also indicate when a treatment shifts from the Goldilocks Zone into overtreatment.

Additional warning signs include:

- Restlessness (patient changes from relaxed to unsettled, e.g. turning the head from side to side after lying still)
- Coolness or moistness of the skin (a change noticed during or after treatment)
- Faintness, weakness, or dizziness (often noticed when changing position)

DEALING WITH OVERTREATMENT IN THE CLINIC

If you notice any of the signs above and suspect overtreatment:

1. Remove the needles as you would for needle shock.
2. If the patient can sit upright, treat DU 14 with a moxa stick, Ontake, or cone moxa.

[Note: In the Toyohari Association, DU 14 is the primary point for recovery from wrong treatment or overtreatment.]

3. If the patient feels faint:
   a. Have them lie with knees bent to bring blood to the head.
   b. In the supine position, use REN 4.
   c. If the knees are bent and REN 4 is difficult to access, use ST 36 as a practical alternative.

OVERTREATMENT AND MENGEN

Sometimes, overtreatment can wrongly be interpreted by practitioners and patients as a favourable healing crisis, often described by forgiving patients with phrases such as: "I must be getting rid of toxins," "No pain, no gain," and "Things have to get worse before they get better."

Sometimes patients have a genuine healing crisis following treatment—a temporary worsening of symptoms that precedes recovery. This is called *mengen* (瞑眩) in Japanese herbal medicine traditions. While *mengen* can occur, it is uncommon and tends to follow a fixed pattern:

- A temporary reaction or symptom appears.
- The reaction lasts less than twenty-four hours.
- It is followed by sustained improvement in the main complaints.

By contrast, overtreatment reactions can include:

- Fatigue that lasts more than twenty-four hours.
- Worsening of current symptoms beyond twenty-four hours or the temporary appearance of other symptoms.
- Poor sleep.

Fatigue may occur as a temporary post-treatment response—it sometimes takes extra energy for the body to integrate changes—but it can also result from overtreatment. If the fatigue lasts more than twenty-four hours, it should be considered overtreatment.

Another common sign is poor sleep on the same day. If your patient reports this at the next session, take it as a clear cue to reduce the dosage.

If the patient experiences these kinds of reactions, you can assume your treatment exceeded "the individual's limit beyond which unnecessary side effects arise".[200]

[200] Manaka, Y., Itaya, K., & Birch, S. (1995). *Chasing the Dragon's Tail: The Theory and Practice of Acupuncture in the Work of Yoshio Manaka*. Brookline: Paradigm Publications. p. 116.

CASE STUDY 9: EXHAUSTION AND HOT FLUSHES

[Note: This case is presented in a more anecdotal style than our formal case studies. Adapted from *Moxa in Motion*, it is included here to illustrate overtreatment and how to respond to it.]

Lizzie, Female, 65

Occupation: *Retired*

This sixty-five-year-old grandmother was visiting Malaysia to see her new grandson. She had been feeling exhausted for several years. She also had many hot flushes, especially at night. Her first treatment was with a Manaka pattern called NIP 1, which used eight needles and four cords at Step 1.[201] *It's a treatment sometimes given for fatigue resulting from kidney weakness. Additionally, for symptom relief at Step 4, I used okyu (small-cone moxibustion) at LI 10, REN 12, and ST 36 (three cones). Ontake was given on the back for Step 2 (rolling on the back with a heated piece of bamboo) instead of kyutoshin.*

She returned the following week, saying she had felt completely wiped out for two days and had been sleeping very long hours. The first night, her hot flushes were worse than ever. Following these two lousy nights, her energy picked up, and her flushes were much reduced.

Clearly, this was overtreatment. I had overestimated how much treatment she could take. Nevertheless, the treatment was on the right track, as she was feeling better. For the next treatment, the dosage was much reduced. The ion-pumping time was halved, and okyu was repeated with one cone on each point. The Ontake time was reduced by 75%. She had a much better week following this, feeling invigorated and energetic.

—Oran Kivity

---

201 NIP stands for normal ion pumping and uses eight points connected by four ion-pumping cords. NIP 1 and NIP 2 will be covered in Vol. 3.

REFLECTIONS

If a master practitioner such as Akihiro Takai can admit that most adverse reactions in his practice were due to overtreatment, we can forgive ourselves for getting it wrong in a first session. By the second, however, we should aim to get it right. Even if we fail, the reactions to early sessions must serve to calibrate future treatments. Getting it wrong routinely is less forgivable.

> *I always mark a big red 'S' on the notes of sensitive patients, so that even if I don't see them for years, when they do come, I'm reminded to treat them with special care.*
>
> —Oran Kivity

Keeping good case notes is crucial for safe and effective practice. Case notes help us track how patients respond over time, spot patterns we might otherwise miss, and adjust our treatments with greater precision. They also protect us from repeating past mistakes—in dosage, technique, or point selection—and allow us to resume treatment seamlessly even after long gaps between sessions. In short, good notes make us better practitioners and augment our ongoing judgment of dosage.

INSENSITIVITY, BLOOD STASIS, AND PROGNOSIS

There is one additional type of patient to consider when determining dosage: those with blood stasis. In the context of Manaka's stimulus-reaction graph, they can sometimes appear as the opposite of a sensitive patient in that they may require stronger stimulation. But this is not because they are less sensitive in the way we've been using the term. In fact, they often respond quickly during treatment, with marked hara changes or strong bodily reactions. The difficulty lies elsewhere: because of the underlying blood stasis, these changes don't hold. Physiological shifts may fade quickly, and the same imbalances are liable to return by the next session.

Manaka wrote extensively about blood stasis and treated it as a prognostic indicator rather than a measure of sensitivity. It frequently makes conditions more stubborn and slower to resolve, despite good immediate reactions. Indicators of blood stasis include a history of multiple surgeries, advanced age with liver meridian pathologies or high blood pressure, and intractable conditions such as psoriasis. Dermatological signs of blood stasis include purple complexion, brown or dark patches on the skin, moles, petechiae and vascular spiders. Patients with extensive sun exposure—such as farmers, fishermen, outdoor labourers, or extreme athletes—may also present in this way.

For these patients, the Goldilocks Zone may require a different strategy. You might consider longer needle retention, more points, or stronger applications such as 100% style *tonnetsukyu* (burning the moxa all the way down), higher numbers of moxa points, or methods that address the blood directly, such as *kyukaku* (cupping) and *shiraku* (bloodletting).

At the same time, it's important to recognise that sensitivity and prognosis can overlap. A highly sensitive patient with a poor prognosis—for example, due to advanced blood stasis—can be one of the most challenging clinical situations you will face.[202]

MODERATING DOSAGE IN STEPS 1–4

As practitioners of acupuncture, moxibustion, and other meridian therapies, we have an extensive repertoire of techniques and methods for treating both the root and the branch. If root and branch treatments are like the two wheels on the front axle of a car, as discussed in Chapter 2, they are in a direct relationship with one another, and each is important.

In the case of elderly or sensitive patients, it makes sense to plan treatments with particular care. A strong root treatment should be balanced with lighter work on the branch. Likewise, a major branch treatment must be adjusted to the patient's level of sensitivity. For example, *shiraku* (bloodletting) should be used with great caution in sensitive patients.

---

202 All these important topics—blood stasis and prognostication, cupping and bloodletting—will be covered in Vol. 3.

STRATEGIES FOR REDUCING DOSAGE

As Manaka's model of treatment shows, the simplest way to reduce dosage is to shorten the duration of treatment. This might mean reducing Step 1—retaining the IPC for 2–5 minutes instead of the usual 10, or shortening the whole session so that the patient is off the table in 20 minutes instead of 45.

Another option is to select lighter techniques. We can use non-insertive ion-pumping methods instead of needling at Step 1. These include silver spike points (SSP) and electrostatic adsorbers (see Chapter 17). We can also use shallow needling at Steps 2 and 4, using finer needles and fewer points.

These practical adjustments should always be framed within the gradualist principle outlined earlier: start low and build up slowly. Table 15.1 summarises ways to reduce dosage within each of the Four Steps.

Table 15.1: Strategies for reducing dosage at each step.

STEP	OPTIONS
1	**Reduce duration of IPC:** • If you normally retain the cords for 10 minutes, shorten the retention time to 5 minutes on the first visit. • If you normally retain for 5 minutes, shorten to 2–3 minutes. • If signs of overtreatment appear in subsequent visits, reduce the duration further.
2	• Shorten treatment duration. • Choose 1 pair of back-*shu* points instead of 2. • Burn 1 moxa ball on each needle instead of 2. • Keep moxa balls at the smaller end of the 1–2 cm range. • Use longer needles or insert less deeply so the moxa sits farther from the skin, producing less heat. • Use shallow needling with a heat lamp instead of *kyutoshin*. • Use shallow needling without heat. • Use non-insertive methods to achieve the aims of Step 2, such as Ontake or moxa cones.
3	• Apply Sotai without moxa. • Omit Step 3 entirely.
4	• Use non-insertive methods such as *ryu* (provided the patient has no allergic reaction to the ball or tape). • Reduce the number of isophasal points from 3 to 2 or just 1. • Instruct the patient to remove takeaways earlier. • Omit Step 4 entirely.
Direct moxibustion	• Select fewer points. • Burn fewer cones on each point. • Remove cones when 50% burnt instead of 80%. • Prevent the patient from feeling heat.

CASE STUDY 10: HOT FLUSHES AND INSOMNIA

Sarah, Female, 43

Occupation: English teacher

PRESENTING CONDITION

Sarah had reached menopause about a year earlier, somewhat earlier than average. She reported troublesome hot flushes and ongoing insomnia.

RELEVANT HISTORY

- Fatigue
- Pain in the coccyx
- Some elbow stiffness
- Left shoulder pain
- Light sleeper, easily woken
- Appears frail and sensitive; describes strong reactivity to external energies

PALPATION

- Upper right quadrant and lower left quadrant

TREATMENT 1

Diagnosis: CS

Step 1: CS with IPC and SSP (1 minute)
Step 2: Ontake on bladder line, focused on BL 18 and BL 27
Step 3: N/A
Step 4: *Okyu*—1 cone per point on ST 36, SP 6, and *Shitsumin* bilaterally

TREATMENT 2 (3 WEEKS LATER)

Patient Response
Sleep improved for 10 days. Tailbone pain reduced. Energy and joint pain improved.

PALPATION

Midline tenderness, subcostal tightness, jump reaction on right ASIS

[Note: Reactions at right ASIS instead of right ST 25–ST 27 can also relate to Mixed Yin.]

Diagnosis: Mixed Yin

Step 1: Mixed Yin with IPC + SSP (3 minutes)
Step 2: Ontake—bladder line and puffy sacrum
Step 3: N/A
Step 4: *Okyu*—1 cone each on REN 4, ST 36, SP 6, and *Shitsumin* (7 cones on the less sensitive side)

TREATMENT 3 (4 WEEKS LATER)

Patient Response
Sleeping much better. Feels stronger. Hot flushes have reduced but are starting to return. Tailbone pain much improved. Energy strong. Some anxiety and rash appeared.

Diagnosis: Ren Dai (left-belt)

Step 1: Ren Dai with IPC + SSP (TB 5 on left)
Step 2: Ontake—repeat
Step 3: N/A
Step 4: *Okyu*—repeat

TREATMENT 4 (2 WEEKS LATER)

Patient Response
Tired from teaching. Feels trapped at work. Hot flushes increased this week. Energy still good.

Diagnosis: Ren Dai (left-belt)

Step 1: Ren Dai with IPC and SSP (TB 5 on left)
Step 2: Ontake—repeat
Step 3: N/A
Step 4: *Okyu*—3 cones per point: HT 6, KID 7, ST 36, SP 6

TREATMENT 5 (4 WEEKS LATER)

Patient Response
Feels like she is ovulating. Wakes 3x/night to urinate. Slightly blurry vision. Sleep is light.

PALPATION

Upper right quadrant, lower left quadrant, midline tenderness

Diagnosis: K3L

Step 1: K3L with IPC + SSP
Step 2: Ontake on either side of spine and sacrum
Step 3: N/A
Step 4: *Okyu*—3 cones per point on ST 36 and SP 6

CONCLUSIONS AND REFLECTIONS

Sarah was a post-menopausal woman presenting with fatigue, insomnia, and textbook signs of counterflow qi (red face and cold feet). Her treatment began with CS and evolved through Mixed Yin to Ren Dai and eventually K3L.

She was clearly a sensitive type: treatments began with one-minute IPC and one cone of *okyu* per point. These were gradually increased to three-minute IPC and three cones. She responded well to Ontake as a rhythmic, non-invasive form of heat therapy—whereas *kyutoshin* may have been too strong.

Shitsumin is traditionally treated on the less sensitive side. Burn one cone on each side and ask the patient which felt warmer. Treat the side where the patient feels less warmth.

PLANNING A TREATMENT AND TASTING SOUP

Stephen Birch teaches that treatment should be planned and mapped out in your mind before inserting the first needle. It is easy to make mistakes if you simply try one technique after another as they occur to you. Successful treatment requires the harmonious planning and combination of different elements and methods.

One of Oran Kivity's early teachers, German trainer Barbara Kirschbaum, used a delightful analogy: treatment is like making soup. You begin with a basic recipe, but keep tasting, adjusting with a little salt here or a bit of spice there. Treatment is a combination of similar flavours, but you need to be aware of the dosimeter and how the patient reacts to each new taste. In practical terms, this means taking the pulse and palpating the skin. If the pulse deteriorates or the skin becomes moist, add moxa at DU 14 or stop treatment altogether. In addition, palpation, pressure pain, symptoms, and patient response can indicate whether the treatment is on track or veering off course.

Manaka, as well as other masters such as Takai, also stressed that when patients present with many diverse symptoms, we should focus only on root treatment. This is a critical point. Some patients arrive with a long shopping list of symptoms, expecting an acupuncture point for each one. This is Western thinking: one drug for the first symptom, another drug for the next, and a third drug for the side effects of the first two.

In TEAM thinking, when a patient presents with multiple symptoms, it is generally better to prioritise root treatment, especially if the patient's overall condition is poor. Without addressing the root cause and improving their general health, any symptomatic changes are likely to be limited or short-lived. Strengthening the patient's overall condition first encourages the body to resolve many symptoms naturally, often with little additional intervention. Once the patient's general health improves, symptomatic treatments can then be added as needed to address any remaining issues.[203]

As patients get stronger, you can change the emphasis of treatment. Start with root treatment and gradually introduce branch treatment for one particular symptom.

Another important consideration is patient expectation. Some patients become more demanding at the end of a session and request that you treat their remaining symptoms.

"Can you do anything for my shoulder?"
"Did you do anything for my knee today?"

All the authors have experience of this situation, which always seems to happen at the end of a session.

> *Many years ago, before I began studying JAAM, with its emphasis on dosage, I was treating a gentleman who, at the very end of the session, said, "Oh, by the way, is there anything you can do for my tight shoulders?"*
>
> *These days, palpating the neck and shoulders is an integral part of my diagnostics. I would already have noticed this tension and gauged whether treatment had released it. But as a younger and less experienced practitioner, I had him sit up and placed some cups on his shoulders. He instantly fainted—not a pleasant experience for him or for me. Fortunately, after removing the cups and putting him in the recovery position, he came round immediately.*

---

203 Birch, S. (2019). 'Treating the Patient, Not the Symptoms: Acupuncture to Improve Overall Health—Evidence, Acceptance and Strategies', *Integrative Medicine Research*, 8(1). pp. 33–41. https://doi.org/10.1016/j.imr.2018.07.005

> *In thirty-four years of practice, that is the only time a patient has fainted on me, and it was a salutary lesson: do not be led by the patient, and always explain that symptoms mentioned at the end of a session will be evaluated and, if still necessary, addressed at the next visit. This was a perfect example of overtreatment.*
>
> —Marian Fixler

To stay in the Goldilocks Zone, it is essential to maintain firm boundaries with demanding patients. Many arrive expecting that, despite years of other therapies failing, acupuncture should deliver results in forty-five minutes. It helps to explain that treatment often reaches its peak effect after two or three days and that they need to wait and see. Most patients can accept this, especially if you explain the concepts of dosage and overtreatment.

CONCLUSION

It is the natural urge of every healer to want to help as much as possible. It is also the natural urge of most patients to try to get the most they can out of a session. These two drives can conspire against successful treatment, especially in the closing minutes of the session. Enough is better than too much.

Recalling that 90% of adverse reactions in Takai's practice were due to overtreatment, it seems clear that incorporating the Goldilocks Zone is the single most important step you can take to reduce the risk of things going wrong in your own practice. Even so, once the concept is understood, it takes time to be fully integrated into practice. As Table 15.1 shows, adjusting the dosage is a delicate, multifaceted task, requiring constant engagement throughout the session—much like a master chef tasting the soup at every stage of preparation.

Michio Murakami, a senior instructor in the Toyohari Association, explained that a course of treatment is like a journey: we want to bring our patients from Point A, the starting point, to Point Z, the finish line.[204] It is human nature to want to get them there as quickly as possible. Yet we should be content if, in one session, we move only from A to F. The journey can always continue from F in the next session.

In addition to twenty-first-century cultural expectations of instant results, there is a constant tension between our temptation to give more and our duty to give less. When we feel the urge to do too much, we can steady ourselves with Murakami's simple wisdom and strengthen our resolve to limit our treatments.

SUMMARY

This chapter introduced several key concepts around dosage:

- **Goldilocks Zone:** Every patient has a zone of treatment that is neither too much nor too little, but just right.
- **Overtreatment:** Most adverse reactions arise from giving too much; a gradualist approach reduces the risk of overtreatment.
- **Sensitive patients:** The very young, elderly, chronically ill, or emotionally vulnerable need special care and reduced dosage.
- **Judging strength:** The jitsometer and dosimeter are mental tools to estimate robustness and set dosage.
- **Feedback:** The pulse, palpation, pressure pain, symptoms, and patient response can indicate whether the treatment is on track or veering off course.
- **Changing states:** Even robust patients may present as unusually sensitive due to stress, illness, or fatigue.
- **Root and branch:** Both are essential components of treatment, but they must be balanced carefully according to the patient's sensitivity. When patients are highly sensitive or present with multiple symptoms, it is better to focus on the root alone.

---

204 Kivity, O. (2009). *Lecture on Dosage* by Michio Murakami. Toyohari Summer School, Tokyo. Personal notes.

WHAT'S NEXT

Our second and final chapter of cases focuses on moxibustion in Step 4 to show how the authors wove dosage into their treatments.

CHAPTER 16

CASE STUDIES PART 2: INTEGRATING MOXIBUSTION AND DOSAGE

In the previous chapter, we explored how treatment dosage must be tailored to each patient, balancing sensitivity and robustness, and taking into account the type of stimulation applied. We also studied the principles and methods of moxibustion, and how these techniques can fulfil different roles within the Four Steps.

This chapter brings those threads together in clinical practice. Here are seven cases, each offering a distinct clinical picture. Pay particular attention to how the treatments were shaped by both the moxa strategies introduced earlier and a careful consideration of dosage.

As with the previous case studies, you may wish to pause with pen and paper as you read and reflect on questions such as:

- How would you connect the cords, based on the diagnosis?
- How did the Step 2 treatment complement Step 1? How would you approach Step 2 yourself?
- How was Step 4 constructed? Which moxa techniques were chosen, and how was the dosage adjusted to match the patient's sensitivity or robustness?

These cases are designed to help you integrate the concepts from the dosage and moxa chapters into real-world practice. As you revisit them over time, you will notice subtleties and connections that may escape a first reading. We encourage you to return to them slowly, reflectively, and more than once.

CASE STUDY 11. CHRONIC KNEE PAIN AND FATIGUE

Hannah, Female, 38

Occupation: Massage therapist; runs a clinic

PRESENTING CONDITION

Hannah presented as stressed and irritable, having spent the last 3 to 4 years building a business under a heavy workload. She reported chronic right knee pain that had persisted on and off since the age of 17, following a fall from a heavy horse onto tarmac. The pain mostly followed the gall bladder meridian and was sometimes accompanied by swelling. Stretching provided some relief. She also reported extreme fatigue.

RELEVANT HISTORY

- Ovarian cancer in early 20s; major surgery and strong chemotherapy. Large vertical scar below the navel to the pubic bone
- Mother passed away 2 years prior to her cancer diagnosis
- Experienced chronic fatigue for approximately 10 years following cancer treatment

PALPATION

- Midline tightness above the navel
- Tightness to the left of the navel, across the waistline, and down the rectus abdominis
- LU 1 and LU 2 areas are tight.

TREATMENT 1

Diagnosis: Ren Dai (left-belt)

Step 1: Ren Dai (left-belt) with IPC (5 minutes)
Step 2: BL 23 (more reactive than BL 22), BL 27, and GB 30 on right with *kyutoshin* on the needles
Step 3: N/A
Step 4: *Okyu* on GB 33 and eyes of the knee points on the right knee

TREATMENT 2 (FOLLOWING WEEK)

Patient Response
Knee much improved (less aching, though still tight). Very relaxed after treatment. Had not drunk coffee all week. Sleep improved, waking more refreshed.

Step 1: Ren Dai (left-belt) with IPC (5 minutes)
Step 2: BL 23, BL 27, GB 30 right with *kyutoshin*
Step 3: N/A
Step 4: *Okyu* on ST 35 (only tender point around knee); light needling around GB 21 for neck/shoulder tightness; *okyu* on BL 14, BL 15, BL 17–3 cones per point

TREATMENT 3 (FOLLOWING WEEK)

Patient Response
Knee greatly improved (even after gardening/carrying heavy planters). Better energy levels. Much calmer overall (moxa on the back particularly helpful). Arrived late, limited treatment time.

Step 1: Ren Dai (left-belt) with EA (electrostatic adsorbers) (1 minute)
Step 2: No time for back treatment
Step 3: N/A
Step 4: *Okyu* on GB 33/GB 34 right until pressure pain cleared; scar treatment using *teishin* on vertical abdominal scar; empishin on SP 6 (Day 27 of cycle) for dysmenorrhoea support

TREATMENT 4 (FOLLOWING WEEK)

Patient Response
28-day menstrual cycle (usual 31–32 days) with less pain/bleeding. Felt slightly tired during period. Knees remained entirely pain-free.

Step 1: Ren Dai (left-belt) with IPC (5 minutes)
Step 2: BL 23 with *kyutoshin*
Step 3: N/A
Step 4: *Okyu* on BL 14, BL 15, BL17 (5 cones each); *teishin* treatment around occiput

CONCLUSIONS AND REFLECTIONS

Hannah's pattern remained stable throughout the course of treatment. This was a Ren Dai (left-belt) pattern, as the Dai Mai reactions presented on the left rather than the right. This presentation is the exception to the REDLLL rule. TB 5 is needled on the left to release reactions around the left ST 25, so LU 7 is needled on the right.

Step 4 branch treatments were applied simultaneously with Steps 1 and 2 on the front and back, showing once again that the Four Step protocol is more pragmatic than linear. As a safety measure, *okyu* was applied to the back only after the *kyutoshin* had burned down. The number of direct moxa points was adjusted based on the degree of pressure pain.

Okyu was applied to upper thoracic points (e.g. BL 14, BL 15, BL 17) for their calming effect.

GB 30 was needled with *kyutoshin* on the affected side due to reactivity and its empirical link to knee pain.

A *teishin* (non-inserted, blunt-tipped needle) was used to treat tension at the occiput and soften the long abdominal scar. This treatment is not part of the MSA canon. However, it was included to support qi and blood circulation in the lower abdomen.

For more discussion of electrostatic adsorbers and their role in Step 1, see Chapter 17.

CASE STUDY 12. CHRONIC INFLAMMATION AND FATIGUE

Jennifer, Female, 41

Occupation: Teacher

PRESENTING CONDITION

Jennifer presented with a long-standing tendency towards fatigue, was prone to viral infections, and had chronic inflammation. She reported ongoing muscle and nerve pain, poor appetite, and persistent insomnia.

RELEVANT HISTORY

- Headaches
- Swollen glands and sore throat
- Dizziness
- Mouth ulcers
- Cold hands and feet
- Irregular bowel movements

PALPATION

- Tightness above the navel
- Very flaccid and cool below the navel
- Right LU 1 and ST 12 very reactive
- Bilateral ASIS tenderness

TREATMENT 1

Diagnosis: YQR

Step 1: YQR with IPC and SSP (15 minutes)
Step 2: *Okyu*—3 cones on BL 17, BL 18, and BL 20, bilateral
Step 3: N/A
Step 4: *Okyu*—3 cones on REN 12, LI 11, and ST 36, bilateral

TREATMENT 2 (FOLLOWING WEEK)

Patient Response
Reported increased abdominal movement and bowel activity. Energy levels improved. Better resilience under stress.

Diagnosis: YQR

Step 1: YQR with IPC and SSP (15 minutes)
Step 2: *Okyu*—3 cones on BL 17, BL 18, BL 20, and BL 23, bilateral
Step 3: N/A
Step 4: *Okyu*—3 cones on REN 12, REN 6, LI 11, and ST 36, bilateral

TREATMENT 3 (FOLLOWING WEEK)

Patient Response
She felt significantly energised for about 36 hours, describing the effect as "like a tonic", with a noticeable improvement in her overall sense of well-being. However, she overexerted herself afterwards and experienced a partial relapse, though not to her original baseline.

Diagnosis: YQR

Step 1: YQR with IPC and SSP (15 minutes)
Step 2: *Okyu*—3 cones on BL 17, BL 18, BL 20, and BL 23, bilateral
Step 3: N/A
Step 4: *Okyu*—3 cones on REN 12, REN 6, LI 11, and ST 36, bilateral

TREATMENT 4 (FOLLOWING WEEK)

Patient Response
Took longer to feel better post-treatment, but energy was good on treatment day. Brief recurrence of mouth ulcers resolved quickly. Described a 'toxic release' sensation following treatment that subsided.

Diagnosis: YQR

Step 1: YQR with IPC and SSP (15 minutes)
Step 2: *Okyu*—3 cones on REN 12, REN 6, KID 3, LI 11, and ST 36, bilateral
Step 3: N/A
Step 4: *Okyu*—7 cones on DU 14

TREATMENT 5 (FOLLOWING WEEK)

Patient Response
No toxic sensations. Energy remained strong throughout the week. Mouth ulcers did not recur. Digestion improved. Hands warmer, feet still cold.

Diagnosis: YQR

Step 1: YQR with IPC and SSP (15 minutes)
Step 2: *Chishin* at BL 23 and BL 25, bilateral with infrared (FIR) lamp on back; additional retained needles at KID 3 and SP 6, bilateral
Step 3: N/A
Step 4: *Okyu*—7 cones on DU 14; home therapy: nightly hot foot soaks

CONCLUSIONS AND REFLECTIONS

Jennifer presented with a consistent YQR pattern. Direct moxa was selected over needle moxa due to her slender build. Her viral load and immune sensitivity led to noticeable but manageable treatment reactions. She experienced reliable energy gains and quick symptom reduction in most areas—especially digestion, energy, and stress resilience. Sleep remained unaffected throughout treatment.

She also learned to pace herself better, avoiding overexertion during high-energy periods. Her cold extremities were addressed by *chishin* at KID 3 and SP 6, along with home-based warm foot soaks.

She completed the series feeling stronger and arranged to return for follow-up in four to six weeks.

CASE STUDY 13. STROKE RECOVERY AND MOBILITY ISSUES

Nissim, Male, 43

Occupation: Salesman

PRESENTING CONDITION

Nissim presented with an unsteady gait and weakness in his left leg, the result of a stroke he had suffered 4 years earlier. He had been hospitalised for 2 months following the stroke, which involved cerebral bleeding. The clot was not surgically removed but was gradually absorbed by the surrounding tissue.

RELEVANT HISTORY

- Grogginess, leg numbness, weakness, and limping when fatigued
- Frequent dizziness, but no headaches
- Shoulder stiffness and tightness
- Severe fungal infection on the big toenail of the unaffected (right) leg: nail is black and thick

PALPATION

- Upper right quadrant
- Left lower quadrant

TREATMENT 1

Diagnosis: CS

Step 1: CS with IPC and SSP (5 minutes)
Step 2: Ontake on bladder line, focusing on BL 18 and BL 27
Step 3: N/A
Step 4: *Okyu*—ST 36 bilaterally and 7 long cones on the affected toenail

SUBSEQUENT TREATMENTS (TREATMENTS 2–7, WEEKLY)

Patient Response
Patient began showing immediate improvements: stronger gait, improved energy, and reduced dizziness. Weekly treatments followed a similar protocol:

Step 1: CS with IPC and SSP (10 minutes)
Step 2: Ontake or occasionally *kyutoshin*
Step 3: N/A
Step 4: *Okyu* on ST 36 and the toenail

TREATMENT 8 (4 WEEKS LATER)

Patient Response
Left calf and ankle tight/stiff. Fatigued from late nights over holiday season. Healthy pink nail visible at cuticle, fungal nail growing out.

PALPATION

- Belly cold below navel
- Midline tight
- Upper right quadrant
- Lower left quadrant

Diagnosis: K3L

Step 1: K3L with IPC and SSP (10 minutes)
Step 2: *Kyutoshin* on BL 18 and BL 23
Step 3: N/A
Step 4: *Kyutoshin* on tightest point of left calf

TREATMENT 9 (1 WEEK LATER)

Patient Response
Left leg significantly stronger; Nissim is planning to go jogging. Dizziness has not returned since first treatment. No visible nail changes yet, but surrounding skin on the toes and medial aspect of the foot has improved. Upper back still tight.

PALPATION

- Upper right quadrant tight
- Left ASIS elicits jump reaction

Diagnosis: CS

Step 1: CS with IPC and SSP (10 minutes)
Step 2: Ontake—repeat
Step 3: N/A
Step 4: *Okyu*—repeated as before, plus several tight/tender upper back points

CONCLUSIONS AND REFLECTIONS

Nissim had experienced a severe stroke, and four years later, his recovery had plateaued. Initial abdominal findings showed a CS pattern, commonly linked to liver disharmony and qi/blood stagnation. The IPC treatment addressing structural imbalances in the octahedron, the gentle blood-moving effects of the Ontake moxibustion, and *okyu* at ST 36 were central to restoring movement and energy.

The fungal toenail—indicative of poor circulation—was addressed using *okyu* while the IPC were in place. Seven cones were applied per session. He never felt any heat, as the fungal layer was so thick, but clear signs of recovery were visible after three months.

It's a little surprising that the upper right quadrant symptoms remained obvious each week. Often, these improve permanently with regular treatment. In this case, we suspect that the patient, while vegetarian and quite engaged with spiritual practice and meditation, may also have been drinking more than he admitted, which may have been affecting the liver and subcostal reactions.

CASE STUDY 14. INFERTILITY

Amina, Female, 34

Occupation: Urban planner

PRESENTING CONDITION

Amina had been trying to conceive for 2.5 years. She had undergone 5 cycles of Clomid and 3 rounds of intrauterine insemination (IUI) with hormone injections. At the time of treatment, she was about to begin in vitro fertilisation (IVF). An ovarian cyst had been identified on her right ovary but had since resolved, and she had been cleared for treatment.

RELEVANT HISTORY

- Polycystic ovaries
- No previous pregnancies
- Irregular periods and acne
- On the contraceptive pill for over 10 years

PALPATION

- Midline tightness above the navel
- Tightness across the left waist and around the left ASIS

TREATMENT 1

Diagnosis: Ren Dai (left-belt)

Step 1: Ren Dai (left-belt) with IPC (5 minutes)
Step 2: Direct moxa on BL 19 + BL 23
Step 3: N/A
Step 4: Direct moxa on SP 6

TREATMENT 2 (FOLLOWING WEEK)

Patient Response
Follicles growing on both sides. Slight bloating and mild headache. Embryo transfer postponed due to PCO.

Diagnosis: Ren Dai (left-belt)

Step 1: Ren Dai (left-belt) with IPC (10 minutes)
Step 2: *Kyutoshin* on BL 18 + BL 23
Step 3: N/A
Step 4: Light *chishin* needling on BL 17 + direct *okyu* on REN 4 and SP 6

Follow-up: No cyst. Embryo transfer imminent.

TREATMENT 3 (12 WEEKS LATER)

Patient Response
14 follicles collected; 11 fertilised; 4 top-quality blastocysts frozen. Period day one.

PALPATION

- Midline tightness above the navel
- Tightness across the left waist and right belt, equal both sides.
- LU 1–LU 2 tighter on the left

Diagnosis: Ren Dai (right-belt)

Step 1: Ren Dai (right-belt) with IPC (10 minutes)
Step 2: *Kyutoshin* on BL 23 + BL 27 (tight points)
Step 3: N/A
Step 4: Intradermals on SP 6 (left) + SP 10 (right) for menstrual pain

TREATMENT 4 (3 WEEKS LATER)

Patient Response
Less menstrual pain. Sleep improved. Started down-regulation with hormone injections—some insomnia. Mild cold with dry throat and slight chest mucus.

Diagnosis: YQR + YWD

Step 1: Ren Dai (right-belt) with IPC (10 minutes)
Step 2: Cupping around BL 12–BL 13 + *kyutoshin* on BL 27
Step 3: N/A
Step 4: Direct *okyu* on SP 6 + light needling on DU 23

TREATMENT 5 (3 DAYS LATER)

Patient Response
Cold resolved. GP confirmed no bacterial infection. Continuing down-regulation.

PALPATION

- Midline tightness above the navel
- Tightness across the left waist and around the left ASIS

Diagnosis: Ren Dai (left-belt)

Step 1: Ren Dai (left-belt) with IPC (10 minutes)
Step 2: *Kyutoshin* on BL 18 + BL 23
Step 3: N/A
Step 4: Light needling on BL 17

Treatment continued through the stimulation phase to build the endometrium ahead of the frozen embryo transfer. The pattern remained consistent. Branch treatment supported the womb lining and promoted qi and blood circulation to the lower abdomen. Direct moxa was applied to SP 6, BL 17, and *josen* (*shiqizhuixia*, M-BW-25).

[Note: This point is just below L5 and is often puffy.]

CONCLUSIONS AND REFLECTIONS

Amina's first IVF cycle resulted in a positive pregnancy test. Although the eight-week scan appeared normal, the twelve-week scan showed growth had stopped at nine weeks, and the pregnancy ended with medical management.

Further testing identified a chromosomal abnormality—Turner syndrome—likely attributable to the sperm. Three months later, Amina resumed frozen embryo treatment. She received treatment throughout the cycle, resulting in a successful pregnancy and the live birth of a healthy baby.

CASE STUDY 15. HIP AND GROIN PAIN

Patricia, Female, 48

Occupation: Music teacher

PRESENTING CONDITION

Patricia presented with left hip and groin pain. It was caused by a groin sprain sustained 6 years earlier during yoga practice. The pain was sharp and radiated down to her knee, often accompanied by a twisted, cramping sensation or a feeling of cold. An MRI had revealed synovitis in the hip joint. In the days leading up to her first visit, she experienced several episodes of sleep paralysis, a condition that had been dormant for the past year. She also had a history of restless legs syndrome, previously diagnosed at a sleep clinic. In general, she reported low energy. Given her history of reactive arthritis and fluctuating joint pain, she had been monitored for inflammatory markers and rheumatoid factor by her GP, though previous tests had been inconclusive.

RELEVANT HISTORY

- Reactive arthritis following 2 urinary infections
- Osteophyte in hip and femoral head deterioration (MRI 4 months ago)
- Sulphasalazine taken for 3 months (4 months ago) with no improvement; discontinued due to side effects
- Shingles (1 year ago) in lumbar region, worsened groin pain
- Mild chronic fatigue syndrome (5–7 years ago)
- Nervous breakdown at age 15
- Endometriosis
- She'd had difficulty coming to terms with her father's death 3 years earlier, describing their relationship as "joined at the hip".
- History of an emotionally controlling marriage
- Extensive history of various therapies

PALPATION

- Midline tightness above the navel
- Weakness below the navel
- Tightness across the right waistline
- Bilateral trapezius tension
- LU 1–LU 2 tension (greater on left)
- ST 12 tightness
- Tight lower quadratus muscles on back
- Depression around DU 4

TREATMENT 1

Diagnosis: Right YWD and YQR

Step 1: Ren Dai (right-belt) with electrostatic adsorbers (EA) (1 minute)
Step 2: N/A
Step 3: N/A
Step 4: Direct *okyu* on LIV 5 (groin pain point)—7 cones; pain released with pressure test. *Okyu* on ST 36–7 cones

TREATMENT 2 (FOLLOWING WEEK)

Patient Response
Felt very relaxed after treatment and had a good night's sleep. Hip felt more stable with reduced raw sensation into groin. Reported 'electric shock' sensations on the lateral hip. Energy felt more robust. Complexion appeared brighter.

Step 1: Ren Dai (right-belt) with EA (1 minute)
Step 2: N/A
Step 3: N/A
Step 4: Direct *okyu* on ST 36; warm bamboo applied along gall bladder meridian around left hip and liver meridian on right lower leg. Hip felt more open after treatment.

TREATMENT 3 (FOLLOWING WEEK)

Patient Response
Sleeping well and feeling rested. Blood test showed no inflammatory markers. Felt more stable, centred, and less exhausted. Two nights prior to treatment had a jabbing pain down to the knee on the left outer hip (after physio exercises). Overall sense that hip is more open and energy is circulating better.

PALPATION

This week, the abdominal pattern was reversed. The midline was still tight, but the Dai Mai was more reactive on the left.

Diagnosis: Ren Dai (left-belt)

Step 1: Ren Dai (left-belt) with EA (1 minute)
Step 2: N/A
Step 3: N/A
Step 4: Warm bamboo applied to hip and contralateral shoulder. Yellow empishin placed on left ear—outer hip point was more reactive than inner.

TREATMENT 4 (FOLLOWING WEEK)

Patient Response
Outer hip pain cleared the day after treatment. Some days entirely pain-free. Tolerated press tack in ear and reported it felt beneficial.

PALPATION

This week, the abdominal pattern changed. Upper right quadrant tightness, lower left quadrant pressure pain and jump reactions. The midline was still tight.

Diagnosis: K3L

Step 1: K3L with IPC (5 minutes)
Step 2: *Kyutoshin* on BL 23 and BL 27 area
Step 3: N/A
Step 4: Warm bamboo over areas corresponding to hip; direct *okyu* on ST 36

CONCLUSIONS AND REFLECTIONS

From the initial intake and clinical observation, there were many indications that this patient would prove sensitive: a long and complex medical history, emotional trauma from both adolescence and more recent years, and consistently low energy. Treatment, therefore, needed to be applied with a very low dose. Electrostatic adsorbers (EA) were used instead of needles with IPC, and these were retained for only a short time. By treatment 4, she was stronger and IPC were used for the first time.

Because of the patient's significant mental and emotional issues, Emotional Freedom Technique (EFT) was incorporated into the sessions, and she was also taught how to practise it at home. This often took up much of the session time, so there was not always time to proceed with Steps 2–4.

Altogether, she received ten treatments at weekly or fortnightly intervals, of which four are described in detail above. At times, Ontake moxa was also applied while the IPC were in place, particularly around GB 29 and GB 34 on the left side. With regular moxa, the sensation of coldness in the hip disappeared.

She experienced one flare-up lasting several days, aggravated by a long drive to Scotland, which subsequently settled. Further checks showed no inflammatory markers or rheumatoid factor, and her lymphocyte count returned to normal.

For more discussion of electrostatic adsorbers and their role in Step 1, see Chapter 17.

CASE STUDY 16. MIGRAINES AND SLEEP DISTURBANCES

Sophia, Female, 31

Occupation: Mental health charity worker

PRESENTING CONDITION

Sophia presented with migraines characterised by flashing lights and a pounding sensation in her head. The migraines began when she was 18. The pain was bilateral and located in the temporal region. Her shoulders were tight. The migraines had recently worsened, with 4 episodes occurring in the previous 2 weeks. She was working full-time and studying part-time, and reported phases of poor sleep.

RELEVANT HISTORY

- Father had migraines
- History of cystitis

PALPATION

- URQ and LLQ tight
- Midline tightness
- LU 1 and LU 2 areas tight
- KID 16 tight on left

TREATMENT 1

Diagnosis: K3L (combination of YQR and CS)

Step 1: K3L with IPC (5 minutes)
Step 2: BL 18 + BL 27 with *kyutoshin*
Step 3: N/A
Step 4: BL 10 + BL 14–both very tight points—light *chishin* needling

TREATMENT 2 (2 WEEKS LATER)

Patient Response
Had 1 mild migraine. Sleep improved. Mid-back tightness reduced.

PALPATION

- Midline tightness much better
- Upper right and lower left quadrant reactions

Diagnosis: CS

Step 1: CS with IPC (5 minutes)
Step 2: BL 18 + BL 27 with *kyutoshin*
Step 3: N/A
Step 4: *Chishin* light needling—GB 21 + BL 14.

TREATMENT 3 (2 WEEKS LATER)

Patient Response
No migraines. Good sleep. Conscious of upper back tightness.

Diagnosis: CS

Step 1: CS with IPC (5 minutes)
Step 2: BL 20 (tighter than BL18) + BL 27 with *kyutoshin*
Step 3: N/A
Step 4: GB 21 + BL 14

TREATMENT 4 (2 WEEKS LATER)

Patient Response
No migraines all month. Better stress management. Less menstrual cramping.

PALPATION

- Midline tightness
- Upper right and lower left quadrant reactions

Diagnosis: K3L (5 minutes)

Step 1: K3L with IPC
Step 2: See Step 4 below
Step 3: N/A
Step 4: BL 14 + GB 21 light needling. As the period was due, bled vascular spider around *josen* (*shiqizhuixia*, M-BW-25) + wet-cupped BL 27 right.

[Note: Manaka had unique ideas about blood stasis and prognosis. Bloodletting is an important part of his approach. These topics will be covered in Vol. 3.]

TREATMENT 5 (4 WEEKS LATER)

Patient Response
No migraines. Upper back sore from studying. Less painful menses.

Diagnosis: K3L

Step 1: K3L with IPC (5 minutes)
Step 2: BL 27 with *kyutoshin*
Step 3: N/A
Step 4: *Okyu* on upper thoracic points (T4, T6, T7) + BL 17. Cupping around BL 13 tight area

CONCLUSIONS AND REFLECTIONS

Sophia's presentation alternated between CS and K3L, and treatment focused on consistent approaches at root and branch levels. *Okyu* on the upper back provided a calming effect and helped relieve stress. Over time, her migraines did not recur, and she reported better stress management and quality of life. She returned two years later, still free of migraines, for pregnancy support.

CASE STUDY 17. XEROSTOMIA AND SEVERE LEG PAIN

Emma, Female, 79

Occupation: Retired academic programme manager

PRESENTING CONDITION

Emma presented with xerostomia, which she described as a "hairy tongue". She also reported severe pain in the left frontal thigh and gluteal region, rating it as "15 out of 10". In addition, she experienced persistent fatigue.

RELEVANT HISTORY

- Left throat cancer surgery (this year)
- Atrial fibrillation
- Bilateral knee replacements (6 years ago)
- Hysterectomy at age 36
- Nocturia
- Hearing aids / poor hearing
- Hypothyroidism

PALPATION

- Midline tightness above the umbilicus
- Significant weakness below the umbilicus
- KID 16 tender on palpation
- Mild ASIS tenderness
- Bilateral trapezius tension
- LU 1–LU 2 tension (greater on left)
- ST 12 tightness
- Tight lower quadratus muscles on back
- Depression around DU 4

Diagnosis: YQR

TREATMENT 1

Step 1: YQR + IPC (7 minutes), followed by cranial work and scalp massage
Step 2: *Chishin* at BL 23, BL 25, BL 43, GB 12, and DU 17 with infrared (FIR) lamp on the lower back
Step 3: N/A
Step 4: *Okyu* on DU 4; warm *enshin* on neck, posterior torso, and legs

[Note: An *enshin* is a rounded rubbing tool used for very gentle surface stimulation. In this instance, it was warmed up on a small, portable room heater. See Figure 3-2.]

TREATMENT 2 (2 WEEKS LATER)

Patient Response
Reported increased saliva, significant pain reduction (from 15/10 to 7/10), and improved energy. Noted mental stress and ruminating about the U.S. elections.

PALPATION

- REN 17 tender
- Right SP 21, LU 1–LU 2 tension
- Tight, right subcostal
- Right KID 16 tender
- Tight midline above umbilicus, weak below

Diagnosis: Mixed Yin

Step 1: Mixed Yin + IPC (7 minutes)
Step 2: *Chishin* needling at BL 23, BL 25, BL 43 with infrared (FIR) lamp on back, GB 12, SP 6, and DU 17
Step 3: N/A
Step 4: Warm *enshin* on neck, posterior torso, and legs

TREATMENT 3 (3 WEEKS LATER)

Patient Response

Continued increased saliva. Pain reduced to 5/10 in thigh and gluteal region.

PALPATION

- Midline tightness above the umbilicus
- Significant weakness below the umbilicus
- KID 16 tender on palpation
- Mild ASIS tenderness
- LU 1–LU 2 tension (greater on left)
- ST 12 tightness

Diagnosis: YQR

Step 1: YQR + IPC (7 minutes), followed by cranial work and scalp massage
Step 2: *Chishin* needling at BL 23, BL 25, BL 43, GB 12, and DU 17 with infrared (FIR) lamp on back
Step 3: N/A
Step 4: *Okyu* on DU 4; warm *enshin* on neck, posterior torso, and legs

TREATMENT 4 (2 WEEKS LATER)

Patient Response
No longer experiencing thigh and gluteal pain. New complaint: left lateral knee pain, rated 4/10.

PALPATION

- Left LU 1–LU 2 and KID 16 tender on palpation
- Left ST 25 tender
- Bilateral ASIS tender

Diagnosis: YQR + YWD (belt reactions on the left, not the right)

Step 1: Ren Dai (left-belt) and IPC (7 minutes)
Step 2: *Chishin* needling at BL 23, BL 43, BL 18, BL 20 with infrared (FIR) lamp on low back
Step 3: N/A
Step 4: Taught Korean hand microsystem massage for left knee pain

FOLLOW-UP:
Patient left a voicemail: "I feel so much better today. No pain! Thank you."

CONCLUSIONS AND REFLECTIONS

Emma was an elderly patient presenting with debilitating pain, fatigue, and xerostomia following recent cancer surgery. Initial YQR findings included widespread tightness and deep abdominal weakness, with concurrent upper respiratory and back reactivity.

Treatment was gentle and supportive, combining IPC with cranial work, warm *enshin*, and targeted *chishin* needling. Cone moxa on DU 4 contributed to grounding and energy support, while shifts in the diagnosis from YQR to Mixed Yin and eventually Ren Dai (left-belt) reflected the evolving nature of her symptoms.

Over four treatments, Emma's severe pain reduced dramatically and ultimately resolved. Salivation improved, energy increased, and new symptoms, such as knee pain, were effectively addressed with minimal intervention. This case demonstrates the capacity of light stimulation protocols to ease complex chronic symptoms, even in elderly patients with multifactorial health issues.

CLOSING THOUGHTS

Several themes stand out in this chapter. First, dosage is always relative—treatments were continually adjusted to match each patient's level of sensitivity or robustness. Gentle stimulation proved effective in some cases, while others tolerated stronger interventions. The key was not in following the linear Four Step protocol but in gauging the right dose: not too little, not too much, but just right.

Second, the Four Steps provided a shared framework, yet each author treated in their own individual way. *Okyu*, Ontake, and *kyutoshin*; *enshin*, *chishin*, and takeaways were all applied differently according to context and patient need. Differing polarity methods, such as IPC, SSP, or EA, were also deployed to reinforce the treatment and extend its effects.

Third, these cases highlight the importance of adaptability. Sometimes Step 4 treatments were carried out alongside root work; at other times they were given instead of, or after, other steps. The common factor was a responsiveness to palpatory findings and patient feedback, ensuring that dosage and technique were always aligned with what the body could handle.

Taken together, these cases show how dosage awareness and moxibustion enrich the Manaka system, bringing flexibility, precision, and depth to Step 4. The framework remains the same, but the practitioner's skill lies in adjusting the strength, timing, and method of stimulation to help patients achieve real and lasting change.

WHAT'S NEXT

Before we close, there are a few final pieces to set in place. The concluding chapter looks at more aspects of fine-tuning: using different polarity agents, organising your workflow, and offering final advice for carrying Manaka's wisdom into your own practice.

CHAPTER 17

PUTTING IT ALL TOGETHER

The purpose of this chapter is to continue the fine-tuning begun in earlier chapters. First, we'll examine additional polarity agents—some presented by Manaka in *Chasing the Dragon's Tail*, others developed more recently—and compare their performance at Step 1 in terms of dosage and workflow.

Second, we'll revisit the Four Steps. Until now, we've worked with them as a linear progression, but practice is rarely so neat. Here, we'll explore how to integrate the steps into a practical and flexible workflow, highlighting the options and their respective pros and cons.

If we think of our readers as musicians, then so far you've learned your scales and perhaps a handful of songs. Now it's time to explore interpretation—how to play those songs in different ways, and why you might choose one variation over another, depending on the context.

To begin, let's return to Step 1. Up to now, we've described it mainly in terms of needles and IPC, but polarity can also be established in other ways. Some of these methods come from Manaka's own toolkit; others are contemporary innovations. Each brings a different balance of dosage, workflow, and patient comfort. By broadening our view of Step 1, we can make more informed choices for various clinical situations and fine-tune treatments with greater flexibility.

ALTERNATIVE POLARITY AGENTS AT STEP 1

SILVER SPIKE POINTS (CONTEMPORARY MSA)

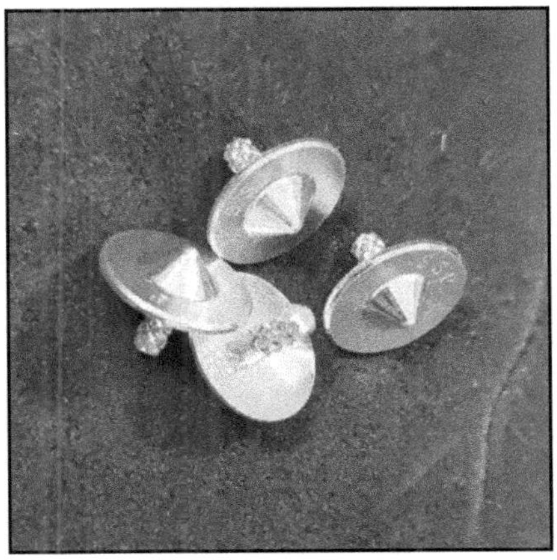

Figure 17-1: Silver spike points or silver terminals.

Our first variation is a contemporary development: silver spike points (SSP). This is the name you'll see in catalogues from suppliers such as Sankei in Japan, but it's a slightly awkward translation from Japanese—*spike* isn't the most inviting term. Since these electrodes really function as terminals for conducting current, a softer and more descriptive name would be silver terminals. In this book, we'll introduce them as SSP, so readers can easily recognise and scurce them, while keeping *silver terminals* in mind as a friendlier alternative.

SSP are small, rounded silver electrodes that can be taped to the skin at the master and coupled points and then connected with an IPC. They look a little like miniature spinning tops, with a rod on one side and a blunt cone (the so-called spike) on the other. The electrode is taped to the skin with the spike pressing gently on the point and the rod facing upwards as an attachment point for the IPC clip.

This setup enables polarity treatment without the need for inserted needles. SSP make things simple for practitioners and comfortable for patients. Treatment times are typically five to ten minutes, comparable to those of IPC with needles. Manaka did not use them, but in contemporary MSA practice, they are flourishing. They are routinely used by both Oran Kivity and Paul Movsessian, as well as many of their students in Australia, Brazil, and Indonesia.

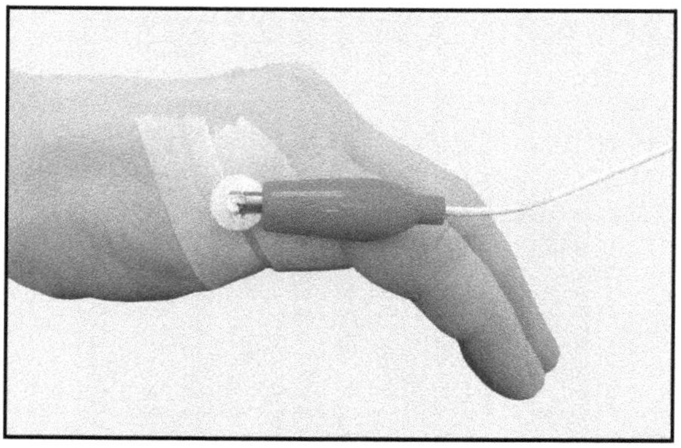

Figure 17-2: The placement of SSP is quick and painless.

GENERAL RULES

Once clipped in place, SSP function much like IPCs with needles. They are location-sensitive: if there is no change at the related primary area and point, you can reposition them, just as you would with a needle. This is quick, painless, and easily done while the patient lies relaxed.

In practice, SSP are useful because they make Step 1 polarity treatment accessible to patients who prefer not to be needled. They are straightforward to apply, easy to adjust, and, as many practitioners have found, very effective.

ELECTROSTATIC ADSORBERS

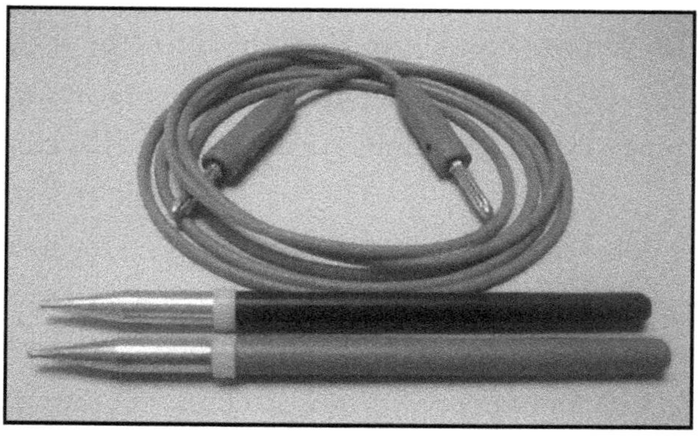

Figure 17-3: The ends of Dr Manaka's electrostatic adsorbers are designed with rounded tips, like teishin, and, like teishin, are touched lightly to the skin.

Electrostatic adsorbers (EA) look very different from IPC. They consist of two blunt-tipped metal rods connected by a copper cable. Built into the circuit is a highly sensitive ceramic capacitance device that withdraws static electrical charges caught or stored in the body's tissues. When the probes are touched to the skin, they 'adsorb' these charges.

By placing oppositely directed diodes in each of a pair of these rods, they are given a very slight positive–negative polarity. Manaka noted that they are simple to use, stating, "Not only are they free of sterilisation problems, but their application is extremely simple, needing only to be touched to the relevant points."[205] Although it's true that EA do not need to be sterilised like inserted needles, in the light of modern clinical practice, we would still suggest cleaning the tips of the probes with alcohol wipes between patients.

Some modern EA, such as those in Figure 17-2, utilise probes made of different metals, adding another layer of polarity effects. EA can be used in the Step 1 treatments presented here, though they come into their own when applied with polar channel pairs—an alternative Step 1 root treatment that we will explore in the next volume.

GENERAL RULES

First, locate the points, perhaps marking them with a pen, and then hold or rest the tips of each probe lightly on the skin. There is no need for pressure—just enough contact to prevent slipping and to make the connection. The probes are held perpendicular to the skin, and unlike with needling, there is no attempt to follow meridian flow.

After 30–60 seconds, remove the probes and retest the abdominal reactions. If there is some improvement, you can repeat the placement for slightly longer, but Manaka did not retain the EA for more than two minutes per side.

With EA, the key benefit is brevity. They should be retained up to a maximum of two minutes. This means Step 1 can be completed quickly. If your preference is to create more time for later steps, or to see more patients per hour, EA are a useful option. Additionally, patients find them very comfortable.

---

205 Manaka, Y., Itaya, K., & Birch, S. (1995). *Chasing the Dragon's Tail: The Theory and Practice of Acupuncture in the Work of Yoshio Manaka*. Brookline: Paradigm Publications. p. 125.

SHARED RULES FOR POLARITY AGENTS

The same safety guidelines that we learned with needling and IPC apply to treating with SSP and EA. Always remove jewellery before treatment and never insert other needles while polarity devices are in place. If a patient shows any negative reaction, discontinue immediately—such reactions are extremely rare, especially with EA.

CHECKING AFTER APPLICATION

Whichever polarity agent you choose, the principle is the same: apply for a short period, then test the results. Table 17.1 compares the three.

Table 17.1: Comparing post-application checks.

POLARITY METHOD	PROCEDURE
IPC with needles	Check the abdomen roughly 30 seconds after placing the final clip. If the abdomen is changing slowly, consider relocating one or more of the needles. Alternatively, hover your little finger and thumb over the black and red clips, respectively.[206]
IPC with SSP	Check the abdomen roughly 30 seconds after placing the final clip. If the abdomen is changing slowly, consider relocating one or more of the SSP, or hold your little finger and thumb over the black and red clips, respectively.
EA	Retain for 30–60 seconds, then recheck. If the results are positive, reapply at the same points. Modify locations if necessary. Retain for a maximum of 2 minutes in total.

[206] Stephen Birch's so-called *wuwu* technique: see Chapter 6.

These simple test–retest loops help you confirm the effectiveness of Step 1 before moving on in your workflow. By checking promptly and adjusting when needed, you ensure that the polarity agent you've chosen is achieving its goal and providing a solid foundation for the subsequent steps. We can now turn to the wider workflow and the choices you can make to balance dosage, root and branch treatment, and the best use of available time.

WORKFLOW

So far in this book, we've discussed the Four Steps as distinct entities, which should be performed in a linear sequence. A linear progression is certainly a helpful model as you are starting out in MSA. The discussion below should help you as the Four Steps become familiar and comfortable; there are several shortcuts where you can treat steps concurrently, rather than sequentially.

Moreover, it will help you fine-tune your treatments, placing different weight on root and branch, for example, or different polarity agents, depending on your treatment focus.

Having explored alternative polarity agents for Step 1, let's now consider how to integrate all Four Steps into a flexible, efficient workflow that adapts to patient needs and clinical constraints.

STEP 1

COMPARING DIFFERENT POLARITY AGENTS

With a choice of three different polarity agents, you might wonder how to choose between them. Much depends on personal preference and intention. In Chapter 2, we introduced a secondary goal for Step 1: to relax the body and mind. The combined outcome of Steps 1–3 is the release of tension from the body. Researchers in the United States have described a relaxation effect that can induce a wide range of beneficial psychophysiological changes in patients.[207]

---

207 Dusek, J. A., & Benson, H. (2009). 'A Model of the Comparative Clinical Impact of the Acute Stress and Relaxation Responses', *Minnesota Medicine*, 92(5). pp. 47–50.

With IPC, where the treatment duration can be as long as ten minutes, the patient often sinks into a more relaxed state. The shorter duration of treatment with EA is insufficient to achieve the same level of relaxation. Stephen Birch, only partly in jest, says that he likes to trigger this relaxation effect by "pinning the patient to the table". Once the needles are in and the cords attached, the patient has no option but to relax. This process is encouraged by limiting conversation, giving them tacit permission to drift away.

Using IPC with SSP also keeps patients still for an equivalent amount of time. In practice, using SSP is less fiddly and more comfortable for patients than needles. If comfort and ease are the only considerations, they are the better option, but dosage may also be a factor (see Chapter 15).

PERFORMING STEP 4 WITH STEP 1

Another advantage of IPC treatment—whether with needles or SSP—is that the ten-minute retention creates a window to administer other treatments, such as small-cone moxibustion or Ontake. In this way, you can combine Steps 1 and 4, making the most of your time by performing two steps concurrently rather than consecutively.

We've discussed how to perform small-cone moxibustion, but any moxa treatment in your playbook can be applied while the cords are in place. These include small-cone moxibustion, large-cone moxibustion, a moxa stick, a moxa box and Ontake, or HOT (Hirata Ontake Therapy). Many of these methods will be covered in subsequent volumes.

DOSAGE

We have seen that comfort and ease of use are important factors in choosing a polarity agent, but dosage also plays a decisive role. Shallow needling with IPC tends to deliver a stronger signal than non-insertive methods, such as SSP or EA. Birch suggests that this greater stimulation moves qi and blood more effectively, making it more suitable for chronic conditions where long-term stagnation is an issue.

With robust patients, we can spend more time on branch treatments, whereas with sensitive patients, we should focus more on the root treatment, sometimes to the exclusion of any branch treatment. Thus, if you intend to devote more time to symptoms, it makes sense to use EA to complete Step 1 quickly. For sensitive patients, lower doses are called for: SSP or EA with shortened durations. In some cases, only a few seconds with EA may be required.

ALTERNATIVES AT STEP 1

In Vol. 2, we will explore another of Manaka's unique treatment approaches: the polar channel pairs at Step 1. This approach sometimes involves needling the *jing*-well points and clipping the IPC to the needles—a demanding procedure for both the patient and the practitioner. Manaka developed the electrostatic adsorbers specifically as a more comfortable alternative. However, he rarely used them for the Eight Extraordinary Vessels.

That said, in contemporary practice, some practitioners *do* use them at Step 1. Birch notes that while they can be effective, the abdominal changes they produce are often less marked than those achieved with IPC.

Table 17.2: Comparing ion-pumping tools.

PATIENT TYPE	STRONGER METHODS (IPC WITH NEEDLES)	GENTLER METHODS (SSP / EA)
Robust	Suitable for all patients, with adjustments made to treatment duration as needed. May affect qi and blood more than non-insertive methods, so useful in chronic conditions.	EA can be used to complete Step 1 quickly with a mild dose, leaving more time and allocating more of the overall treatment dosage to branch work.
Sensitive	Use with caution; shorten retention if used at all.	SSP are a good choice. Shortened duration is essential. If using EA, duration may be only a few seconds. Focus on root treatment only (limit or exclude branch treatment).

These dosage guardrails help you make informed choices at Step 1, balancing strength, sensitivity, and treatment priorities.

STEP 2

We've explored a number of ways to apply Step 2:

- *Kyutoshin* warm needle
- *Chishin* shallow needling
- *Chishin* shallow needling with a heat lamp
- *Okyu* small-cone moxibustion

As always, dosage shapes our choices—not just of the treatment method, but also of the number of points and rounds of moxa. With weaker patients, we do fewer of both; with more robust patients, we needn't be afraid to do more. Not too much, not too little, but just right!

As in Step 1, we can incorporate techniques from Step 4, allowing us to perform them concurrently. For example, apply *chishin* at GB 20 and GB 21 before doing *kyutoshin* on the back-*shu* points—an economical way to treat katakori (tight shoulders). The correct order is *chishin* first, *kyutoshin* second. The reverse order risks the patient jumping as you palpate and insert the *chishin* while moxa is burning on the needles. *Kyutoshin* requires forethought and vigilance.

By the same token, if doing *chishin*, then there is no harm in adding *okyu* concurrently. If, however, you're doing *kyutoshin*, avoid *okyu* while the moxa on the needles is burning. We discussed this idea in Chapter 13, but it's worth repeating here in the context of Step 2 sequencing. To perform *okyu* and *kyutoshin*, one option is to set up the moxa on the needles in the lower back, then perform *okyu* on the upper back. Once you've finished the *okyu*, you can light the *kyutoshin*. Patients often find it deeply relaxing to experience two contrasting heat sensations in sequence.

In later volumes, we will further expand our Step 2 repertoire, including needling yang points, cupping, large-cone moxibustion, Manaka's wooden hammer and needle, and Ontake.

STEP 3

We've learned one simple Sotai method for structural adjustment, which can be performed with or without moxa. It isn't essential to include this step in every treatment, but it can be helpful when there are right–left differences on the back.

For obvious reasons, Step 3 cannot be done concurrently with other steps. The patient should be free of needles and IPC. If you are doing Prone Leg Flexion (PLF), moxa can be applied to BL 18.

It is unusual to do PLF at any time other than after Step 2. Later volumes will introduce additional Sotai techniques, including some that can be performed immediately after Step 1 in the supine position.

STEP 4

Manaka's isophasal treatment was his preferred way of performing Step 4. It is designed as a low-dosage treatment that works harmoniously with the other three steps. Because it usually requires range-of-motion tests, it is applied once all needles from Step 2 have been removed.

Occasionally, you may encounter a patient in such acute pain that you need to address it immediately. In such extreme cases, Brenda Loew reports placing a takeaway tool in the ear at the start of treatment, before Step 1, without provoking the counterflow qi reactions one might expect from metal on the skin during ion pumping. Ear acupuncture can have a dramatic effect on pain and is worth considering as an emergency option to put a distressed patient at ease.

Symptom relief is not confined to Manaka's isophasal treatment, nor is it limited to Step 4. You can add moxa during Step 1, or combine needles and moxa during Step 2, provided you monitor dosage with your jitsometer assessment. At this stage, you are free to draw on your own clinical experience and healing skills, but keep in mind that Manaka's recommendations were designed to work as part of his overall system.

If your patient is strong, you can include a fair amount of symptom relief. If your patient is weak, the focus should remain on the root treatment, or root treatment plus one predominant symptom. What you should not do is chase every symptom with an equivalent branch treatment—this will quickly lead to adverse reactions. In practice, economy and self-restraint are important considerations: a little symptom relief can be powerful, but over-treating undermines your good intentions.

Taken together, the Four Steps can be applied flexibly—sometimes consecutively, sometimes concurrently—depending on dosage, intention, and the patient's condition.

SUMMARY

- **Alternative polarity agents:** Step 1 does not need to be applied with needles. SSP and EA offer alternative options, each with different effects and emphases on dosage, workflow, and patient comfort.
- **Workflow and flexibility:** The Four Steps are taught sequentially, but clinical reality is rarely so neat. Treatments can be adapted, overlapped, or shortened depending on priorities. With experience, root and branch can be balanced more fluidly, and concurrent treatments can save time without compromising results.
- **Shared principles:** Whatever the polarity agent, the rules remain the same—palpate, apply, check, and adjust.
- **Dosage and choice:** Stronger methods (IPC with needles) may be better for chronic stagnation; gentler methods (SSP) suit sensitive patients, and EA suit busy clinics or focusing on branch treatment. Choosing the right agent means weighing strength, sensitivity, comfort, and available time.

THINGS TO COME

That's all, folks! Congratulations, you have completed MSA Level 1! In many ways, Level 1 is the hardest of the Manaka trainings because it asks you to absorb so many new ideas. Learning acupuncture is like learning a new language, and learning Manaka's octahedral model is like taking on a challenging new dialect at the same time. It needs time for these new concepts to bed in and become routine.

At first, practising MSA might feel both exciting and daunting. But if we strip this book down to its fundamentals, you've learned eight basic patterns. That's like learning eight songs. MSA may appear to be a rigid sequence with its Four Steps, but within the framework of the octahedral model, it offers ample scope for creativity and imagination. If you keep singing those same eight songs, two things will happen: you'll become an expert at performing them—and eventually, you'll grow restless and want something more challenging.

Subsequent books will build on this foundation. We'll continue to use the octahedral model, not only with new ion-pumping treatments at Step 1, but also with whole-body moxa treatments at Step 1 that can replace ion pumping entirely. We'll explore Manaka's use of the Chinese clock, cover new branch treatments such as specialised Japanese cupping and microbleeding techniques, and examine his meridian frequencies—applied with a wooden hammer and needle, and expanded into meridian frequency moxibustion with Ontake. Your repertoire of songs will expand.

Dr Manaka was a remarkable figure, towering over the field of acupuncture and lighting the way for others. His system is unique in so many ways. From our perspective as practitioners, it is easily testable and repeatable. The feedback methods are immediate and straightforward. From the patients' perspective, the system has a genuine 'wow' factor: they can feel the abdomen change within seconds of ion pumping. Abdominal and point palpation engage them in the process, enabling them to participate in the treatment in a fully embodied way.

TESTING THE WATER OR JUMPING IN

Marian Fixler and Oran Kivity have both studied and taught MSA together. They have found that there are two ways to learn this system. One approach is to integrate the ideas gradually with what you already do—much like testing the water with your toes. The other, which they both chose, is to jump straight in. The best way to learn Manaka is to grasp the system with both hands and immerse yourself in it—chasing the dragon's tail!

> *For me,* Dragon *was, at first, an intimidating book. I picked it up in a London bookshop and put it straight back on the shelf, thinking it looked far too scientific for me. And yet, once Stephen had explained the principles of the octahedral model in class, I devoured it. It was an intellectual white-knuckle ride that I couldn't put down. I read it on the bus, I read it in the clinic, and I read it in bed. Perhaps that just shows my nerdy credentials, and clearly, that book is not for everyone.*
>
> —Oran Kivity

We hope that *this* book inspires you in the same way that Manaka inspired each of us—Brenda, Marian, Oran, Paul, and Stephen—by giving you a simpler foundation text than *Chasing the Dragon's Tail* to guide your first steps along the Manaka path.

Good luck on your journey!

ABOUT THE AUTHORS

MANAKA'S CHILDREN

A few years ago, I was in Tokyo for a Toyohari conference, accompanied by Koki Takemoto, my assistant at that time. Koki had been studying MSA with me for more than a year and knew the way I worked more intimately than anyone else. Proud of his progress, I was very much looking forward to introducing him to my teacher, Stephen Birch. When the moment came, I strode up to him and surprised all three of us by saying, "Hey, Steve, meet your grandson!" Momentarily perplexed, Stephen rose to the occasion and greeted Koki with a joke of his own.

Teasing though I was, there was truth in Koki's designation as grandchild. Manaka was Birch's mentor, and Stephen, in turn, revolutionised my understanding of acupuncture—not just mine, but also that of Brenda Loew in the United States, Paul Movsessian in Australia, and Marian Fixler in the United Kingdom. Working on this book with him was an inspiration; he made our two-dimensional explanations three-dimensional. Dr Manaka would be proud of him. We are all Manaka's children now, and Koki has quite a few aunts and uncles—you can meet the family below.

—Oran Kivity, Taiwan, 2025

Oran Kivity

British acupuncturist Oran Kivity trained in Europe, China, and Japan, and has been in continuous practice since 1987. He specialises in Japanese methods and, with Marian Fixler, co-founded Toyohari UK, the British branch of the Toyohari Association of Japan. He lectured in acupuncture at the University of Westminster and the Northern College of Acupuncture, and was the founding editor of *Keiraku Chiryo—International Toyohari News*. He is the author of six books, including *Moxa in Motion with the Ontake Method* and *Hirata Zone Therapy with the Ontake Method*.

Now based in Taiwan, Oran supports authors in the acupuncture field through his imprint, Sayoshi Books. He practises, writes, coaches, and teaches from the southern port town of Kaohsiung, where he lives happily by a river, near a lake, and close to the sea.

Stephen Birch

Stephen Birch is an acupuncturist, author, and researcher who has been instrumental in bringing Japanese acupuncture traditions to the West. He trained in the United States, then studied extensively in Japan under Dr Yoshio Manaka and other leading masters, becoming one of the foremost authorities on Japanese acupuncture and moxibustion.

He also completed a PhD in acupuncture research at the University of Exeter in the United Kingdom. He is the author and co-author of several influential texts, including *Chasing the Dragon's Tail*; *Extraordinary Vessels*; *Hara Diagnosis; Japanese Acupuncture: A Clinical Guide*; *Understanding Acupuncture; Shonishin: Japanese Pediatric Acupuncture*; and *Restoring Order in Health and Chinese Medicine*.

Stephen has taught internationally for more than three decades, shaping the practice of thousands of acupuncturists worldwide. He is the president of the non-Japanese branches of the Toyohari Association and continues to lecture, research, and publish widely on Japanese methods of diagnosis and treatment. Away from work, he has a passion for rare tequilas and reputedly keeps a vast collection at home.

Marian Fixler

Marian Fixler qualified in 1991 and, after seven years of practising Traditional Chinese Medicine, shifted to Japanese acupuncture following training with Stephen Birch. Since then, she has worked in private practice and in varied clinical settings, including an NHS GP surgery, alcohol services, and the HIV/AIDS field. Marian has published numerous articles, including research demonstrating the efficacy of Japanese acupuncture for chronic conditions.

She taught for many years as a senior lecturer at the University of Westminster and as a guest lecturer at other colleges. She has organised training in Manaka-style acupuncture in the United Kingdom, hosted international teachers, and is a senior faculty member of the Toyohari Meridian Therapy Association, teaching widely across Europe. When not working, Marian loves wild swimming—especially in winter—and walking in nature with her springer collie, Hiro.

Brenda Loew

Brenda Loew received her acupuncture licence in 1991 and her doctorate in 2023. She has more than thirty-five years of clinical and teaching experience in the United States and Canada.

She co-founded the Toyohari Association of North America, where she is president emeritus and core faculty, and has trained extensively in Japan with senior Toyohari teachers. Based in Seattle, she serves on the faculty of the University of Washington Department of Family Medicine's Osher Centre for Integrative Health and is also adjunct faculty at Bastyr University and the Middle Way Acupuncture Institute.

Thanks to Stephen Birch, she specialises in Japanese acupuncture—particularly MSA, Toyohari, and Shonishin paediatric therapy—and is committed to bringing our ancestors' wisdom into modern practice, moving away from reductionist models towards Living Systems thinking. Outside of work, she enjoys meditation, films, coffee, matcha, powwows, 'yarning' with colleagues, and the natural beauty of the Pacific Northwest, the unceded sacred ancestral land of the Salish People who protect the connection to land, sea and sky.

Paul Movsessian

Paul Movsessian has over forty years of clinical and teaching experience in Traditional East Asian Medicine, specialising in Japanese acupuncture, moxibustion, Manaka System Acupuncture, and Sotai. Trained in Australia, he continued postgraduate studies in Japan before lecturing extensively in Australia, the United States, Canada, and New Zealand. He has published articles and research papers, taught at universities and private colleges, and now delivers his courses worldwide through webinars.

Paul is recognised as a key influence in introducing Japanese acupuncture and moxibustion to Australia, serving for many years as a consultant to institutions and associations seeking to understand these systems in contrast to Traditional Chinese Medicine. He runs a successful clinic in the Blue Mountains, Australia, and in his spare time enjoys beekeeping and raising Japanese Bantam chickens.

FEEDBACK

Thank you for reading *Manaka Made Simple*.

Books improve when readers share what worked, what didn't, and what they'd like to see in future volumes. If you found the material useful or enjoyed the way it's presented, please consider leaving an honest review online. Reviews make a huge difference—they enable other practitioners to discover the book and help us to create even better future editions.

Thank you.

—Oran Kivity, Stephen Birch, Marian Fixler, Brenda Loew, Paul Movsessian

BIBLIOGRAPHY

A

Akabane, K. (1986). *Hinaishin Ho (The Intradermal Needle Method).* 12th ed. Yokosuka: Ido no Nippon Sha.

Auteroche, B., Gervais, G., Auteroche, M., Navailh, P. & Toui-Kan, E. (1992). *Acupuncture and Moxibustion: A Guide to Clinical Practice*. Edinburgh: Churchill Livingstone.

B

Baek, S. (1990). *Classical Moxibustion Skills in Contemporary Clinical Practice.* Boulder, CO: Blue Poppy Press.

Becker, M. (n.d.). Japanese Direct Moxa: Extra Foot Points. Unpublished manuscript. Available at: *https://www.scribd.com/document/869096355/Moshe-Becker-Moxa-Points-Foot*

Birch, S. (1989/1990). 'Acupuncture in Japan: An Introductory Survey. Review'. *NAJOM*, Part 1, 6; Part 2, 7; Part 3, 8; Part 4, 9.

Birch, S. (1992). 'Naming the Un-Nameable: A Historical Study of Radial Pulse Six Position Diagnosis'. *Traditional Acupuncture Society Journal*, 12.

Birch, S. (1997). *An Exploration with Proposed Solutions of the Problems and Issues in Conducting Clinical Research in Acupuncture*. PhD thesis. University of Exeter.

Birch, S. (1997). 'Forming a Prognosis—Perspectives from the Works of Japanese Acupuncturists: A Preliminary Compilation of Ideas'. *NAJOM*, 4(10).

Birch, S. (1997). *An Introduction to the Use of Palpation Methods in the Practice of Acupuncture and Moxibustion in Japan, with a Focus on Hara Diagnosis/Abdominal Palpation*. Course handout. Anglo-Dutch Institute for Oriental Medicine.

Birch, S. (1997). *Japanese Acupuncture and Moxibustion: A Brief Overview*. Course handout. Anglo-Dutch Institute for Oriental Medicine.

Birch, S. (2009). 'Dr Manaka Yoshio's Insights and Contributions to the Field of TEAM'. *NAJOM* (Special Issue: In Memory of Dr Manaka Yoshio), 16(47).

Birch, S. (2009). 'Filling the Whole in Acupuncture. Part 1: What Are We Doing in the Supplementation Needle Technique?' *European Journal of Oriental Medicine*, 6(3).

Birch, S. (2009). 'Filling the Whole in Acupuncture. Part 2: What Are We Doing in the Supplementation Needle Technique?' *European Journal of Oriental Medicine*, 6(3).

Birch, S. (2011). *Shonishin: Japanese Pediatric Acupuncture*. Stuttgart: Thieme Medical Publishers.

Birch, S. (2013). 'Traditional Needling Techniques as Practical Constructions from Reading Historical Descriptions'. *European Journal of Oriental Medicine*, 7(3).

Birch, S. (2016). *Shonishin: Japanese Pediatric Acupuncture*. 2nd ed. Stuttgart: Thieme Medical Publishers.

Birch, S. (2019). 'Treating the Patient, Not the Symptoms: Acupuncture to Improve Overall Health—Evidence, Acceptance and Strategies'. *Integrative Medicine Research*, 8(1). *https://doi.org/10.1016/j.imr.2018.07.005*

Birch, S., Cabrer, M., & Rodriguez, M. (2025). *Restoring Order in Health and Chinese Medicine: Studies of the Development and Use of Qi and the Channels*. 2nd ed. London: Sayoshi Books.

Birch, S., & Felt, R. (1999). *Understanding Acupuncture*. Edinburgh: Churchill Livingstone.

Birch, S., & Ida, J. (1998). *Japanese Acupuncture: A Clinical Guide*. Brookline: Paradigm Publications.

C

Caudet, F. (2023). *Isaburo Fukaya: The Master of Japanese Moxibustion*. Tarragona: Okyayasan Books.

Chant, B., Madison, J., Coop, P., & Dieberg, G. (2017). 'Beliefs and Values in Japanese Acupuncture: An Ethnography of Japanese-Trained Acupuncture Practitioners in Japan'. *Integrative Medicine Research*, 6(3). *https://doi.org/10.1016/j.imr.2017.07.001*

Chant, B., Madison, J., Coop, P., & Dieberg, G. (2017). 'Contact Tools in Japanese Acupuncture: An Ethnography of Acupuncture Practitioners in Japan'. *Journal of Acupuncture and Meridian Studies*, 10(5). *https://doi.org/10.1016/j.jams.2017.08.006*

Chen, K., & Ciu, Y. (1991). *Handbook to Chinese Auricular Therapy*. Beijing: Foreign Languages Press.

Cheng, X. (ed.) & Deng, L. (1987). *Chinese Acupuncture and Moxibustion*. Beijing: Foreign Languages Press.

D

Dale, R. (1999). 'The Systems, Holograms and Theory of Micro-Acupuncture'. *American Journal of Acupuncture*, 27(3–4).

Dawkins, R. (1976). *The Selfish Gene*. Oxford: Oxford University Press.

Deadman, P., Al-Khafaji, M., & Baker, K. (1998). *A Manual of Acupuncture*. East Sussex: Journal of Chinese Medicine Publications.

Devitt, M. (2015). 'The Legend of Waichi Sugiyama, the Father of Japanese Acupuncture'. *Meridians: The Journal of Acupuncture and Oriental Medicine*, 2(4).

Dusek, J. A., & Benson, H. (2009). 'Mind-Body Medicine: A Model of the Comparative Clinical Impact of the Acute Stress and Relaxation Responses'. *Minnesota Medicine*, 92(5).

E

Eckman, P. (ed.) (1988). *Koryo Hand Acupuncture*. Seoul: Eum Yang Maek Jin Pub Co.

F

Fratkin, J. (1999). 'The Emergence of Japanese Style Acupuncture'. *California Journal of Oriental Medicine (CJOM)*, 10(1), Winter.

Fukaya, I. (1982). *Kadenkyu Mongatari: Family Recipes in Moxa Therapy*. Tokyo: Sankei Publishing Company.

Fukushima, K. (1991). *Meridian Therapy*. Tokyo: Toyo Hari Medical Association.

H

Hashimoto, K., & Kawakami, Y. (1983). *Sotai: Balance and Health Through Natural Movement*. Tokyo: Japan Publications Inc.

Hecker, H., Steveling, A., & Peuker, E. (2005). *Microsystems Acupuncture: The Complete Guide: Ear–Scalp–Mouth–Hand*. Stuttgart: Thieme.

Hua, B. X. (1994). *Chinese Auricular Therapy*. Beijing: Scientific & Technical Documents Publishing House.

I

Ido-no-Nippon (1986). *500th Special Issue*, 45(4).

Irie, S. (1980). *Fukaya Kyu Ho*. Tokyo: Shizensha.

K

Kazuo, T. (2002). 'Examination on the Immunological Effects of Moxibustion Treatment'. *North American Journal of Oriental Medicine*, 9(25).

Kivity, O. (2018). 'Japanese Acupuncture: What's So Unique?' *European Journal of Oriental Medicine*, 9(2).

Kivity, O. (2020). *Moxa in Motion with the Ontake Method: Rhythmic Moxibustion Methods from Japan for Mind-Body Healing*. London: Sayoshi Books.

Kivity, O. (2021). *Hirata Zone Therapy with the Ontake Method: Repurposing the Lost Art of Japanese Dermatome Moxibustion for Contemporary Practice*. London: Sayoshi Books.

Kivity, O. (2025). *Lecture on Fukaya Kyu by Felip Caudet, Jakarta, Indonesia*. Personal notes.

Kivity, O. (ed.) (2007). 'Kikei Nuggets'. *Keiraku Chiryo—International Toyohari News*, 1(3).

Kobayashi, A., Uefuji, M., & Yasumo, W. (2007). 'History and Progress of Japanese Acupuncture'. *Evidence-Based Complementary and Alternative Medicine*, 7(3). *https://doi.org/10.1093/ecam/nem155*

M

Manaka, Y. (2009). 'The Concept of Meridians from a Systems Perspective'. *NAJOM* (Special Issue: In Memory of Dr Manaka Yoshio), 16(47).

Manaka, Y., Itaya, K., & Birch, S. (1995). *Chasing the Dragon's Tail: The Theory and Practice of Acupuncture in the Work of Yoshio Manaka*. Brookline: Paradigm Publications.

Manaka, Y., & Urquhart, I. (1972). *The Layman's Guide to Acupuncture*. New York: Weatherhill.

Matsumoto, H. (1994). 'Acupuncture and Moxibustion in Japan'. *NAJOM*, 1(2).

Matsumoto, K., & Birch, S. (1986). *Extraordinary Vessels*. Brookline: Paradigm Publications.

Matsumoto, K., & Birch, S. (1988). *Hara Diagnosis: Reflections on the Sea*. Brookline: Paradigm Publications.

Matsumoto, K., & Euler, D. (2008). *Kiiko Matsumoto's Clinical Strategies: In the Spirit of Master Nagano*. Vol. 1. Brookline, MA: Kiiko Matsumoto International.

McCann, H., & Ross, H. (2015). *Practical Atlas of Tung's Acupuncture*. Germany: Verlag Muller & Steinicke.

Miyawaki, K. (1976). *Yin Yo Rokugyo Setsu no Shinjutsu: Yin Yang Six Phase Acupuncture Treatments*. Tokyo: Soikai Sha.

Miyawaki, K. (1990). 'Abdominal Diagnosis of the Extraordinary Vessels'. *Keiraku Shinryo*, 242(3–4).

Mizutani, J. (1998). *Practical Moxibustion Therapy*. Vancouver, BC: NAJOM

S

Shanghai College of Traditional Medicine (1985). *Acupuncture: A Comprehensive Text*. Seattle: Eastland Press.

Shimizu, K. (1986). 'Pressure Pain Points, Diagnosis and Treatments'. *Ido-no-Nippon*, 45(4).

Shinma, H. (2015). *The Treasure Book of Points: Fukaya Kyu*. Tokyo: Shinma.

Shiozawa, F. (1976). 'Treatment Effect of Empishin'. *Ido-no-Nippon*, 35(11).

Shudo, D. (1990). *Japanese Classical Acupuncture: Introduction to Meridian Therapy*. Seattle: Eastland Press.

Shudo, D. (2003). *Finding Effective Acupuncture Points*. Translated by S. Brown. Seattle, WA: Eastland Press.

U

Unschuld, P. U. (1986). *Medicine in China: Nan Ching, the Classic of Difficult Issues*. Berkeley: University of California Press.

Unschuld, P. U., & Tessenow, H. (2011). *Huang Di Nei Jing Ling Shu: The Ancient Classic on Needle Therapy*. Berkeley: University of California Press.

W

Wang, J. Y., Robertson, J., & Van Buren, K. (2008). *Applied Channel Theory in Chinese Medicine: Wang Ju-Yi's Lectures on Channel Therapeutics*. Seattle: Eastland Press.

Wexu, M. (1985). *The Ear—Gateway to Balancing the Body: A Modern Guide to Ear Acupuncture*. New York: Aurora Press.

Y

Yang, J. (1601/1963 reprint). *Zhen Jiu Da Cheng (Great Compendium of Acupuncture and Moxibustion).* Beijing: Renmin Weisheng Chubanshe.

Yasui, H. (2010). 'History of Japanese Acupuncture and Moxibustion'. *Journal of Kampo, Acupuncture and Integrative Medicine*, Special Edition.

Young, M. (2014). *The Moon over Matsushima - 'the Single': Clinical Moxibustion Treatments*. Kindle edition. Available at: *https://www.amazon.co.uk/dp/B00N98FXE8*

Young, M. (2023). *The Moon over Matsushima: Insights into Moxa and Mugwort.* 2nd ed. London: Sayoshi Books.

VIDEO RESOURCES

Japanese Acupuncture Today. (2015). Episode 2: Moxibustion [Video]. Interview with Sascha Gröbe and Merlin Young. Available at: *https://www.youtube.com/live/uvFZFJrOoDE*

Japanese Acupuncture Today. (2018). Episode 3: 'Harikyu' [Video]. Panel discussion with Birch, Mizutani, Loew, and Kivity. Available at: *https://youtu.be/aoN3bwXmacY*

Japanese Acupuncture Today. (2022). Episode 7: 'Making Moxa—Inside Yamasho' [Video]. Site visit to Yamasho with Oran Kivity. Available at: *https://youtu.be/D44d9AS_Ltk?si=V9e3_BHL2BJhLdUf*

MANAKA MADE SIMPLE VOL. 2 (IN DEVELOPMENT)

In Vol. 1, you learned the foundations: how to recognise the primary patterns and adapt them to different clinical situations. Vol. 2 takes you further. You'll deepen your understanding across all four steps, explore the polar channel pairs and open-point cycles, learn refined moxa and *okyu* methods, discover new Sotai protocols, and work with Manaka's meridian frequencies. Your clinical repertoire will expand considerably, giving you the tools to treat more complex cases with confidence.

ALSO BY SAYOSHI BOOKS

Exceptional books on acupuncture, moxibustion, and East Asian medicine

Sayoshi Books is dedicated to publishing high-quality books for practitioners and students of East Asian medicine. Our books bridge traditional knowledge with modern clinical insights, offering practical guidance and deep expertise.

Moxa in Motion with the Ontake Method: Rhythmic Moxibustion Methods from Japan for Mind-Body Healing

—Oran Kivity

A ground-breaking exploration of rhythmic moxibustion methods from Japan using Ontake Warm Bamboo, integrating traditional knowledge with innovative applications for pain relief and systemic balance.

Also available in Chinese and Polish. Translations into Bahasa Indonesia, French, Portuguese, Spanish, and Japanese will be available in early 2026.

Hirata Zone Therapy with the Ontake Method: Repurposing the Lost Art of Japanese Dermatome Moxibustion for Contemporary Practice

—Oran Kivity

An exploration of the dermatome moxibustion system developed by twentieth-century Japanese masters Kurakichi Hirata and Yoshio Manaka, repurposed for contemporary practice with Ontake Warm Bamboo. This practical guide will teach you to create immediate and powerful therapeutic effects.

Also available in French

The Moon over Matsushima: Insights into Moxa and Mugwort (Second Edition)

—Merlin Young

The definitive book about moxibustion, exploring its history and linking traditional East Asian practices with emerging scientific research on transient receptor potential ion channels.

Restoring Order in Health and Chinese Medicine: Studies of the Development and Use of Qi and the Channels

—Stephen Birch, Miguel Angel Cabrer Mir,
Manuel Rodriguez Cuadras

An in-depth study of the dynamics of qi, the development of the channels, and how to apply classical principles to contemporary acupuncture practice.

The Lost Art of Jôsetsu-Hô Moxibustion: Finding Effective Moxa Points with String Measuring

—Felip Caudet, Hideo Shinma

The first translation into English of Caudet's seminal work in Spanish. A detailed exploration of the Jôsetsu-Hô string-measuring method, detailing ways to locate effective moxa points for enhanced therapeutic results.

Other Titles by Sayoshi Books

While Sayoshi Books primarily focuses on East Asian medicine, we also took the opportunity to republish this deeply personal memoir.

Daughter of the Waves: Memories of Growing Up in Pre-War Palestine

—Ruth Jordan

Ruth Jordan's award-winning autobiography is a vivid, witty, and poignant account of her childhood in British Mandate Palestine. Growing up in a seaside suburb of Haifa, she captures a nation in its formative years, navigating its struggles and transformation into statehood. Originally published in 1982, this timeless memoir is today more relevant than ever, providing a fresh perspective on Palestine through the eyes of someone who was actually there.

Discover more at **sayoshibooks.orankivity.com**

INDEX

C

D

E

F

G

H

I

J

K

L

M

N

O

R

S

T

U

V

W

X

Y

Z

www.ingramcontent.com/pod-product-compliance
Ingram Content Group UK Ltd.
Pitfield, Milton Keynes, MK11 3LW, UK
UKHW051451290926
15471UKWH00008B/1136

9 781068 381423